Mental Health and Relationships from Early Adulthood through Old Age

This unique text encourages young adults to reflect on their prospective longevity for setting goals and making decisions, become aware of the aspirations and concerns of other generations, and consider personal direction in relation to peer group norms. The sources for learning about mental health and relationships include a blend of academic research, insights from literature, student interviews with older and younger relatives, and personal observations.

Stages of adulthood including early adulthood, middle adulthood, retirement age, and old age, are described showing how people can pursue individual growth and nurture the mental health of relatives throughout life. The main themes of younger and middle-aged adults include stress, parenting, peer socialization, family conflict, career readiness, domestic abuse, intergenerational relationships, and mental health. In addition, the educational needs of older adults focus on mental health, family caregiving, grandparenting, physical and social health, problems of younger generations, retirement, loneliness and social isolation, elder abuse, death, grief, and recovery.

All chapters conclude with a section about *Generational Perspectives Activities,* assignments with agenda for class and family discussions, problem-solving scenarios, key concepts, and criteria for self-evaluation. This will be of interest to undergraduate and graduate college students enrolled in lifespan courses offered by family studies, educational psychology, human development, counselling, social work, gerontology, nursing, and business.

Paris S. Strom is a Professor of Educational Psychology at Auburn University in Auburn, Alabama. Paris currently teaches child, adolescent, and adult development courses to undergraduate and graduate students. He is the author of over 100 journal articles and books about the learning process throughout the human lifespan.

Robert D. Strom is a Professor Emeritus of College of Education at Arizona State University. His teaching, writing, and research focus on lifespan development and mental health to support families. He is the author of over 200 articles and textbooks. Robert and Paris are a father-and-son team.

Mental Health and Relationships from Early Adulthood through Old Age

Paris S. Strom and Robert D. Strom

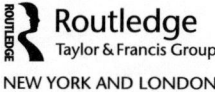
Routledge
Taylor & Francis Group

NEW YORK AND LONDON

Designed cover image: Cover Design by Paris S. Strom Copyright © 2024

First published 2024
by Routledge
605 Third Avenue, New York, NY 10158

and by Routledge
4 Park Square, Milton Park, Abingdon, Oxon OX14 4RN

Routledge is an imprint of the Taylor & Francis Group, an informa business

© 2024 Paris S. Strom and Robert D. Strom

British Library Cataloguing-in-Publication Data
A catalogue record for this book is available from the British Library

ISBN: 978-1-032-51133-7 (hbk)
ISBN: 978-1-032-49770-9 (pbk)
ISBN: 978-1-003-40126-1 (ebk)

DOI: 10.4324/9781003401261

Typeset in Times New Roman
by MPS Limited, Dehradun

Access the Support Material on: www.routledge.com/9781032511337

Contents

PART IV
Old Age (Ages 80+)   225

Introduction
Thinking about the Future

The Future and Longevity

Americans, on average as of 2023, can expect to live about 80 years or perhaps longer if they were born in the present millennium (Arias et al., 2021; Huet, 2024). This extension of the lifespan has redefined the scope of human development and presents unfamiliar and difficult challenges for policy makers, health care providers, employers, educators, religious institutions, families, and individuals. Education for longevity should begin during early adulthood (ages 20–40) when the emergence of ideals is common, students become able to objectively examine the views of others, can explain reasoning for their own opinions, and show a willingness to participate in self-evaluation. The knowledge base for learning about mental health and relationships throughout the lifespan is drawn from academic research, non-academic reports based upon interviews with other generations, and observations of peers. The four stages of adult life to be examined in this book will include early adulthood (ages 20 to 40), middle age (ages 40 to 60), retirement (ages 60 to 80), and old age (ages 80+).

Learning about Adult Development

Introducing the challenges of growing older resembles a method used by anthropologists to explore the lives of people in non-industrialized and little understood societies. The scientists travel to remote locations where they observe tribal life, witness the customs and rituals, identify gender role expectations, catalogue lessons taught to children, and summarize socially desirable behavior. After extensive fieldwork, the anthropologists return home to report about overall impressions and provide details regarding the newfound knowledge. These firsthand accounts often correct false assumptions and beliefs that were previously held about a specific community of strangers.

Consider a more familiar situation where learning from those who are older is necessary to become informed about how their goals and concerns resemble and differ from young adults. The United States is an age-segregated culture where most people identify with their own age-group (tribe). Conversations with peers of the same generation are more pleasing because they reflect greater agreement based on mutual exposure to ideas and events that happened while growing up. When social and technological changes accelerate, there are bound to be disruptions in role expectations, conversations with other age groups decline, and increased misunderstandings arise about the communities of strangers represented by other age cohorts.

DOI: 10.4324/9781003401261-1

In this connection, most parents realize young adults have experiences their relatives are too old to know firsthand but should learn about through conversations with daughters and sons as they share situations and events unprecedented for their age group (Minkin & Horowitz, 2023). The social distancing that separates generations explains why young adults more often look for advice and encouragement from friends who have been exposed to similar conditions than looking to their parents or grandparents for guidance. If each generation could be persuaded to recognize the others as essential sources to learn from, the quality of life could be improved for everyone.

Mindset for Longevity Planning

Several conditions contribute to a productive mindset for thinking about the future. Being able to anticipate and evaluate possibilities is an important asset. A team of psychologists and philosophers co-authored *Homo Prospectus* (Seligman et al., 2016). Their contention was that motivation to think more often about the future is a transition in public behavior that appears to be essential for mental health of all generations in longevity societies. Devoting greater attention to planning for the future has also been a topic explored by Douglas Rushkoff, a media theorist. In *Present Shock: When Everything Happens Now,* Rushkoff (2014) pointed out that looking toward the future, a practice that was far more prevalent when the average lifespan was shorter, has greatly declined in favor of 'presentism,' living for the moment.

When students define themselves mainly as consumers, they focus on the present, getting what is wanted as soon as possible instead of exercising patience and showing a willingness to delay gratification. People who lack long-term goals are more influenced by the daily deluge of social media reports that combine past, present, and future events in a confusing sequence. One goal for the development of digital technology was to outsource memory, to free people so they could place greater emphasis on current events. However, the excessive dependence on mobile devices and non-stop messaging from persuasive media has made it difficult for people to stay focused, establish attainable goals, and try to prevent further loss in the concept of community necessary for cohesion and to support harmonious relationships among generations.

For these reasons, the first recommendation for a mindset to foster longevity planning is to resist the narrow definition of self as a consumer in favor of a more comprehensive impression as an individual who is guided by personally chosen values and governed by a sense of purpose. A second recommendation is to recognize it is possible for people to control their pace of living. Although young adults expect a longer life than their parents, many report they constantly feel hurried, even by peers who insist on quick responses to text messages. When people are rushed, one predictable consequence is the feeling of frustration. Another loss is a decline in reflective thinking, an important factor for intelligent decision making.

The pervasive complaint about being hurried should be counterbalanced by a realization there are some goals that cannot be reached quickly. To possess a healthy long-term outlook students should practice being tolerant of ambiguity, recognize doubt does not have to be overwhelming, and develop a willingness to show patience (Kellerman & Seligman, 2023). The risk for those who are mainly present-oriented is that this orientation limits them to a pursuit of short-term goals. In turn, they generally insist on receiving constant feedback about most aspects of their behavior. However, for goals that involve long-term planning, greater time and effort must be invested before it becomes sensible to evaluate progress. This situation presents a significant problem for individuals who crave reassurance, cannot wait to find out the results of their efforts, and consider it difficult to accept delay in almost every circumstance. An important factor is allowing students to choose some of their own goals that can be used later as criteria for self-evaluation.

A third recommendation for a productive mindset is to adopt flexible thinking because this motivates learning about aging from men and women further along in their own longevity journey. These adults can identify predictable situations to anticipate and obstacles to overcome. This book is intended to increase the sources of insight young adults can count on to help them plan for an extended lifespan. These learning sources, mostly from outside the school, include parents, grandparents, siblings, aunts, uncles, cousins, and neighbors.

Goals and Motivation in a Hurried Society

Many people express regret that time is getting away from them. Because there does not seem to be enough time, they generally conclude their tasks must be done more quickly in order to keep up. James Gleick (2000), author of *Faster: The Acceleration of Just About Everything*, urged the recognition, "… that neither technology nor efficiency can acquire more time for you because time is not a thing you have lost. It is not a thing you ever had. It is what you live in. You can drift in its currents or you can swim" (p. 280).

The impression that time is slipping away is illustrated by nightly arguments in families where young children want plenty of time to look at pictures and listen to stories read by parents at a pleasant and relaxing pace. Sometimes children protest by telling parents, "You're reading too fast." In such cases, the child's request for "I want another story" is still being heard as mother exits the bedroom. Speeding up the bedtime ritual might cause guilt for some parents but they rationalize that life in an accelerated context dictates rushing ahead to finish the next task on a relentless to-do list that, at the end of the day, could still include responding to e-mails, paying bills, and obtaining relief from stress by watching television.

Young adults can expect greater longevity than their older relatives. Nevertheless, they commonly express disappointment because the social environment causes them to feel hurried. This familiar complaint urges a sensible recognition that some goals cannot be attained quickly. To acquire the long-term outlook they need, students must be able to accept incompleteness in performing some tasks. The point is that when someone focuses only on the present instead of acquiring a balanced view of time, their narrow outlook restricts them to pursuit of short-term goals. This is demonstrated by individuals who insist on continuous feedback about most aspects of their behavior. However, for long-term planning, greater time and effort should be invested before it is reasonable to evaluate progress. Students should be encouraged to set some goals that can later be applied as criteria for self-evaluation.

The slower pace that characterized yesterday's world encouraged expectations for a more predictable future. In contrast, the contemporary scene causes students to experience stress, feel overwhelmed, and often suffer from anxiety regarding school performance, express doubts about career choice, worries related to their readiness for employment, concerns about keeping friends, establishing intimacy while realizing that some relationships do not last, and selecting a balanced plan for living instead of continually overscheduling themselves (Schulte, 2015). Feelings of uncertainty are beneficial if they stimulate curiosity and creative thinking. But if there is too much uncertainty, the consequent anxiety can produce emotional disturbance.

Educators should counteract the common habit of young adults to respond to situations quickly without much thought. One way to do this is for students to engage in tasks that require reflection, concentration, and deliberation instead of speedy interaction. Thinking is adversely affected when conditions needed to promote learning are rushed. When students are expected to reach goals in less time than necessary for their learning, frustration is the consequence. If the classroom schedule does not include sufficient time for students to discuss ideas and consider questions, meaningful conversations and listening skills are in jeopardy (Turkle, 2021). Efforts to fast track instruction and shorten time to practice necessary skills guarantee some students will fall behind, others will perform poorly, and groups will be unable to solve complex problems.

Similarly, when the schedule to process data is abbreviated, students may reject reflective thinking in favor of hasty methods of information processing. Instead of delaying judgment until a range of possibilities have been generated and carefully examined, people accustomed to being rushed adopt impulsive thinking and reach premature conclusions. Many obstacles associated with pressures to hurry thinking undermine cognitive development (Katz et al., 2021).

Memory and Creativity

We could remind each other about effects caused by the science fiction novel *1984*. George Orwell (1949/1983) intended his story to be a memory of the possible future, about what could happen to a society instead of limiting ourselves to being influenced only by recalling events that happened in the past. The events described in Orwell's novel remain vivid for people across time and are recognized as a source of insight, guidance, and planning. This is the power of forward memory so, instead of supposing our scope of memory is limited to recalling mistakes made in the past, forward aspects of memory could help people avoid repeating mistakes that have yet to happen.

Scientists have not conceived of a memory function that implicates the future, enables people to look ahead to ensure desirable events and situations are thought about more often so they become more likely to happen. The concept of a forward-oriented memory is dismissed because it is a logical contradiction. Memory studies have always focused on what is recalled about the past. We feel certain that memory can only make us aware of what has already taken place. When faced with the task of looking ahead we refer to other cognitive assets like intuition, insight, and imagination, mental abilities that help identify possible ways to shape a future we want to eventuate. This book goes beyond the memory of older age groups as a single basis to inform students about the future of aging because the elder perspective can be only partially correct in an era of rapid change. The vision of youth must also be shaped by creative thinking.

Consider science fiction stories that portray undesirable futures as examples of forward memory, warnings meant to trigger reflection and to motivate actions to bring positive change. Situations in fiction have to make sense within the context of a story because events in the real world often seem senseless, reflecting an environment where good people are exposed to danger and suffering while corrupt people profit from mistreatment of others. The expectation for equity and fair play is frequently challenged by the reality of daily life.

The older a person is, the shorter their future. Consequently, many older people avoid thinking about the end of life. A novel motivator to encourage young people to look ahead and implicate their forward memory is the Tikker wrist watch. This non-traditional clock provides a continual reminder that time is our most valuable asset. The watch is designed to acknowledge that life is truly short so we should make every moment count. This watch provides the time of day, calculates normal life expectancy for age of the owner, and displays a running countdown of estimated time s/he has left as a reminder to make wise choices to enhance personal legacy. Everyone should make decisions that ensure enough time is spent with loved ones, engage in physical exercise, perform community service, pay attention to spiritual development, and focus on self-improvement.

Stories in literature, movies, and television sometimes include flashback scenes meant to inform the audience about events or situations that took place at an earlier time. The narrative of this book attempts to envision aspects of tomorrow by combining the memories shared by older people along with instances of flashing forward to make known conditions readers might expect to encounter during their journey to the future.

The goals of a storyteller are to present imaginary or real-life examples that illustrate how some concept or method relates to a particular situation. Readers enjoy stories, pay attention to the processes of events and often remember key elements of a tale longer than the related factual information. Whether storytellers read from a book or report, describe events in a movie or a television program, reveal an incident someone shared with them, or communicate a personal observation, their stories can help others make connections that increase the value of a lesson, grasp concepts that previously appeared unclear, and realize why certain issues require greater attention. The potential impact of stories on awareness, comprehension, and relationships are difficult to gauge but the magic is there for those who experience it. This book includes stories that are meant to reinforce the importance of principles along with their practical application.

Sources of Knowledge

Insights for this book have been drawn from the literature on educational psychology, developmental psychology, medicine, technology, social work, nursing, gerontology, anecdotal experiences of middle age and older adults, augmented by creative intuition of young adults. Collective resources are prescriptive, intended for individual consideration about personal application. The benefits that can be expected from merging an academic and public sourcing strategy are reciprocal learning, exposure to unfamiliar ways of seeing situations and events, recognizing potential to teach and learn from classmates by sharing the outcomes of interviews, and being able to compare personal opinions with the impressions of other age groups. Gaining awareness about age diversity improves readiness for successful employment and can increase appreciation for conversations with the outsiders from other age groups. In this book, research questions are posed, traditions are challenged, new ideas and reforms are explained, proposals are encouraged, and uncertainties acknowledged. Fictional conversations and stories are told as a way to stimulate thinking and motivate wonder.

This book will refer to five adult generations when they are implicated in the text. Table 1 shows the age span boundaries for each generation as defined by the Pew Research Center (Dimock, 2019).

Table 1 Five Generations by Age as of 2024

Generation Z	Millennials	Generation X	Boomers	Silent
Ages 12–27	Ages 28–43	Ages 44–59	Ages 60–78	Ages 79–96
Born 1997–2012	Born 1981–1996	Born 1965–1980	Born 1946–1964	Born 1928–1945

Discover Generational Perspectives

No book can offer sufficient insight to fully describe or interpret aspects of longevity. Therefore, the *Generational Perspectives Activities* section provided at the end of each chapter expands personal outlook. These *Activities* are meant for individual exploration and self-selected assignments in cooperative learning teams. The *Activities* consistently include (a) agenda for team discussion; (b) questions for interviewing people of other age groups and family roles, such as parents or grandparents; (c) problem-solving scenarios with options for decision making; (d) group reviews of chapters; and (e) issues for self-evaluation. College students can respond to some of these questions based on personal experience but other questions require involvement with roles students have yet to assume such as being a parent or a grandparent. These inquiries require referral to guidance sources who are older than the peer group.

Determine Your Resources

We recommend that each student team consisting of four to five members conduct an assessment to determine the resources they can collectively count on to represent future stages of development. Access to different age groups is needed; for example, you will be talking to and learning from young adult parents (who have preschoolers), middle-aged people (whose children are in elementary or secondary school), and retired people, grandparents, and older adults.

   Children are a basic focus for men and women of all age groups. The common mission of parents is to take care of younger family members. Fulfilling this responsibility provides a sense of purpose, growth of compassion, and expansion of maturity. Accordingly, for each of the four age group stages (early adulthood, middle age, retirement, and old age), two of the four chapters in each part of the book describe adult concerns about children and adolescents that require considerable time and attention. Linking personal development with the well-being of younger and older relatives is a necessary step to actualize prospects for maturity.

Students Choose Assignment Activities

Teams should examine the *Generational Perspectives Activities* for the chapter they will read next. The usual practice is for teachers to assign the same homework activities to all students. In contrast, for this book, individual students choose their own homework activities with team approval and later share what they have learned independently with teammates and the teacher. Discuss and decide on the activities each teammate will be accountable for and expect them to report to the team. This practice fosters valuable peer teaching. Rely on critical thinking in the selection of tasks and allow for some activities to be performed by more than one teammate. Some of the chapters include more activities than a team prefers to pursue. In that case, skip some activities which are not chosen. Avoid overloading yourselves; this is necessary to support wise time management.

Sometimes students may decide to change resources for a designated Activity. To illustrate, an Activity might designate interviewing grandparents but the team prefers to find out how parents feel about the topic. Some reasoning and problem-solving tasks may not identify a source so decide for yourselves. A reminder is that while reasoning and problem solving continue to be relevant throughout life, these mental abilities are among the first to decline with aging. All teammates should interview their parents and grandparents about reasoning and problem-solving tasks and compare generational perspectives. Student reliance on a balanced emphasis of age group resources usually means more can be gained in understanding other generations.

Guidelines for Interviews as Sources of Learning

Newspaper reporters, television commentators, talk show hosts, and podcast providers rely on interviews and polling as methods to make known detailed experiences of eyewitnesses to incidents, learn expert views on special topics, and find out how ordinary people view ideas, situations, and public policy. No one can represent the full range of how other people of their age, family role, or cultural background view events and situations. Nevertheless, there can be benefit in discovering impressions of people whose age is older or younger than your own. One effective method to explore aspects of the future is called action research, conducted by students who interview older and younger generations, and report what they learned to teammates and the classroom teacher. The purpose of student generational reporting is to acquire a broader outlook than when they are limited to peer opinions. Teacher assignments to students should require some conversations with older and younger generations as sources of learning. Ignoring these out-of-school advisors diminishes the scope of learning. The following recommendations should enhance the benefits of interviews by young adults.

1 Provide the informants (parents, grandparents, other relatives, neighbors, or teachers) an opportunity to read the agenda questions for their interview in advance so they can reflect ahead of time. This strategy can reduce anxiety and offers an orientation for the conversation. Students are likely to think of additional questions as they listen to responses. Such follow-up questions can clarify and encourage elaboration for aspects of experience.

2 Tell the individual or group the amount of time scheduled for their interview. Being informed about the schedule helps participants think about the length of their explanations. If all goes well and the person(s) interviewed are in agreement, the conversation can be extended.

3 Students are familiar with pressures to be hurried. This familiar pattern should be abandoned in favor of reliance on patience and resolve to avoid rushing those being interviewed. Allow everyone the time they need to explain themselves. After posing a question, wait for reflection. People feel more comfortable when they are not hurried, and their comments will likely be more thoughtful and revealing.

4 Thank participants for their cooperation. State that you would like to take notes. Always ask for permission if you want to use a recording device. Recognize that some people are unwilling to fully express themselves when comments are recorded. Respect their wishes.

5 Consider using group interviews. For example, you could choose a senior center or assisted living facility, places where older people live or congregate. Two teammates should work together and begin by contacting the facility director to introduce themselves and share the agenda questions that elders will be asked during an interview. Then the director can identify potential volunteers and contact you by text about a day and time convenient for interested seniors to meet in their community living room. A similar method could apply to group interview of older adults at a church or synagogue.

6 Unless the agenda questions are meant to be progressive, allow informants to choose the order to answer based on their own priorities.

7 Tell participants that if they feel uncomfortable about any agenda question and prefer not to answer, their recommended response is "I pass on that one."

8 If someone wishes to respond in a language other than English, arrange for an interpreter to help.

9 Interview people who you feel comfortable with in a setting that is safe, private, and free from distractions to retain focus. An option is for two teammates to do the interview with one person asking questions and the other person taking notes.

10 Assure the person interviewed that her/his name will not be revealed in any form. The sources of all comments in your reports should be confidential and names should be anonymous. The interviews would not be posted digitally online or played for others to hear. Also, the summary of the interviews made by the team would be shared verbally with the classmates for purposes of learning from the collective interviews.

11 When interviewing children or adolescents in their home, obtain parent permission.

12 When an interview is over, tell the person(s) if their answers presented insights for you. Then ask if there is anything else s/he would like to share about the topic. Often informants appreciate hearing student responses to some of the same questions they have just been asked. This is a good way to enable reciprocal intergenerational learning.

13 Soon after an interview, while the conversation is fresh, review your notes and summarize the ideas that will be presented to teammates and the teacher.

14 After results are reported to teammates, it is helpful to tell ways your interview might have been improved. Reflective reporting is a helpful way to enhance self-evaluation skills.

If you have any questions about ensuring conditions that are safe and private for interviews, ask your instructor.

References

Arias, E., Tejada-Vera, B., Ahmad, F., & Kochanek, K. (2021, July). *Provisional life expectancy estimates for 2020*. (Report No. 015). U.S. Department of Health and Human Services, National Vital Statistics System. https://www.cdc.gov/nchs/data/vsrr/vsrr015-508.pdf

Dimock, M. (2019, January 17). Defining generations: Where Millennials end and Generation Z begins. *Pew Research Center, 17*(1), 1–7. http://www.pewresearch.org/fact-tank/2019/01/17/where-millennials-end-and-generation-z-begins/

Gleick, J. (2000). *Faster: The acceleration of just about everything*. Vintage.

Huet, E. (2024). *The believers.* Bloomberg Businessweek: Special Issue, The Longevity Issue, pp. 12–17.

Katz, R., Ogilvie, S., Shaw, J., & Woodhead, L. (2021). *Gen Z, explained: The art of living in a digital age*. The University of Chicago Press.

Kellerman, G., & Seligman, M. E. P. (2023). *Tomorrowmind: Thriving at work with resilience, creativity, and connection – now and in an uncertain future*. Atria Books.

Minkin, R., & Horowitz, J. (2023, January 24). *Parenting in America today*. Pew Research Center. https://www.pewresearch.org/social-trends/2023/01/24/parenting-in-america-today/

Orwell, G. (1983). *1984*. Harcourt Brace. (Original work published 1949)

Rushkoff, D. (2014). *Present shock: When everything happens now*. Penguin.

Schulte, B. (2015). *Overwhelmed: Work, love, and play when no one has the time*. Picador.

Seligman, M. E. P., Railton, P., Baumeister, R., & Sripada, C. (2016). *Homo prospectus*. Oxford University Press.

Turkle, S. (2021). *The empathy diaries*. Penguin.

Part I
Early Adulthood (Ages 20–40)

1 Student Stress and Mental Health

Prevalence of Stress among Generations

The 2022 *Stress in America* survey was conducted online in the United States on behalf of the American Psychological Association (2022). Subjects included 3,192 adults (age 18+). This national data gathering examined sources of stress, intensity of anxiety, and the ways people in various age groups respond to stress. Inflation was reported as a source of stress for the majority of adults (83%), who stated that the economy (69%) and money (66%) are a significant source of stress. The data show a clear generation gap. Generation Z (born 1995–2012, ages 12–29 in 2024) reported higher levels of financial stress than other generations; 46% of respondents under the age of 35 said they were so stressed they cannot function. An *American Opportunity Survey* by McKinsey & Company (Dua et al., 2022) found that in terms of their financial security, nearly half of the Generation Z respondents were concerned about the stability of their job and not having enough money to cover living expenses for more than two months. In addition, they believed their salary is insufficient for a good quality of life.

The American College Health Association (2022) surveyed 14,746 males, 35,531 females, and 3,443 transgender students for a total of 54,204 participants from 129 post-secondary educational institutions. Participants were asked to identify factors that negatively impacted their academic performance. The most often reported problem was procrastination (males 49.3%, females 49.7%, transgender 65.1%). Results also indicated that some of the participants had an ongoing or chronic medical condition diagnosed or treated in the last 12 months; the two most prominent medical conditions included stress (males 31.7%, females 46.7%, transgender 63.8%) and anxiety (males 24.2%, females 40.5%, transgender 59.6%).

Health and Resilience

People differ in their sources of stress and extent to which they are influenced by external pressures. The weight of external stressors is not the only factor that requires consideration. Another variable is how people view their situation (Iles-Caven et al., 2023). At one pole of vulnerability are individuals who seem stress resistant, with ability to cope with considerable pressure, and still carry on effectively. At the opposite pole are individuals who appear to break down whenever they have to manage even slight stress (Nowicki, 2016). According to Fricchione et al. (2022), individuals who appear stress resistant share certain characteristics. They are aware their environment includes negative forces but do not become preoccupied by them, and remain open to making changes in personal behavior. In addition, they perceive situations that are unfamiliar as

DOI: 10.4324/9781003401261-3

opportunities for growth, want to be involved when they believe their actions could make a difference, and consider themselves as in charge of most of the things that happen to them.

The way someone perceives a situation can be more important than the objective reality. According to Abramowitz and Blakey (2020), people who can readily adapt to new conditions while also being able to retain their sense of control show greater tolerance for stress. Resilience is the ability to restore balance after a difficult experience and integrating it into the total life perspective (Ruderman et al., 2022). According to Southwick et al. (2023), resilient people strive toward a good outcome without feeling overwhelmed by risks that could threaten development. They have doubts and uncertainties like everyone else but possess the ability to recover quickly from setbacks or disappointments that may cause others to quit. The resilient are flexible, share faith, hope, and optimism regarding the future. Resilience can be observed in students from hostile environments who beat the odds, and become healthy adults recognized for achievement.

Masten (2015) led a 45-year longitudinal study of 205 ordinary students from the public schools in Minneapolis. The goal was to trace the resilience of these students over a long period of time. When Project Competence was initiated in 1976, the 8- to 12-year-olds were in grades 3–6. They are now in their 50s and 60s. Follow-ups have been carried out every few years with a 90% retention rate of the original participants. In her book *Ordinary Magic,* Masten described obstacles and protective influences for these students. An important finding was that individuals who overcame risks early in life such as poverty and family instability had access to greater protection and more resources than less successful peers lacking the same access to external assets.

Stuart Lustig (2021), senior medical director for Cigna Health, reported that resilience is a skill that everyone has to some extent from an early age. Resilience is at highest levels when children are young but, as they become teenagers, resilience levels drop sharply, as much as 50% by the time people are 18–23 years old. This resilience curve is alarming because it has also revealed that Generation Z is the least resilient of all generations and seems the loneliest based on observations by professionals serving them at Cigna Heath.

Cost of Sustained Stress

The perspective of an individual mediates how stress is perceived. However, when stress is sustained it can erode an individual's capacity to cope with adversity and maintain resilience. The relationship of psychological stress to biological aging was first examined by Epel et al. (2004). Their investigation centered on *telomeres*, genetic structures at the end of each of the 46 chromosomes. Similar to the caps on the end of shoelaces, telomeres function to prevent strands of DNA from unraveling and can thereby promote genetic stability. Each time a cell divides and duplicates, some portion of the DNA telomeres shrink by a few basic pairs. Cells reproduce themselves often to strengthen host organs, grow, or fight disease. However, as people age, their telomeres shorten and, after many rounds of division, the DNA has diminished to such an extent that a cell can no longer further divide or properly carry out its function. Blackburn is credited with the discovery of an enzyme called *telomerase* that helps replenish some portion of the telomeres (Blackburn & Epel, 2017). Blackburn received the Nobel Prize in physiology and medicine in 2009 for studies showing how chromosomes are protected by telomerase with implications for cancer and longevity.

Blackburn and Epel (2017) studied a group of young mothers who had disabled children. These mothers, who met in a weekly support group, shared the difficult caregiving task that they were obliged to continue for an indefinite period. The research hypothesis was that long-term exposure to the extraordinary psychological stress experienced by these mothers would in time influence length of their telomeres. Blood samples from 39 mothers caring for a child suffering from chronic type disorders, like autism and cerebral palsy, were compared with blood samples of 20 mothers who took care of children without disabilities. White blood cells, fundamental to the immune system response for any type infection, were examined with attention to telomeres. Results revealed that the blood cells of mothers who had spent years taking care of their disabled child were genetically 9–17 years older than mothers of the same chronological age who had less demanding caregiver responsibilities. The longer the mothers had taken care of a disabled child, the shorter their telomeres and lower their telomerase activity.

Using a self-rating scale, mothers reported the extent to which they were overwhelmed by daily tasks, and how often they found themselves unable to control issues of importance to them. Mothers who saw themselves as experiencing heavy stress had significantly shortened telomeres compared to those who felt more relaxed, whether or not they were raising a disabled child (Blackburn & Epel, 2017). This was the first investigation to quantify the physiological cost of feeling highly stressed and underscores the need to discover ways to manage pressures that impose a toll on the body. It is sad these women who gave so much of themselves to help a loved one had to pay such a high cost in terms of their mental and physical health.

One implication from this research is the need to obtain relief from certain stressors that cannot be eliminated. This means arranging a schedule so attention can include personal needs such as getting enough sleep, participation in a social network, physical exercise, and having time to pursue personal interests. Epel's (2022) continuing project with mothers of children with disabilities is evaluating a broad array of possible interventions including yoga, meditation, and cognitive therapy to assess effects on telomere length and perceived stress as well as determine what could be done to preserve the capacity for resilience. Mothers in general experience the combined stress of multiple responsibilities of caring for their children, satisfying an employer, managing a household, looking after a husband, and sometimes caring for their aging parents. Learning to relax is a lesson more parents should exhibit so their children get to observe effective ways for managing stress.

Social Status and Stress

A common belief is that the amount of stress someone experiences depends upon their social status. By this reasoning the company president, store manager or school principal are exposed to greater stress than other employees for whom they are responsible. But is this an accurate impression? Marmot (2005, 2015, 2020) examined nearly 28,000 British Civil Service employees for 40 years. All subjects in the study were assigned a rank that identified their relative standing in the status hierarchy. They all had job stability and equal access to the government health care system. Marmot discovered that high status employees were far less likely to present elevated levels of stress and cholesterol. They also had cleaner arteries, fewer heart attacks, and lower index of disability than colleagues whose rank in the hierarchy was beneath their own.

These counter-intuitive outcomes suggest that improvement of social environments can contribute to better physical and mental health (Marmot, 2015, 2020). School principals face daily challenges of management related to students, teachers, staff, parents, and larger community. Teachers also feel extensive demands that require taking work home after school. Students occupy the lowest status within the school hierarchy so they lack input to needed considerations for institutional changes they believe would improve instruction and achievement. Young adults often experience stress older relatives are unaware of or underestimate but often have power to diminish. Within a socially responsive environment where voices of students are heard, Strom and Strom (2024) contend that students can contribute a unique perspective about institutional effectiveness and should be assured the faculty will consider their ideas and suggestions.

Stress Management

Symptoms of Stress

The symptoms of student stress that receive the most attention from teachers and parents are aggressive actions, destruction of property, bullying, stealing, and other anti-social conduct. However, according to mental health professionals, these conditions are not the main symptoms of stress. Such behaviors are bothersome and inform others that someone is experiencing stress and needs help. These individuals may feel threatened and overburdened but they continue to struggle and, given support, might become able to manage stress. Severe symptoms of stress include depression, withdrawal, and resignation. Students presenting these behaviors have quit (Myers & Twenge, 2022).

Effects of Depression

Depression is a serious mental health threat to all age groups. The Mayo Clinic (2023) explains this is not just a matter of being moody or having to deal with a difficult environment; instead individuals have abandoned hope so they quit trying to adjust to situations they view as overwhelming. According to the National Institute of Mental Health (2023), adult prevalence of depressive episodes was highest among individuals aged 18–25 years old (18.6%). Corresponding rates were considerably lower for those 26–49 years old (9.3%) and people age 50+ (4.5%) (Strom et al., 2022). Despite fairly equal rates of depression in childhood, rates change during adolescence when females become nearly twice as likely to suffer depression. Damour (2019) attributes higher risk for females to hormonal changes related to puberty, menstruation, pregnancy, and menopause. Even though depression can be treated, less than one-third of young people who need help get care.

Depression involves elevating and lowering of mood that can negatively influence how individuals feel, think, and behave. When brain chemicals such as serotonin and dopamine are imbalanced, depression can become chronic and require antidepressant medications to bring chemicals into balance. O'Connor and Pirkis (2016) summarized evidence demonstrating how depressed students are more likely than peers to engage in high-risk behaviors like underage drinking, illegal drug taking, driving drunk, and early sexual intercourse. One danger of being preoccupied with problems experienced at the present time is the loss of ability to place these events within the context of a longer time perspective. During periodic depression, it can be motivating to reflect on past achievements as a way to restore self-confidence and sustained effort. Young adults should think about the consequences of disappointing events in a longer time frame that includes the future instead of only the pain of the moment (Thompson, 2022). When people become unable to disengage from their current troubles, some become depressed and, in despair, conclude that suicide seems their only choice (Knapp, 2020).

Anxiety and Uncertainty

Abramowitz and Blakey (2020) described anxiety as the feelings of uncertainty that arise when an unfamiliar situation or event is anticipated. In prior generations, a slower pace of change meant that feelings of certainty were more pervasive, the future seemed to be more predictable so anxiety was less common. Certainty has great appeal to people in modern societies where daily affairs present considerable uncertainty. People worry about what is going to happen next and have doubts about what can be expected (Kurth, 2018). Schulte (2015) observed young adults have to manage many challenges. For example, they are concerned about anxiety related to academic performance, uncertainty about career choice, and worries about the cost of higher education. In addition, there are doubts about readiness to qualify for the preferred workforce placement, concerns centered on maintaining friendships, living with parents while going to college, getting along with a romantic companion, establishing intimacy while knowing some relationships may not last, and choosing a balanced lifestyle rather than continually over-scheduling themselves. Feeling uncertain and having doubts is beneficial if it stimulates curiosity and creative thinking. However, when uncertainty becomes excessive the consequent stress can lead to emotional disturbance. Schools and families should help students avoid this dangerous result of anxiety (Brooks & Lasser, 2018; Galanti, 2020; Horowitz & Graf, 2019; Thompson, 2022).

Some of the conditions that stimulate anxiety seem to be the same as being human. As far as we can tell, animals do not lay awake at night thinking about the problems that cause them to dread the following day. Animals do not have to worry about how they can pay rent on the tree where they live, cover the costs of higher education for multiple offspring, or avoid exposure to sexually transmitted disease. In short, animals do not have capacity to imagine, that wonderful attribute unique to the human mind, but can also incline some people to incessantly foresee almost every conceivable hazard. People worry because of awareness that mankind has a future and what happens tomorrow is less certain than it was for men and women living in earlier times.

Hope and Optimism

Optimism, the expression of hope, is considered an element of emotional intelligence that can have enormous effect on ability to manage frustration. Keefer et al. (2018) reported the way individuals explain their failures and successes to themselves mediates how they process their frustration. An optimistic self-explanatory style enables someone to view failure as a temporary setback, an outcome they have the power to change by increasing their time studying, reading more carefully, and paying attention while taking notes from teacher presentations. A pessimistic self-explanatory style causes people to believe failure reflects personal shortcomings over which they lack control and should accept instead of making vain efforts to improve their behavior. Seligman (2018) studied 500 freshmen at University of Pennsylvania; results of this research showed students' scores on a measure of optimism was the best predictor of grades in the first year of college.

There is evidence that cognitive orientation has an influence on emotions and behavior. The key factor seems to be reliance on accurate thinking more than positive thinking. Goleman and Davidson (2018) documented that resilience is supported in schools and by families where lessons are provided about the importance of hope, optimism, assertiveness, and flexibility. This strategy can improve the outlook on life, motivate better academic performance, and diminish probability of depression. Seligman (2018) conducted 19 international studies involving 2,000 students from ages 5 to 18. Students were taught to think more realistically and flexibly about their daily problems. The emphasis was on slowing down the problem-solving process, clarifying goals, retrieving data without an undue emphasis on speed, and generating possibilities to attain their purposes. The results of the intervention showed that optimism rates rose and rates of depression declined by half. The conclusion was fostering emotional wellness improves mental health and performance.

College Students Living with Parents

Strom and Strom (2005) examined the social dynamics of college students living at home with their parents. The purposes for these interviews were to detect obstacles and benefits experienced by both generations. Participants included 166 students (87 males and 79 females) and 218 of their parents (127 mothers and 91 fathers). Results showed the most common student complaints about living at home with parents were lack or privacy, and being denied the freedom of personal space enjoyed by friends who lived in an apartment or dormitory. Being financially dependent also fostered some frustration. Living at home with parents while attending college usually means more arguments with parents than during high school. Frequent disputes relate to sharing a car, the bathroom, contents of the refrigerator, and dissimilar sleep time schedules. Listening to loud music and watching television that older relatives dislike can be bothersome. Taking a girlfriend or boyfriend into the bedroom and closing the door can motivate family conflict.

Some parents reported they did not want to listen to complaints about the demands of school and faculty. These parents often forfeit a possible role of confidant by reacting with comments that shut down interaction, such as, "You are lucky to be able to attend college. I never had the opportunity." A more reasoned response is to recognize that stresses at school, with peers, and on the job ought to be shared. Students generally rely on a trusted friend (49%) or relative (26%) willing to listen without judgment. This situation presents possibilities to provide feedback on behavior and suggest alternatives for dealing with daily dilemmas. These conversations can be satisfying and occur more often when students are young adults attending college than when they are still going to high school. In effect, parents whose children stay home while going to college have more time to teach some important life skills and young adults are usually more ready to learn about these lessons.

Mothers and fathers try to reduce stress by allowing children to live at home without paying rent, having free and healthy meals, access to transportation, and laundry privileges. Young adults should acknowledge these are important contributions of parents. Most parents expressed disappointment that their children who advocate for global equality seem unable to recognize what this means in a practical sense by sharing domestic chores at home and by considering the needs of loved ones who live with them. Females, more than males, reported that getting along with parents was more stressful;

they believed parents could reduce the stress they impose by adopting more reasonable school expectations instead of assuming their child should outperform peers. McConville (2020) explained that daily examples of how parents manage frustration, cope with setbacks and failures are observed by students while in college more carefully than when they were attending high school.

Parents recognized division of household labor has become more equitable than it was in previous generations when domestic tasks were much more gender-oriented. Paula, a middle-aged mother, is pleased by what she sees as a slow shift in the right direction. When she was growing up the chores for her brothers were shoveling snow and mowing the grass. The boys complained when parents sometimes asked them to also wash dishes since they felt this was women's work. The brothers bribed their sisters, promising to pay them for doing the dishes on their behalf. Paula says her brothers still owe her $825,000 because none of them ever paid their debt.

Acknowledging the transition of adolescents to grownup is demonstrated by parents who explore their individual goals, values, and concerns while also becoming informed about student generational norms. Knowing about the fears, worries, priorities and concerns of young adults can motivate parents to treat them as adults. Parents who welcome a chance to learn from young adult children have much to gain. When both parties are growth-oriented and prepared to learn from each other, they can invite feedback about personal progress in reaching the goals they have chosen for personal success. When customary hierarchical authority in the family is augmented by greater friendship, both of the parties are more inclined to seek advice from one another (Strom & Strom, 2005).

Some parents are disappointed about having a financially supportive role longer than previous generations. They compare their own independence when they were the same age as their children are now. But, in those days, a college degree was less needed for employment. The current labor market reality should motivate parent adjustment to their revised role that fits the times. Such a responsibility may contradict some of the plans parents made earlier to be free of noise and disruption when their children would be old enough to move out. One father summed up his discontent, "This was to be the time when my wife and I could rediscover each other, have constant access to our car and bathroom, and spend more money on ourselves than always putting children first."

Self-Identification as LGBT

According to the U.S. Census Bureau, lesbian, gay, bisexual, and transgender adults (ages 18 to 65+) reported twice the rate of mental health problems as non-LGBT adults (Marlay et al., 2022). These challenges include anxiety, depression, persistent feelings of sadness, hopelessness, family rejection, and suicidal thoughts. The significance of the survey results showed that the younger adult respondents (ages 18 to 29), whether LBGT or non-LGBT, struggled more with both anxiety and depression symptoms, but younger LGBT adult respondents struggled the most.

Stress of College Students

We surveyed college students about their stress and ways others could reduce the unnecessary demands placed on them (Strom et al., 2021). The participants were

351 college freshmen and sophomore students; the response rate was 78%. The 210 females and 141 males identified themselves as White 51%, Black 9%, Hispanic 25%, Asian 8%, and Other 7%. Most of these students were single (86%), and lived at home with their parents (69%). Besides going to school 31% worked full-time, 46% had part-time job, and 23% were unemployed. Students completed the online College Stress Poll including 17 multiple-choice items about the following questions:

What sources of stress do you experience in the classroom and outside of school?

How do you process the feelings that arise whenever you have to manage stress?

What are the main signals students rely on to let them know that they are stressed?

What kinds of events cause the students to worry about things that result in stress?

How have parents taught daughters and sons to manage daily conditions of stress?

What can teachers, parents, and peers do to reduce the undue stress students feel?

How do the students rate themselves in getting enough sleep during week nights?

What are the conditions in which students believe they demonstrate resilience?

What factors do students include in their definition of how to become successful?

How important do students believe their own decisions are in influencing stress?

How often do students feel optimistic about their future in school and at work?

What do students think teachers and parents should know about young adult stress?

How do dating and romantic relationships contribute to stress of students?

Implications for Self

About half (49%) the college student participants acknowledged poor time management was stressful. Time management skills are needed in order to reach personal goals. People whose priorities receive enough attention are more able to govern what happens to them. In this connection students felt their decisions were often hurried and prevented good judgment. This impression was reinforced by poll comments that personal schedules were always or often rushed. When students do not have time to consider relevant information or generate alternatives for solving problems, they are inclined to reject reflective thinking in favor of hasty information processing methods. Instead of delaying decisions until a broad range of options have been examined, individuals accustomed to being rushed are inclined to reach premature conclusions. This is a high cost for compressing the time needed for learning. Time management should be a continuous lesson taught by teachers and relatives as a method to support mental health.

Spending many hours a day phoning or texting friends, and engaging with e-media are distractions from the main student responsibility to invest most of their time on learning. Establishing rules during adolescence that limit amount of time youth are permitted to communicate with friends is a practical way courageous parents support self-regulation and academic performance.

Most people would prefer that life reflect personal decisions. However, in a rapid-paced environment with competing priorities and information overload, some decisions are based on impulse, stress, and expedience. Students should be able to observe mature behavior that helps them realize the health benefits that accompany time management. Individuals with this ability commonly avoid taking on too many responsibilities, breaking promises made to others, ignoring people and activities that matter most, and have a calendar that reflects a reasonable distribution of time. When parents cannot provide a healthy example of time management, daughters and sons often repeat the same pattern, overscheduling themselves and experiencing the stressful results of being unable to control their lives.

When asked to identify sources of stress outside the classroom and home, the most prominent issues were job-related (60%). Some students are poorly informed about what it takes to meet dual obligations of satisfying an employer and obligations to faculty. Taking too many courses in a semester is a common mistake as students overestimate how well they can perform in both sectors. A majority of students felt that they could benefit from the following workshops: time management (62%), understanding stress and effects on individuals (59%), and exercising and meditation for stress reduction (58%). In addition, less than half were interested in attending a workshop about college tuition costs and loans (42%).

Implications for Faculty

The most common worries of students were getting good grades (77%), uncertainty about their future (64%), and figuring out suitable career prospects (44%). Nearly half (48%) expressed disappointment about how some teachers explained ideas, concepts and ways to solve problems. A majority reported feeling stressed because they did not understand content presented in some courses.

Educators are usually surprised when their instruction is considered hard to comprehend. Asking students to reveal confusion by raising their hands in class seldom results in a response because this is seen as a reason for embarrassment; they do not want to be regarded as incapable. For example, a one-time demonstration about solving a mathematics problem is usually insufficient. A more effective teaching strategy is to make online presentations of class lessons that students identify as difficult and then post the step-by-step process on the school learning management system.

Faculty at this college should inform students that not being able to understand concepts can usually be corrected with tutoring support. The purposes of tutoring are to detect errors by observation, identify procedures to remediate mistakes, arrange for guided practice, monitor progress, and provide feedback about achievement. Student denial of academic deficits can sometimes reflect misleading evaluation practices (Rey, 2019). There is evidence that many teachers have low expectations but give high grades regardless of student performance level. Grade inflation is a problem at all levels of education (Buckley et al., 2018). This is a serious mistake because it hides deficits in learning, condones poor performance, and promotes self-confidence that is unwarranted. College students could assume that even though they do not comprehend some of their lessons, the grades they were given in high school implied tutoring was not needed.

There was agreement among the poll participants that teachers should diminish stress by joint planning to avoid overloading individual students, make group assignments so that the collective load can be shared, and allow mistakes without influencing grades. Students believed teacher performance could improve by becoming more informed about stress. They felt that free workshops offered on topics like understanding stresses faced by students, methods to help students cope with stress, recognizing effects of stress, and how to manage their own stress on the job would be helpful.

Implications for Parents

Students reported that relatives could reduce the amount of stress they impose by having more reasonable expectations for achievement. Parent expectations for students to do better than classmates was reported as a common source of stress. Students looked to parents for guidance on how to avoid becoming overscheduled, and provide a personal example of time management that supports productivity as well as relaxation. Students recommended that their school provide free workshops for parents focused on identifying stresses of young adults, ways to support students in coping with stress, and learning how to cope with their own stress in the role of a parent.

Some students reported that their parents had not taught them how to cope with stress. This outcome leads to the conclusion that parents should ask daughters and sons to identify events that are stressful for them and find out how they responded to such situations. Males and females reacted to their stress differently. To diminish stress, males were more likely to play video games (59.6%) than females (9.5%). Parents were recognized for teaching their children at home about showing patience, balancing work and play, and avoiding overscheduling.

Everyone needs resilience. Development of resilience is frequently hampered by self-centeredness. Parents should think about how their own behavior contributes to this deficiency because they have unreasonable academic expectations and discourage students from being able to admit personal limitations. *Narcissism* is defined as excessive self-admiration, shown by an inflated self-impression. The *Narcissism Personality Inventory* was first administered by authors Raskin and Terry (1988). Since then, more than 16,000 students have completed the inventory. Myers and Twenge (2022) found that two-thirds of college students agreed their generation is more self-centered and narcissistic than previous generations.

This hyper-individualistic orientation of narcissism is thought to be the result of a non-stop promotion of student self-esteem, that is independent of achievement, by parents constantly telling their children they are special, protecting them from recognizing or acknowledging their academic failures, and consequently preventing the development of resilience needed to recover from setbacks when things go wrong.

Students whose parents cause them to believe they always perform well lack ability to process criticism from teachers or cooperative learning colleagues. As a result, defensiveness is a common hindrance to acquiring the teamwork skills valued by employers. Getting anonymous feedback from peers and learning to objectively process their criticism are valuable lessons that should be reinforced by parents who realize a need to perform well with co-workers on the job and cooperative teams in school (Turkle, 2015).

Implications for Peers

The most prominent method for students to cope with stress was having conversations with friends more often than seeking advice and emotional assurance from parents or faculty. Nearly half of the student participants (49%) reported a preference to process their stress by talking with friends. They thought friends could diminish stress by, "Respecting my need to make decisions that fit my goals" (61%), "Not interrupt me when I schedule time to study" (41%), and "Not pressure me to quickly answer text messages" (26%). "Tutoring me if I have problems" was seen as another way classmates could reduce stress while contributing to academic achievement (33%).

Given the powerful influence of peers, educators should recognize their corresponding obligation to continually encourage healthy norms of group behavior for cooperative learning teams. The classroom teacher role is changing as the students become more willing to assume greater responsibility to provide tutoring and emotional support for peers. In addition, the school goal to enable student appreciation for interdependence is more likely to be reached by reliance on peer teaching than when everyone has to count on their classroom teacher as the single source of instruction. Peers can also teach how to treat others, an essential lesson in social development.

Students can benefit from reflection about the meaning of friendship. One definition of friendship is to always favor the best interests of someone who we care about, share feelings and ideas with them, and offer advice meant to support growth and maturity. Thinking of friendship in nurturing ways means that real friends would not approve of having a friend deny academic deficits but instead encourage tutoring if they know help is needed. Peers should also support healthy qualities like showing resilience following a failure in class, being optimistic about the future, and recognizing personal accountability for most situations. Friends motivate peers by complimenting the healthy behaviors they observe.

Conclusion

Stress is recognized as a widespread concern and represents a significant obstacle to mental health of college students and negatively impacts their academic performance. Stress and mental health are linked. The pressures young adults experience are evident from personal reports about uncertainty, anxiety, stress, and depression. Optimistic thinking of resilient individuals motivates them to effectively manage unfamiliar challenges, maintain a positive outlook, and continue to persevere when tasks become difficult.

Educators should strive to find out what can be done to reduce unnecessary stress and improve conditions that support mental health and academic achievement. Student uncertainty is minimized by presenting easily understood goals for each class lesson, giving clear directions for assignments, considering the likely consequences before making decisions, and showing flexibility rather than rigid thinking.

Some students reveal stress by aggressive behavior and drawing attention to themselves. But the more serious symptoms of stress are depression, withdrawal, and resignation. Educators and relatives should strive to be recognized as sources of support by students who make their stress known to access help.

At every stage in life people are too old or too young to have direct knowledge of some things based on personal experience. Parents of college-age students should try to find out what young adulthood is like in the current environment so they improve their chances to be seen as sources of advice. Similarly, college students should try to learn from their parents about the stress they face in middle age. Fortunately, both parties can enrich their relationship through reciprocal learning. This opportunity for interaction may be the most challenging aspect of maturity for the parents and the greatest test of growing up for the young adults.

Key Concepts

1 People differ in sources of stress they are exposed to and the extent to which external pressures influences them. The weight of an external stressor is not the only factor for consideration. Another variable is how people view their situation. At one pole are persons who appear stress resistant, able to handle considerable pressure and carry on effectively. At the other extreme are individuals who seem to break down whenever they encounter even slight pressure.

2 Stress resistant people recognize negative forces in their environment but are not preoccupied by them, willing to make changes in their behavior, see unfamiliar situations as opportunities for personal growth, feel a need to become involved when they believe that their actions could make a difference, and consider themselves in charge for most of the things that happen to them.

3 Resilience is the ability to restore balance following a difficult experience and integrating it into the total life perspective. Resilient people strive to obtain a good outcome without being overwhelmed by risks that might otherwise threaten development. They have uncertainties like everyone else but recover quickly from setbacks or disappointments that cause others to give up.

4 Resilience is at highest levels during early childhood. In adolescence resilience drops sharply, as much as 50% by the time a person is 18–23 years old. This change is alarming because there is evidence that Generation Z is the least resilient generation and should receive support from peers, parents, and teachers to cope with unprecedented demands.

5 Accurate thinking deserves as much attention as positive thinking. Students in an experimental program were taught to think more realistically and flexibly about their everyday problems. The emphasis was on slowing down the problem-solving process, thinking more clearly, be able to identify goals and retrieve data without a focus on speed, and think of alternative ways to attain their purpose.

6 When parents and grandparents try to protect young adults from the effects of adversity, these forms of protection often have the negative effect of rendering youth less prepared to manage unforeseen challenges everyone will inevitably experience. Exposure to risk is necessary to develop resilience needed to sustain well-being during any stage of life.

7 One outcome of sustained stress is the need for relief from adverse conditions that cannot be eliminated. This means arranging a schedule that enables attention to personal needs like getting enough sleep, participating with friends in a social network, and getting physical exercise, Being healthy also calls for arranging time to engage in community service, being able to pursue the interests of a hobby, and evaluate how well personal goals are being met.

8 The most significant symptoms of stress are depression, withdrawal, and resignation. Students who exhibit these behaviors have quit. Depression is a serious threat to mental health. This is not a matter of being moody or living in a difficult situation but that individuals have given up hope and no longer persist in adjusting to difficult situations they consider overwhelming.

9 A significant danger of being preoccupied by problems that are experienced in the present is a loss of ability to place these difficulties within the context of a longer time frame. When people are unable to disengage from current troubles, some of them become depressed and might reach the dangerous conclusion that the only option is to take their own life, the ultimate withdrawal from what seems insurmountable and irreversible stress.

10 Parents and college students benefit each another by engagement in reciprocal learning and, in the process, develop qualities that can contribute to personal maturity and greater satisfaction. Living at home is often a challenge for both generations that can also enrich their relationship and access to a long-term valuable source of advice and emotional support.

Generational Perspectives Activities

1.1 Team Discussion
1.2 Agenda for Interviews with Parents
1.3 A Scenario: Reasoning and Problem Solving
1.4 Team Chapter Review
1.5 Criteria for Self-Evaluation of Team Members

1.1 Team Discussion

Each team member answers one question.

1 What are the signs that show you are experiencing an excessive amount of stress?
2 What stressful situations are the ones that you consider to be the most bothersome?
3 What methods do you depend on to obtain relief from the daily stress you experience?
4 Who provides your relatives with a healthy example about ways to manage stress?
5 In what ways are you a source of undue stress for other members in your family?
6 What are the main stresses currently experienced by your parents? grandparents?
7 What are some common stresses at your age that older relatives do not recognize?
8 What individual in your family presents the most valuable lessons for resilience?
9 What are some ways friends contribute to the undue stress that you experience?
10 What are some uncertainties that young adults have to manage on a regular basis?

1.2 Agenda for Interviews with Parents

 1 How do worries of young adults differ from your own concerns at their age?
 2 What are some common uncertainties that are experienced by young adults?
 3 How well do schools meet emotional needs of special education families?
 4 What are some gender differences in stress that occur during early adulthood?
 5 What are effective methods to help students avoid becoming overscheduled?
 6 In what aspects of guidance do you demonstrate the most and least patience?
 7 What things do you worry about most in carrying out your role in the family?
 8 How should schools help students who seem unable to cope with frustration?
 9 How should students express their views about reforms needed at their school?
10 How should parents help young adults cope with the stresses they encounter?

1.3 A Scenario: Reasoning and Problem Solving

Problem-solving scenarios present an opportunity to look at situations that might happen for a family and think about possible solutions. Your task is to think about pros and cons of stated choices, generate additional options, identify relevant information that might be missing, learn how teammates view the options, and defend your reasoning about advice you consider best.

On Monday three of Frank's teachers made assignments that are due Friday. There is not enough time available to complete all of this homework. Frank would welcome your advice:

a Talk to one or more of the teachers and ask permission to revise the due date.
b Ask a classmate to go with you to talk to the teacher about the homework due date.
c Put the most effort into classes where more points are needed to get a better grade.
d Accept the fact that unreasonable stress has become a part of normal everyday life.
e Other _____

1.4 Team Chapter Review

Efforts to assess participant learning, provide feedback, and improve quality of instruction is enhanced by a team review of each chapter.

1 What ideas in the chapter changed the way I think about this topic?
2 What insights from the chapter will I try to apply in my relationships?
3 What is the most important point for me presented in this chapter?
4 What are some aspects of this chapter I would like to better understand?
5 What aspects of this chapter do I wish that I had known about earlier?

1.5 Criteria for Self-Evaluation of Team Members

Directions: Check all that apply to you and share your answers with teammates.

 1 The situations that seem most stressful for me are

    a having disagreements with family members
    b taking on more obligations than is reasonable

c making sure that I manage my finances well
d figuring out the career path I want to pursue
e Other _____

2 Some ways I impose undue stress on my relatives are

a asking questions they do not want to discuss
b telling them how to improve their behavior
c having career expectations they do not like
d ignoring budget limits they set for me
e Other _____

3 The methods I rely on to relieve my stress are

a jogging and other physical exercise
b talking to parents or other relatives
c talking to friends about my situation
d prayer and support from my religion
e reliance on video game participation
f Other _____

4 The ways my parents relieve their stress are by

a watching tv or other events like sports
b talking with their friends
c reading books, magazines, or journals
d working to keep up their yard or garden
e I don't know _____

5 Some things I could do to reduce stress of my parents are

a provide help with some of the household chores
b talk and listen to them more often
c get a part-time job to pay for some of my tuition
d avoid comparing my goals with their goals
e spend more time together
f Other _____

6 The stress experienced by my grandparents is

a a topic I have never discussed with them
b a story I have been told by my parents
c a topic they often talk about to me
d Other _____

7 I believe the stress many young adults experience

a is caused by unreasonable expectations of their parents
b reflects uncertainty and worries about the future
c arises because mental health gets little attention
d is related to the continual demands from peers
e Other _____

8 The signs that show me I have too much stress are

   a headaches and stomach aches
   b being short-tempered with others
   c inability to sleep well at night
   d wanting to be alone
   e Other _____

9 The stress experienced by my brothers and sisters is

   a a topic that we do not talk about together
   b shared with me to learn my reactions
   c unknown to me and I have not asked
   d Other _____

10 My grandparents relieve stress by

   a walking and other physical exercise
   b talking to their friends and relatives
   c I don't know
   d church activities, prayer, and bible reading
   e Other _____

References

Abramowitz, J. S., & Blakey, S. M. (Eds.). (2020). *Clinical handbook of fear and anxiety: Maintenance processes and treatment mechanisms*. American Psychological Association. 10.1037/0000150-000

American College Health Association. (2022, Spring). *American College Health Association-National College Health Assessment III: Undergraduate Student Reference Group Executive Summary*, pp. 5–6. https://www.acha.org/documents/ncha/NCHA-III_SPRING_2022_UNDERGRAD_REFERENCE_GROUP_EXECUTIVE_SUMMARY.pdf

American Psychological Association. (2022, October). *Stress in America 2022: Concerned for the future, beset by inflation*. https://www.apa.org/news/press/releases/stress/2022/concerned-future-inflation

Blackburn, E., & Epel, E. (2017). *The telomere effect: A revolutionary approach to living younger, healthier, longer*. Grand Central Publishing.

Brooks, M., & Lasser, J. (2018). *Tech generation: Raising balanced kids in a hyper-connected world*. Oxford University Press.

Buckley, J., Letukas, L., & Wildavsky, P. (Eds.). (2018). *Measuring success: Testing, grades, and the future of college admissions*. John Hopkins University Press.

Damour, L. (2019). *Under pressure: Confronting the epidemic of stress and anxiety in girls*. Ballantine Books.

Dua, A., Ellingrud, K., Lazar, M., Luby, R., & Pemberton, S. (2022, October 19). *How does Gen Z see its place in the working world? With trepidation*. McKinsey & Company. https://www.mckinsey.com/featured-insights/sustainable-inclusive-growth/future-of-america/how-does-gen-z-see-its-place-in-the-working-world-with-trepidation#/

Epel, E. (2022). *The stress prescription: Seven days to more joy and ease*. Penguin Life.

Epel, E. S., Blackburn, E. H., Lin, J., Dhabhar, F. S., Adler, N. E., Morrow, J. D., & Cawthon, R. M. (2004, December 1). Accelerated telomere shortening in response to life stress. *Proceedings of the National Academy of Sciences of the United States of America, 101*(49), 17312–17315. 10.1073/pnas.0407162101

Fricchione, G. L., Ivkovic, A., & Yeung, A. S. (Eds.). (2022). *The science of stress: Living under pressure*. University of Chicago Press. (Original work published 2016)

Galanti, R. (2020). *Anxiety relief for teens: Essential CBT skills & mindfulness practices to overcome anxiety & stress*. Penguin Random House.

Goleman, D., & Davidson, R. J. (2018). *Altered traits: Science reveals how meditation changes your mind, brain, and body*. Avery.

Horowitz, J. M., & Graf, N. (2019, February 20). Most U.S. teens see anxiety and depression as a major problem among their peers. *Pew Research Center*. https://www.nabh.org/pew-research-center-report-most-u-s-teens-see-anxiety-and-depression-as-a-major-problem-among-their-peers/

Iles-Caven, Y., Gregory, S., Northstone, K., Golding, J., & Nowicki, S. (2023, March). The beneficial role of personality in preserving well-being during the pandemic: A longitudinal population study. *Journal of Affective Disorders*, *331*, 229–237. 10.1016/j.jad.2023.03.056

Keefer, K. V., Parker, J. D. A., & Saklofske, D. H. (Eds.). (2018). *Emotional intelligence in education: Integrating research with practice*. Springer.

Knapp, S. J. (2020). *Suicide prevention: An ethically and scientifically informed approach*. American Psychological Association.

Kurth, C. (2018). *The anxious mind: An investigation into the varieties and virtues of anxiety*. The MIT Press.

Lustig, S. (2021). *How can we help children and young adults build resilience?* YouTube. https://www.youtube.com/watch?v=y_RxItYbi84

Marlay, M., File, T., & Scherer, Z. (2022, December 14). *Mental health struggles higher among LGTB adults than non-LGBT adults in all age groups*. United States Census Bureau. https://www.census.gov/library/stories/2022/12/lgbt-adults-report-anxiety-depression-at-all-ages.html

Marmot, M. G. (2005). *The status syndrome: How social standing affects our health and longevity*. Henry Holt.

Marmot, M. G. (2015). *The health gap: The challenge of an unequal world*. Bloomsbury.

Marmot, M. G., Allen, J., Boyce, T., Goldblatt, P., & Morrison, J. (2020, February). *Health equity in England: Marmot review 10 years on*. The Health Foundation. https://www.health.org.uk/publications/reports/the-marmot-review-10-years-on

Masten, A. S. (2015). *Ordinary magic: Resilience in development*. Guilford Press.

Mayo Clinic. (2023). *Depression (major depressive disorder)*. https://www.mayoclinic.org/diseases-conditions/depression/symptoms-causes/syc-20356007

McConville, M. (2020). *Failure to launch: Why your twentysomething hasn't grownup … and what to do about it*. G.P. Putnam's Sons.

Myers, D., & Twenge, J. (2022). *Social psychology* (14th ed.). McGraw-Hill.

National Institute of Mental Health. (2023, July). *Major depression*. National Institute of Health. https://www.nimh.nih.gov/health/statistics/major-depression

Nowicki, S. (2016). *Choice or chance: Understanding your locus of control and why it matters*. Prometheus.

O'Connor, R. C., & Pirkis, J. (2016). *The international handbook of suicide prevention* (2nd ed.). Wiley-Blackwell.

Raskin, R., & Terry, H. (1988). A principal components analysis of the *Narcissistic Personality Inventory* and further evidence of its construct validity. *Journal of Personality and Social Psychology*, *54*(5), 890–902. 10.1037/0022-3514.54.5.890

Rey, V. M. (2019). Effects of engaging students in a remedial course. *Practitioner to Practitioner*, *10*(3), 8–13. https://files.eric.ed.gov/fulltext/EJ1246587.pdf

Ruderman, M. N., Clerkin, C., & Fernandez, K. C. (2022). *Resilience that works: Eight practices for leadership and life*. Center for Creative Leadership.

Schulte, B. (2015). *Overwhelmed: How to work, love and play when no one has the time*. Picador.

Seligman, M. E. P. (2018). *The hope circuit: A psychologist's journey from helplessness to optimism*. Public Affairs.

Southwick, S. M., Charney, D. S., & DePierro, J. M. (2023). *Resilience: The science of mastering life's greatest challenges* (3rd ed.). Cambridge University Press.

Strom, P. S., Hendon, K. L., Strom, R. D., & Wang, C.-h. (2022). High school student stress and school improvement. *School Community Journal, 32*(2), 205–228. http://www.schoolcommunitynetwork.org/SCJ.aspx

Strom, P. S., & Strom, R. D. (2005). Parent-child relationships in early adulthood: College students living at home. *Community College Journal of Research and Practice, 29*(7), 517–529. 10.1080/10668920590953980

Strom, P. S., & Strom, R. D. (2024). *Polling student voices for school improvement: A guide for educational leaders.* Information Age Publishing.

Strom, P. S., Strom, R. D., Sindel-Arrington, T., Rude, R. V., & Wang, C.-h. (2021). Gender differences in stress of community college students. *Community College Journal of Research and Practice.* 10.1080/10668926.2021.1873872

Thompson, D. (2022, April 11). Why American teens are so sad. *The Atlantic.* https://www.theatlantic.com/newsletters/archive/2022/04/amerian-teens-sadness-depression-anxiety/629524/

Turkle, S. (2015). *Reclaiming conversation: The power of talk in a digital age.* Penguin.

2   Taking Risks and Higher Education

National Risk Assessment

Some dangerous risks that young adults encounter include unplanned pregnancy, sexually transmitted diseases, substance abuse, visiting predators online, not getting enough sleep, texting while driving, smoking tobacco, skipping school, dropping out, joining a gang, getting involved with criminal behavior, bringing a weapon to school, cheating, lying to parents and teachers, delay in meeting responsibilities, not studying for tests, ignoring physical exercise, not planning a reasonable schedule, making poor nutritional choices, avoiding tutoring that can overcome academic deficiencies, reckless driving, and being the passenger of a driver who has been drinking. The Centers for Disease Control and Prevention (2023) *Youth Risk Behavior Surveillance System* annually monitors six categories of health-related behaviors that reflect leading causes of death and disability among young people. The categories are (1) behaviors that contribute to unintentional injuries and violence, (2) sexual activity that can result in unintended pregnancy or sexually transmitted diseases, (3) alcohol and substance abuse, (4) addiction to tobacco, (5) unhealthy diet, and (6) insufficient exercise.

The United States Drug Enforcement Administration (2023) has issued a warning that fentanyl is the single deadliest drug threat our nation has ever encountered. Fentanyl is involved in more deaths of Americans under age 50 than any other cause of death, including heart disease, cancer, homicide, suicide, and other accidents. Most of those deaths were attributed to fentanyl mixed with other illicit drugs like cocaine, methamphetamine, and heroin, with many users unaware they were taking fentanyl. Only two milligrams of fentanyl is considered a potentially lethal dose.

Origins of Risk Analysis

Being able to gauge risk is a skill everyone should acquire because this asset can prevent taking foolish risks. Consider what happens when individuals are unable to accurately determine whether the risks they take are reasonable or believe that their personal courage is confirmed by engaging in situations generally shunned by others as being too risky. During the conflict between North and South Korea that began in the 1950s, military leaders began a new policy to protect troops. *Risk analysis* is the practice of monitoring the ability of individuals to accurately gauge risks. Psychological teams were formed to conduct risk analysis with members of air force squadrons (Torrance, 1957). The goal was to identify fighter pilots who should be temporarily withdrawn from the scene of battle.

DOI: 10.4324/9781003401261-4

Before this strategy was adopted, the single consideration for pilots to obtain relief from combat was to have completed a specified number of combat missions. The policy was amended to include risk analysis for pilots who flew too low or too near the enemy response system so their actions potentially jeopardized lives of crew members, aircraft, and the mission. Because of severe stress associated with their assignment, some pilots took on the characteristics of high-risk takers. They were no more courageous than their peers but seemed to lose the fear required to carry out successful bombing runs. Therefore, regardless of whether they had flown a minimum number of flights to justify a furlough, pilots detected by risk analysis as needing relief were reassigned to the hospital for recuperation. The purpose of removing airmen from combat was to help them recover their sense of caution, the normal fear that is needed to perform the dangerous tasks of fighter pilots (Torrance, 1957).

Monitor Risk Assessment

The risk analysis strategy applied by psychological teams has been credited with saving many lives. Subsequent studies have found this strategy to confirm ability to accurately estimate risk is a basic survival skill that sometimes can stop functioning, even among the most intelligent people (Hopkin & Thompson, 2022; Sukel, 2016; Vose, 2018). Everyone should be responsible for continually monitoring this potentially dangerous aspect of behavior in relatives and peers and provide feedback. Schools do not present dangers comparable to a battle field, but they can pose significant risks. Students who leave school before graduation are more likely to become casualties than survivors in the labor force that is increasingly driven by technology and higher education. Just as American fighter pilots required external feedback to detect when their risk assessment ability was impaired, peers, parents, and teachers should provide observational input for individual risk analysis. In particular, it is important to challenge the so-called *personal fable* that causes some youth to suppose they are exempt from harmful risks others wisely choose to avoid (Myers & Twenge, 2019; Sus, 2023).

Youth can behave impulsively when they experiment with novel and stimulating events. Such activities support the self-impression of autonomy and motivate imagined opportunities for physical pleasure. However, their ability to look ahead and calculate dangerous outcomes of some behaviors is limited. This means many students are poorly equipped to evaluate relative risk of appealing situations that can cause trouble for them. Despite making foolish choices and experiencing feelings of invincibility, it is erroneous to suppose youth are irrational. On the contrary, Jensen and Nutt (2016) explained that in terms of brain development cognitive abilities essential for effective reasoning are nearly complete by age 15. Indeed, adolescents are just as capable as adults in logically assessing whether a situation is dangerous. This is why students can get high scores on aptitude measures such as the Scholastic Abilities Test (SAT) that is based on rational deduction and logic (College Board, 2021).

Brain research has determined that the foremost predictor of unsafe decisions by young adults occurs when their ability is outweighed by anticipation of some reward, despite the gravity of a risk. The reward-seeking impulse that originates deep in the brain releases dopamine when some source of pleasure is contemplated, such as sexual relationships, consuming drugs, gaining social status, or being perceived as good looking. Until a fully developed prefrontal cortex becomes available that can impose greater self-control, the willingness to engage in dangerous risk-taking urges careful monitoring by relatives, friends, and educators (Bear et al., 2020).

Many college students are reluctant to ask their older relatives for advice before taking daring risks because this would challenge their feelings of independence. They do not want to be told about a need for moral constraints. Discussions about risk assessment can be more helpful than trying to instill fear or assure students they are trusted unconditionally. There can be greater benefit when, in a safe setting with older family members who care about them, students calmly reflect on possible outcomes of actions not yet taken than to consider damage of poor decisions after the fact. A mature adult with a reputation for willingness to listen is sometimes permitted to review options with a student and anticipate consequences that could be associated with each choice. These conversations provide a chance to monitor risk assessment and urge that all choices should take into account how each possible action might interfere with long-term plans. When students are encouraged to make plans and commit themselves to attaining their goals, it is easier to avoid foolish risks (Cassidy, 2021). Scenarios that feature common risks ought to be routinely assigned as homework to focus discussions between students, parents, and peers. This is an uncommon expectation but could result in more reasonable decision making.

Recognize Growth-Oriented Risks

When students are urged to recognize possible rewards that accompany growth-oriented risks, they usually become more willing to take such chances. To illustrate, setting personal goals is a risk that defines a sense of purpose and enables acceptance of guidance to govern behavior. Giving anonymous feedback to cooperative learning teammates is a risk that can yield awareness and preserve honesty. Giving advice is a risk that reveals the scope and limitations of personal perceptions. Becoming a volunteer is a risk that motivates helping others whose needs could be ignored. Self-assertion is a risk that requires letting others know where we stand about issues of importance to us. Sharing differences of opinion presents the risk of disagreement but also promotes an opportunity of gaining insight from reciprocal learning. Taking elective courses about unfamiliar topics risks exposure to new frames of reference but offers the advantage of broader perspectives. Trusting friends and relatives is a risk that can become a basis for mutual support. Risking spontaneity is a departure from routine that can result in beneficial experiences that could not have been planned (Kellerman & Seligman, 2023).

Risk and Prosocial Behavior

The human brain reaches its full size by age 10 but mature development is incomplete until about age 25–30 (Jensen & Nutt, 2016). The ability to reflect on possible consequences of actions yet to be taken (risk assessment) instead of being governed by the temptation of instant gratification implicates the prefrontal cortex, the last region of the brain to mature. This domain is responsible for a set of mental skills known as *executive functioning* that serve as a management system for the brain. Executive functioning skills promote long-term planning strategies to decide a career, obtain education training, schedule use of time, and monitor personal progress (Barkley, 2020). Being able to focus attention and persevere in getting tasks done is evidence of healthy executive functioning. Greater control of emotional impulses becomes normative as men and women are increasingly able to calculate risk versus reward situations while in their 20s. Focusing attention and being able to ignore distraction is promoted by the prefrontal cortex. Young adults are also influenced by peer pressures to participate in potentially dangerous behavior, such as consuming drugs, unsafe sex practices, and driving habits like texting or being a passenger in a car driven by someone who has been drinking alcohol (Jensen & Nutt, 2016).

The prefrontal cortex also has a role in motivating prosocial behavior, actions taken to help others like volunteering to spend time visiting the residents of a nursing home. Prosocial behavior is defined as doing commendable things without an expectation for recognition or reward (McAdams et al., 2021). Evidence that prosocial development is not taking place is shown when individuals remain self-centered, narcissistic, and willing to ignore wellbeing and mental health of people around them. Giving high priority to prosocial behavior can support personality development for attributes such as fairness and respect for cultural differences. This mindset encourages people to leave behind the traditional practice of demonstrating pride toward members of one's ethnic or national heritage while expressing less concern about the welfare of outsiders.

For the first time in history, most societies possess global awareness that can motivate increased prosocial behavior, broaden the definition of personal identity, and build commitment to collaboration. Young adults are the most prominent subpopulation to provide leadership in advocating for the civil rights of minorities, urging the inclusion of migrant groups, increase gender equity, and increased attention focused on self-correction and accountability. Achieving these favorable personality characteristics is a challenge that calls for revision of social priorities traditionally conveyed to youth by schools, families, and religious institutions. Currently, all public schools in the United States are expected to devise an annual improvement plan. By far the most common plans that have been generated reflect the resolve to develop a broader curriculum that addresses missing elements such as social and emotional learning that can contribute to development of maturity (Whitaker, 2018).

Mistakes and Perseverance

Teachers and parents should encourage students to risk some mistakes and recognize them as necessary for learning. Unfortunately, some students are misled by adult advisors who believe that the best path is to always avoid mistakes, a decision that can render them incapable of generating original ideas. As students advance through the grades, the fear of being wrong means that making mistakes and taking risks become unacceptable. In contrast, creative people of all age groups recognize that being wrong repeatedly may be necessary before discovering a solution for some problems (Goldberg, 2018). Creative people do not become discouraged by their mistakes. Instead, they are motivated by eliminating options that do not produce solutions. If students are not prepared to be wrong, they will not be able to generate ideas that are unique.

The path to creative thinking typically includes side roads that lead nowhere and require backing up, revising assumptions, and mapping out new paths to reach the destination. Terrance Tao, Professor at the University of California at Los Angeles, is a recipient of the Fields Medal for Mathematics, the highest award in his academic expertise. Tao explained that mathematicians participate in a continuous process of trial and error. Someone comes up with a wrong idea and pursues it for a time until realizing it does not work. Then, another idea is put forward and also subjected to trial. Eventually, by process of elimination, a solution is discovered and becomes acceptable. Nobel Prize-winning chemist Harry Kroto at Florida State University expresses a similar opinion about the way problems should be pursued. When asked what proportion of his own experiments are failures, he estimated 95% but qualified his answer that failure is not the right word—you are just finding out what does not work. In the same way, Albert Einstein observed that anyone who claims to have never made a mistake has never tried anything new (Nielsen & Thurber, 2019).

No one succeeds at everything they try the first time so the willingness to acknowledge failure is essential. The first Harry Potter book by J. K. Rowling was rejected 12 times before she found a company willing to contract for her manuscript (Siegel & Bryson, 2018). Theodor Seuss Geisel, affectionately called Dr. Seuss, received 27 denials from publishers regarding his first children's book. He was reading the latest rejection while walking down Madison Avenue in New York City when he saw a friend from college who had recently been hired as an editor at Vanguard Press. Seuss showed the manuscript to his friend and two hours later received his first book contract. Looking back Seuss recalled that if he had walked on the other side of Madison Avenue and not met his friend, he probably would have wound up in the dry cleaning business (Jones, 2019). J. K. Rowling and Theodor Geisel knew that we cannot allow our failures to define us and instead should strive to recover from our setbacks by demonstrating resilience.

Many adults are unwilling to describe their own failures to younger family members. They often reason that if I tell them about my failures they will be aware of my limitations. Certainly, revealing our failures makes us vulnerable but this is a risk worth taking. If instead the goal is to be perceived as a person who rarely or never makes mistakes, younger people will likely conclude that you are unable to comprehend their problems. The advisors that young adults most often choose are older than themselves who have demonstrated a willingness to admit personal shortcomings and describe efforts to overcome them. People who care about us should know about some of our failures or they cannot help us to confront our difficulties (Goldberg, 2018).

Relatives and friends should appreciate the powerful influence of encouragement, admit their own setbacks, resolve to overcome difficulties, and detect behaviors that require correction. These examples build resilience and confidence students need to recognize some challenges are opportunities. When parents and teachers try to protect students from exposure to adversity, their efforts often have the unintended effect of rendering an individual less capable of managing challenges that will inevitably be experienced by everyone. The key appears to be how people learn from mistakes. Without correction, poor choices become habits that can negatively shape behavior. Making mistakes is the way people discover what they are able to do and have yet to learn. Researchers agree that development of resilience requires some exposure to risk (Damour, 2020; Fricchione et al., 2016; Southwick et al., 2023).

Minimize the Cost of Mistakes

Airline pilots learn navigation skills by having extensive practice in a flight simulator. This experience allows beginning aviators to learn from mistakes without exposure to costly consequences that could occur during an actual flight. In effect, pilots can assess the risk of certain maneuvers and then correct their errors without expense. In this way, they can make mistakes without also making headlines. Simulator training is used to prepare astronauts and implicated in video games where players pretend to be race car drivers or downhill skiers who take risks and then correct poor judgment without exposure to physical injury. Because the cost of making mistakes is certain to be low and the feedback needed to improve performance is constant, flight instruction using simulators requires less time, costs less money, and results in better pilot performance ratings. There is abundant evidence that making mistakes is necessary for growth and progress throughout life. From the time infants take their first tumble as they begin to walk, mistakes are an inevitable aspect of living and experience of anyone who is willing to approach tasks that are new or difficult.

Continued effort following mistakes is important to improve performance. The pleasure of success occurs when previous defeats are overcome. In addition, exposure to making mistakes can motivate courage, stamina, and resilience (Duckworth, 2018). Throughout history progress has depended on the sustained efforts of individuals who repeatedly made mistakes but did not consider failures as evidence of inability. Rather, they recognized the need to stay engaged with a task to find answers instead of giving up. Success that follows mistakes sustains motivation and hope to keep trying in meeting the next difficult venture.

Teachers do not have the power to prevent students from making mistakes but can control costs related to mistakes. The reason cost must be kept low is because some mistakes are needed for learning to happen. When students fear making mistakes, they avoid the exploration of new ideas that could produce insights. The belief that success is possible without making mistakes is a contradiction of human experience. Students are more willing to make mistakes when teachers allow them to explore new ways of looking at things without having an influence on their course grade, choose unfamiliar topics for projects, and try innovative ways of reporting by formats like photographs or pod casting. In these situations, students are willing to take a chance, mindful that mistakes they are bound to make can be corrected, are likely to lead to success, and not threaten their report card (Metcalfe, 2017).

Parents have an important role in supporting a realistic perspective on making mistakes. If parents believe that refusing to admit failure is the way to preserve student self-esteem, they try to prevent experiences that are actually needed to grow and cope with events when first tries are not good enough and quitting is a poor choice. The capacity to succeed with school work requires detection of mistakes, resolve to correct them, renewed effort using more suitable methods, and remaining confident about the eventual outcome. These responses help students view new and different tasks as opportunities for learning instead of believing that it is evidence of their incompetence. The resilience to overcome obstacles cannot be acquired without practice and patience. Hooker (2022) observed that students don't take risks if teachers don't take risks. Unwillingness to take risks and view failure as a learning tool can stifle creativity and innovation. This means encouraging mistakes, controlling the cost of errors, and giving corrective feedback are important contributions to thinking (Levine, 2020).

Sharing experiences can reinforce a hopeful attitude that helps students process failures. Most older relatives have failed many times so they have lots of failures to choose from during discussions with students. Teams should discuss these questions in class.

1 In what activities will you risk failure to learn something new?
2 What situations are the ones where you are most likely to fail?
3 Of all your failures, what was the most difficult one to accept?
4 Who usually helps identify your failures and ways to recover?
5 Which friendship failures would you handle differently now?
6 What are some of your plans that turned out to be unsuccessful?

7 What failures bother you less than they bother other relatives?
8 How do you respond to relatives when they experience failure?
9 What failures have you looked back upon with some pleasure?
10 How do family members react when they find out you failed?

Dependence on Continuous Praise

What students become depends in part on feedback they receive about their behavior. When feedback is always praise and excludes corrective criticism, students do not gain an ability to accurately estimate personal failure or assess their progress toward maturity. Adults should consider ways to motivate students to take growth-oriented risks without over-praising them. Giving praise in response to poor performance is not a gift. Encouragement supports persistence in trying to do difficult tasks but praise should be reserved to confirm progress. Parents should strike a balance in telling daughters and sons they love them but offer praise when it is deserved and criticism when warranted (Dweck, 2017; Kakinuma et al., 2022; Zhao et al., 2017).

There is also praise inflation. Positive traits can be so exaggerated that words lose their meaning. It might not seem enough to say that a girl is "pretty" unless describing her as "drop dead gorgeous," or a student is not just "smart" but "a genius." Adults need to distinguish between encouragement and praise. There is benefit in encouraging students if performance is mediocre and providing praise when performance shows improvement. Praise should always be as specific as possible so that students understand what they do well (Vohs & Baumeister, 2017).

Higher Education and Readiness for Employment

Young adults dream of getting a job that will provide middle-class status and a secure financial future. Previous generations were able to reach this goal by finishing high school, getting a job, and working hard. However, employers are agreed that post-secondary education has become a new minimum requirement for placement and promotion within their company (Bonvillian & Sarma, 2021).

Advantages of Attending College

The Association of Public and Land-Grant Universities (2023) reported evidence that having a college degree improves one's employment prospects and earnings. On average, the salaries of bachelor's degree holders are 84% higher than peers who have only a high school diploma. The gap in annual income of recent graduates (ages 22–27) is more than $22,000. Health and safety benefits for living a fulfilling life are also implicated. Bachelor's degree holders are 47% more likely than high school graduates to have health insurance provided by their job. Life expectancy is also longer for those who have attended higher education. Studies suggest that people who have attended at least some college can expect to live seven years longer than those with no postsecondary education (Ma & Pender, 2023).

The decision to continue learning beyond high school usually means choosing one of the nation's nearly 1,200 community colleges. These institutions provide instruction for 10 million students, about 45% of all undergraduates, with tuition rates one-third the cost of tuition at public universities (Community College Research Center, 2021). Community colleges perform a leadership role in offering students their initial training for some economic sectors forecast to create the greatest number of jobs. For example, one-third of new jobs before 2031 are projected to be in the health care fields such as nursing, radiology, physical therapy, and pharmacy (United States Bureau of Labor Statistics, 2022, 2023).

Parent-Student Discussions about College and Employment

A well-defined role for parents is needed to support students as they consider career exploration including possible choices for college (Fiske, 2023). Adolescent polling has found that students prefer to talk with parents about career choices (Minkin & Horowitz, 2023; Strom & Strom, 2024). Students and parents can benefit from examining the *Occupational Outlook Handbook* (*OOH*), available online from the United States Bureau of Labor Statistics (2023). This resource presents employment projections for the 2021–2031 decade.

As young adults look ahead to finding their place in the world of work, they have a great deal to think about—What's the salary? How far away is the job? What are the benefits? Can I do the job? Will this position provide satisfaction? Is it a healthy environment? What is the current employer support for mental health and well-being? The American Psychological Association (2023) conducted a *Work in America Survey* about workplaces as engines of psychological health and well-being involving 2,515 employed adults age 18 and older. A majority (77%) of workers reported being very or somewhat satisfied with employer support for mental health and well-being; over half (59%) strongly or somewhat agreed that their employer regularly provided information about available mental health resources. Results also showed a concern by some employees (77%) who were experiencing job-related stress associated with workplace burnout such as emotional exhaustion (31%), not motivated to put forth one's best effort (26%), irritability or anger with co-workers or customers (19%), and feelings of being ineffective (18%). An overwhelming majority of workers (94%) said it is very or somewhat important to them that their work environment is a place where they feel a sense of belonging. Improving work conditions should be a mutual effort by the employers and employees.

Obstacles to College Graduation

The nation is taking a great risk by failing to develop a long-term comprehensive plan that can provide young adults with cost-free higher education. What is our plan to educate the 14+ million illegal immigrants who continue to arrive? How can we make sure that minority and first-generation students are able to complete their degree, and get a job?

Colleges generally have a poor record of being able to retain students until graduation. Only 64% of college students graduate with a bachelor's degree within 6 years (National Center for Education Statistics, 2022). Results are even worse for low-income first-generation students whose dropout rate is 89%, four times the rate of second-generation students (Quadlin & Powell, 2022). UnidosUS (2020), the largest Hispanic civil rights organization, wanted to determine why so many students leave school without earning a diploma. The plan was to interview current and former college students living in Chicago, Los Angeles, New York, and San Antonio. The goal was to listen to individual experiences, identify obstacles for completing a degree, and assess understanding about tuition and debt.

First, many non-completers reported having to give higher priority to employment than the classroom. Balancing demands of school and a job is not unique to Hispanics. Only 25% of college freshman are enrolled fulltime; most are financially dependent on parents, grandparents, or other relatives. About 45% of college students work 20 or more hours a week. Similarly, most community college students (60%) work 20 hours a week and one-third are employed over 35 hours. Estimates are that 82% of the national population increase between now and 2050 will attribute to immigrants who arrive before then and their descendants born in America. Because of low-income these people will have to work while they also attend school (UnidosUS, 2020).

Second, many dropouts felt unprepared for college level work despite the fact they have a high school diploma or general education equivalency diploma, GED. Only half of all students in the 50 largest cities, where most minorities live, complete high school. That figure is far below the national graduation rate of 82%. Great disparity is also evident when comparisons are made between student achievement in inner city, suburban, and rural schools (National Center for Education Statistics, 2022).

According to the National Research Center on Hispanic Children and Families, the 18.6 million Latino children (ages 18 and younger) represented 26% of the national child population in 2019 (Chen & Guzman, 2021). These students are approximately half of the child population in three southwestern states (New Mexico, California, and Texas) while also exceeding 40% in Nevada and Arizona.

The National Center for Education Statistics (2022) estimates that 64% of undergraduates will finish a bachelor's degree within six years at the same institution. The figures are even more disappointing when it is recognized that Hispanics, the most rapidly growing subgroup, has one of the lowest college completion rates at (46%). In addition, over the past decade, the proportion of Whites with degrees compared to Blacks with degrees has not narrowed but gotten worse (Estrada, 2020; Marcus, 2021; Mineo, 2021).

Student Obligations for Study Habits

More students should think about the risks associated with their poor study habits. Chen (2022) found that, based on college placement scores, many students are poorly prepared for the work expected of them at that level. As a result, such students have to enroll in remedial reading or remedial mathematics classes that do not count toward college credit. Across the nation, 56% of African Americans, 45% of Hispanics, and 35% of Whites are enrolled in remedial classes, often referred to as developmental courses. Yadusky et al. (2020) found that fewer than 10% of students relegated to developmental coursework actually earn a degree in the measured timespan (usually six years). The main cause for academic remediation is inability to comprehend texts that are complex. Rey (2019) explained the unwillingness of students to engage in slower more careful reading is implicated. Many students believe they should not have to take developmental classes because their high school teachers had assigned them high grades.

College Curriculum Reform

Most dropouts quit school as freshmen or sophomores when the general studies requirement prevents them from enrolling in classes directly related to career preference.

If students were allowed to study their preferred career path from the beginning and choose an occupation based on knowledge of personal strengths and labor market forecasts, more of them might remain in school instead of dropping out (Kirp, 2019). However, general studies requirement means students must first perform well in courses they may not be interested in before being allowed to take classes leading to their chosen career. The concept of general studies contradicts what is known about motivation for learning. The elimination of general studies would enable students to finish a degree in less time, perhaps two years, and at much lower cost. England and Australia are among many countries that permit students to move directly from high school to professional studies such as law and medicine. Physicians and attorneys from these countries are considered competent, graduate at a younger age, and encumber less debt (Quadlin & Powell, 2022; Rowe, 2019).

First-Generation Students and Their Parents

Colleges should appreciate the motivational benefits of involving relatives as a student support system. Families are concerned about the future of younger relatives, and they want to help. A defined support role is especially important for those students whose relatives did not attend college. The probability that students will complete requirements for a bachelor's degree rises with education attainment of their parents. The Pew Research Center (Fry, 2021) found that among young adults whose parents did not go to college, only 20% completed a bachelor's degree. For those with at least one parent who completed some college, 34% finished a bachelor's degree. The share rises among adults with one parent who has a bachelor's degree (60%). For students of parents who both earned a degree, 82% have a bachelor's degree. This pattern is consistent across demographic groups.

Given the rapidly growing proportion of first-generation college students, faculty should provide orientation workshops specifically for their parents. The goals of workshops could be to acquaint parents with common obstacles students have to manage, ways school inform students about various majors to prepare for particular careers, efforts to maximize retention, importance of parent encouragement to sustain student motivation, and other ways families can continue to be supportive (Minkin & Horowitz, 2023). Being willing to hear complaints about stress at school, concerns about specific classes or teachers, and learning to adjust to unfamiliar stresses should be recommendations for parents. About 70% of Latino students are the first person in their family to attend college, compared to 48% of white students. This means navigating higher education with less guidance than often comes from families with firsthand knowledge of the experience (UnidosUS, 2020).

A successful example of motivational support for first generation college students is the Hispanic Mother-Daughter Program (Educational Outreach and Student Services, 2023) introduced in 1984 at Arizona State University. The purpose was to change the underrepresentation of women and women of color at ASU. Each year, 7th graders and their mothers (or guardians) are selected as teams to become familiar with how to get prepared for a college education. Monthly workshops are scheduled at the main campus in Tempe on topics such as peer pressure, completing a high school diploma, tutoring opportunities, and forecasts about jobs in the future. By 2023, more than 10,000 Latina students had completed the program. This experience continues to enable females to know that their dream to graduate from college is attainable.

Conclusion

The experience of young adults includes a range of possible risks that might threaten or enrich personal development. Deciding in advance how much risk is acceptable in particular situations clarifies the range of options that are available and eases decision-making. Students make better choices about lifestyle when trusted adults help them monitor their ability to consider possible consequences. Being a careful listener can qualify older relatives to offer feedback in addition to what is provided by peers.

Encouraging growth-oriented risks such as mistake making and confronting difficult tasks is an important function of educators. When students are comfortable trying unfamiliar ways to solve problems, realize failure is an essential part of the learning process, and know they can explore without cost to their grade point, there is greater learning. In contrast, people of every age who stop taking potentially beneficial risks become less able to adjust to change, exhibit more rigid behavior, and show less flexibility in thinking.

Most people rely on praise more than encouragement to motivate student learning. This risky orientation causes students to overestimate their abilities and skills, undervalue the need to work hard, persist in difficult situations, ignore academic deficiencies, seek tutoring, and learn to handle external criticism about personal shortcomings. Students should accept more demanding standards in school and demonstrate greater motivation to study for a global competition.

Helping students recognize failure is usually related to a lack of comprehension that can be overcome by tutoring is an important lesson. Otherwise, some students are inclined to attribute their deficiencies to causes they are unable to overcome. Learning to give criticism to students is a challenge for educators and peers when they offer feedback to teammates. Accepting criticism is a similar challenge that can prevent individuals from finding out deficits they need to focus on. Common guidelines can help students realize criticism can improve behavior and achievement.

Economists contend that the number of college graduates has to increase to maintain a productive economy. Otherwise, unemployment rates for young adults with only a high school diploma will worsen, income disparity between the well and poorly educated will grow, and the nation will lose the advantage of a more talented workforce. Colleges require curriculum reform, having a support role for families, and convincing students to spend much more time studying. An entitlement with free access to college and vocational training seems appropriate based on projections of increasingly larger minority and immigrant populations. This policy could increase career opportunities for more students and support better national economic health.

Key Concepts

1 The ability to accurately gauge risk is a skill everyone should learn and apply. This valuable asset can prevent foolish decisions. Risk analysis is the practice of monitoring the ability of people to accurately gauge risks they face. Being a confidante of students makes it possible to interact with them about possible consequences associated with potential risks they may take.

2 The expectation that success is possible without making mistakes contradicts the history of human experience. When students fear mistakes, they avoid exploration of thinking that could bring improvement in academic performance. When teachers render cost of mistakes low enough so students are comfortable seeing ideas in new ways, there is a corresponding rise in achievement.

3 If parents believe denial of failure is a way to preserve the self-esteem of their son/ daughter, they prevent experiences that are needed to cope with situations when first tries are not good enough and quitting is a poor option. Allowing mistakes, controlling the cost of errors, and giving corrective feedback can be beneficial.

4 The willingness of adults to share personal failure experiences can qualify or disqualify them from being considered by young adults as a source of advice. Generally, grownups suppose that memories they share should feature personal achievement without mention of their failures. But young adults view older people who admit personal failures as more able to understand them.

5 If the feedback students receive is always praise and excludes corrective criticism, they do not acquire an ability to accurately gauge personal progress or advance toward maturity. Adults should consider how to motivate students to participate in growth-oriented risks without reliance on over-praising them. Praise in response to poor performance is an act of deception.

6 General acceptance of the concept of interdependence is needed to recognize that all youth require family and community support to maximize health and achievement. The more sources of support that students have the less likely they are to engage in high-risk behavior and the more likely they participate in prosocial behaviors that contribute to mental health of others.

7 The personal fable describes a significant limitation in risk assessment of adolescents and young adults. Many are inclined to see themselves as invulnerable and will not suffer harmful consequences that might affect others who take the same risks.

8 Low income and minority students are targeted for recruitment by community colleges. In the next two decades, the entire net growth in the labor force will be drawn from groups the public education system has poorly prepared for employment. In 2023, people of color became a majority of the population below the age of 30.

9 The nation's ability to compete globally could improve if college and technical education was an entitlement. This possibility would mean that students of all economic and racial backgrounds could have equal opportunity to acquire schooling needed for job preparation. Students would be free from encumbering a large debt or expectation that relatives have to pay for tuition.

10 Most dropouts quit as freshman or sophomores when the college curriculum ignores their career study interest in favor of required general studies. If students were permitted to focus on their preferred occupation from the start and select careers that accord with job forecasts, more of them might decide to remain in school instead of quit before completing degree requirements.

Generational Perspectives Activities

> **2.1 Team Discussion**
> **2.2 Agenda for Interviews with Parents or Grandparents**
> **2.3 Agenda for Interviews with High School Students about College**
> **2.4 A Scenario: Reasoning and Problem Solving**
> **2.5 Team Chapter Review**
> **2.6 Criteria for Self-Evaluation of Team Members**

2.1 Team Discussion

Each team member answers one question.

1 What lessons have relatives taught that guided your decisions about risk-taking?
2 Who would you ask for advice when considering whether to take a particular risk?
3 How would you describe yourself in terms of willingness to engage in risk taking?
4 What are some of your long-term goals that could be considered significant risks?
5 How do you feel about the costs for students when they make mistakes in classes?
6 How have your teachers encouraged exploration of ideas without affecting grades?
7 How important will perseverance be in enabling you to attain some personal goals?
8 What failures have parents and grandparents told about when they were your age?
9 Who is the most likely person to praise you regardless of whether it is deserved?
10 What are some risks your school should take to improve the quality of learning?

2.2 Agenda for Interviews with Parents and Grandparents

1 What risks did you take during adolescence (ages 10–20) and wish you had not taken?
2 What are some risks you think people should continue taking throughout their lifetime?
3 What do people from your age group consider to be very risky behavior for them?
4 What risks would you suggest should be taken by the college students in your family?
5 What risks do some of your younger relative take that you consider to be troublesome?
6 What risks would you like to take if they would not result in adverse consequences?
7 What are some risks you avoided in the past but looking back wish you had taken?
8 What do you think have been the most significant risks you have taken so far in life?
9 What risks are you more inclined to take than most people who are your same age?
10 Who was the adult who helped you most to assess consequences while growing up?
11 What have you tried to teach younger relatives about their need to make mistakes?
12 What are your observation of the way parents try to interpret the failures of children?
13 What have you told younger relatives about mistakes you made while growing up?
14 What risks do you wish that more schools would take to support student growth?
15 How should colleges change so student training is more in line with employment?

2.3 Agenda for Interviews with High School Students about College

1 What should our nation do about the tuition costs of higher education?
2 How do you feel about attending a technical school to get job training?
3 How do you view living at home with parents while going to college?
4 What changes should colleges make to become more relevant for jobs?
5 What will be your major in college and how did you decide about it?
6 What advice have friends and family given you on choice of a college?
7 What do you think are your academic strengths and learning deficiencies?

2.4 A Scenario: Reasoning and Problem Solving

Problem solving scenarios present an opportunity to consider situations that might occur for a family and think about possible solutions. Your task is to look at pros and cons of choices that are stated, think of additional options, identify relevant information that might be missing, find out how teammates see the options, and defend your reasoning about advice you consider best.

Vernon and his wife Gwen are concerned about their 17-year-old daughter Stacey, a junior in high school. This semester Stacey performed poorly in mathematics. What do you suggest?

a Talk with Stacey about the reasons she sees for poor performance
b Visit with the teachers to request one-to-one tutoring for Stacey
c Penalize Stacey by grounding her until her grades are acceptable
d Explain that you did not like mathematics either but not to worry
e Other _____

2.5 Team Chapter Review

Efforts to assess learning, provide feedback, and improve quality of instruction is enhanced by a group review of each chapter.

1 What ideas in the chapter changed the way I think about this topic?
2 What insights from the lesson will I try to apply in my relationships?
3 What is the most important point for me presented in this lesson?
4 What are some aspects of this chapter I would like to better understand?
5 Which aspects of this chapter do I wish that I had known about earlier?

2.6 Criteria for Self-Evaluation of Team Members

1 My greatest worry about risks for my younger relatives are:

  a sexual behavior that may lead to unwanted pregnancy
  b drinking alcohol and consumption of illegal substances
  c lack of academic motivation and failure in the classroom
  d insufficient physical exercise and fitness consideration
  e Other _____

2 In conversations about risk taking with my friends

  a we never talk about the risks that we encounter
  b they do not seek my advice
  c we rely on each other for advice
  d Other _____

3 The way I respond to my poor academic progress or failure is

  a teachers never inform me regarding this aspect of my performance.
  b have conversations with the teacher and request tutoring.
  c blame my peers for not helping me.
  d blame myself for being a procrastinator.
  e Other _____

4 Looking back, I would have handled some of my friendship problems differently.

  a I would have avoided being with people who were poorly chosen friends.

   b An apology would be given for mistreatment of someone who was a friend.
   c The persons who took advantage of me would be told to get out of my life.
   d I would have talked with my parents about how to deal with difficulties.
   e Other _____

5 Of all my failures, the most difficult to accept were

   a a romantic involvement that never should have happened
   b cheating on tests in order to do better in class competition
   c finding out my abilities did not match my preferred career.
   d lying to my parents about my whereabouts and activities.
   e Other _____

6 When I shared with younger relatives some of my foolish risks

   a they were surprised but more accepting than I expected
   b I would not tell relatives anything about my foolish risks
   c they mentioned some of their mistakes in the same context
   d the respect they had shown me before seemed to vanish
   e Other _____

7 The situations where I remain willing to take risks include

   a finding out new information about computers and technology
   b being prepared to learn from people from other countries
   c understanding how my role in the family is changing
   d acquiring teamwork skills that I need for work
   e Other _____

8 Which of my risks and poor judgments do I look back on with disappointment?

   a Thank goodness some of my career goals were never achieved.
   b I am grateful for not marrying someone who was a consideration.
   c striving to be popular before deciding to focus on schoolwork
   d Joining friends in smoking or taking drugs
   e Other _____

9 My view about students making mistakes in the classroom is

   a teasing from peers and social rejection will be a consequence
   b success is possible only by making mistakes and correcting them
   c mistakes lead to poor self-esteem and undermine self-confidence
   d teachers should make cost of mistakes low to support exploration
   e Other _____

10 Some innovations I hope more colleges would be willing to take include

   a allow students to study their major during their first year of college
   b eliminate the college requirements for taking general studies
   c poll students to determine how they view their conditions of learning
   d trust students to participate in peer and self-evaluation practice
   e Other _____

References

American Psychological Association. (2023). *2023 Work in America Survey: Workplaces as engines of psychological health and well-being.* https://www.apa.org/pubs/reports/work-in-america/2023-workplace-health-well-being

Association of Public and Land-Grant Universities. (2023). *How does a college degree improve graduates' employment and earnings potential?* https://www.aplu.org/our-work/4-policy-and-advocacy/publicuvalues/employment-earnings/

Barkley, R. A. (2020). *Executive functions: What they are, how they work, and why they evolved.* Guilford Press.

Bear, M., Connors, B., & Paradiso, M. A. (2020). *Neuroscience: Exploring the brain* (4th ed.). Jones & Bartlett Learning.

Bonvillian, W. B., & Sarma, S. E. (2021). *Workforce education: A new roadmap.* MIT Press.

Cassidy, S. S. (2021). *Choose possibility: Take risks and thrive (even when you fail).* Mariner.

Centers for Disease Control and Prevention. (2023). *Youth Risk Behavior Surveillance System.* https://www.cdc.gov/healthyyouth/data/yrbs/index.htm

Chen, G. (2022, February 12). *Are high school graduates ready for college? Studies are dismal. Public School Review.* https://www.publicschoolreview.com/blog/are-high-school-graduates-ready-for-college-studies-are-dismal

Chen, Y., & Guzman, L. (2021, September 15). *Latino children represent over a quarter of the child population nationwide and make up at least 40 percent in five southwestern states.* National Research Center on Hispanic Children & Families. https://www.hispanicresearchcenter.org/research-resources/latino-children-represent-over-a-quarter-of-the-child-population-nationwide-and-make-up-at-least-40-percent-in-5-southwestern-states/

College Board. (2021). *The Scholastic Aptitude Test (SAT).* https://www.collegeboard.org/

Community College Research Center. (2021, July). *An introduction to community colleges and their students.* Teachers College, Columbia University. https://ccrc.tc.columbia.edu/media/k2/attachments/introduction-community-colleges-students.pdf

Damour, L. (2020). *Under pressure: Confronting the epidemic of stress and anxiety in girls.* Ballantine Books.

Duckworth, A. (2018). *Grit: The power of passion and perseverance.* Scribner.

Dweck, C. S. (2017). *Mindset: The new psychology of success.* Random House.

Educational Outreach and Student Services. (2023). *Hispanic Mother-Daughter Program.* Arizona State University. https://eoss.asu.edu/hmdp

Estrada, S. (November 3, 2020). *Research roundup: Equity and Black students in higher education.* Institute of Education Sciences, College Completion Network. https://collegecompletionnetwork.org/index.php/news/research-roundup-equity-black-students

Fiske, E. (2023). *Fiske guide to colleges 2024.* Sourcebooks.

Fricchione, G. L., Ivkovic, A., & Yeung, A. S. (Eds.). (2016). *The science of stress: Living under pressure.* University of Chicago Press.

Fry, R. (May 18, 2021). *First-generation college graduates lag behind their peers on key economic outcomes. Pew Research Center.* https://www.pewresearch.org/social-trends/2021/05/18/first-generation-college-graduates-lag-behind-their-peers-on-key-economic-outcomes/

Goldberg, E. (2018). *Creativity: The human brain in the age of innovation.* Oxford University Press.

Hooker, C. (2022). *Ready, set, fail: Using failure & risk-taking to unlock creativity.* X-Factor EDU.

Hopkin, P., & Thompson, C. (2022). *Fundamentals of risk management: Understanding, evaluating and implementing effective enterprise risk management* (6th ed.). Kogan Page.

Jensen, F., & Nutt, A. (2016). *The teenage brain: A neuroscientist's survival guide to raising adolescents and young adults.* HarperCollins.

Jones, B. J. (2019). *Becoming Dr. Seuss: Theodor Geisel and the making of an American imagination.* Dutton.

Kakinuma, K., Nakai, M., Hada, Y., Kizawa, M., & Tanaka, A. (2022). Praise affects the "Praiser": Effects of ability-focused vs. effort-focused praise on motivation. *The Journal of Experimental Education, 90*(3), 634–655. 10.1080/00220973.2020.1799313

Kellerman, G., & Seligman, M. E. P. (2023). *Tomorrowmind: Thriving at work with resilience, creativity, and connection – now and in an uncertain future*. Atria Books.

Kirp, D. (2019). *The college dropout scandal*. Oxford University Press.

Levine, M. (2020). *Ready or not: Preparing our kids to thrive in an uncertain and rapidly changing world*. Harper.

Ma, J., & Pender, M. (2023). *Education pays 2023: The benefits of higher education for individuals and society*. College Board. https://research.collegeboard.org/media/pdf/education-pays-2023.pdf

Marcus, J. (August 13, 2021). *Racial gaps in college degrees are widening, just when states need them to narrow*. The Hechinger Report. https://hechingerreport.org/racial-gaps-in-college-degrees-are-widening-just-when-states-need-them-to-narrow/

McAdams, D. P., Shiner, R. L., & Tackett, J. L. (Eds.). (2021). *Handbook of personality development*. Guilford Press.

Metcalfe, J. (2017, January). Learning from errors. *Annual Review of Psychology, 68*, 465–489. 10.1146/annurev-psych-010416-044022

Mineo, L. (2021, June 3). Racial wealth gap may be a key to other inequities. *The Harvard Gazette*. https://news.harvard.edu/gazette/story/2021/06/racial-wealth-gap-may-be-a-key-to-other-inequities/

Minkin, R., & Horowitz, J. (2023, January). *Parenting in America today*. Pew Research Center. https://www.pewresearch.org/social-trends/2023/01/24/parenting-in-america-today/

Myers, D. G., & Twenge, J. M. (2019). *Social psychology* (13th ed.). McGraw-Hill Education.

National Center for Education Statistics. (2022). *Undergraduate retention and graduation rates. Condition of Education*. U.S. Department of Education, Institute of Education Sciences. https://nces.ed.gov/programs/coe/indicator/ctr

Nielsen, D., & Thurber, S. (2019). *The secret of the highly creative thinker: How to make connections others don't*. Laurence King.

Quadlin, N., & Powell, B. (2022). *Who should pay? Higher education responsibility, and the public*. Russell Sage Foundation.

Rey, V. M. (2019). Effects of engaging students in a remedial reading course. *Practitioner to Practitioner, 10*(3), 8–13. https://eric.ed.gov/?id=EJ1246587

Rowe, M. (2019). *The way I heard it*. Gallery Books.

Siegel, D., & Bryson, T. (2018). *The Yes brain: How to cultivate courage, curiosity, and resilience in your child*. Bantam.

Southwick, S. M., Charney, D. S., & DePierro, J. M. (2023). *Resilience: The science of mastering life's greatest challenges* (3rd ed.). Cambridge University Press.

Strom, P. S., & Strom, R. D. (2024). *Polling student voices for school improvement: A guide for educational leaders*. Information Age.

Sukel, K. (2016). *The art of risk: The new science of courage, caution, and chance*. National Geographic.

Sus, V. (2023). *Ten personal fable examples*. https://helpfulprofessor.com/personal-fable-examples/

Torrance, E. P. (1957, May). Group decision-making and disagreement. *Social Forces, 35*(4), 314–318. 10.2307/2573319

UnidosUS. (2020). *A path forward for Latinos: Laying the groundwork for equity in higher education*. https://unidosus.org/wp-content/uploads/2021/07/unidosus_apathforwardforlatinos_121720.pdf

United States Bureau of Labor Statistics. (2022, September 8). *Employment projections—2021–2031*. [USDL-22-1805]. [News release]. https://www.bls.gov/news.release/pdf/ecopro.pdf

United States Bureau of Labor Statistics. (2023). *Occupational outlook handbook*. https://www.bls.gov/ooh/correct in text

United States Drug Enforcement Administration. (2023). *Fentanyl awareness*. U. S. Department of Justice. https://www.dea.gov/fentanylawareness

Vohs, K. D., & Baumeister, R. F. (2017). *Handbook of self-regulation: Research, theory, and applications* (3rd ed.). Guilford.

Vose, D. (2018). *Risk analysis: A quantitative guide* (3rd ed.). Wiley.

Whitaker, T. (2018). *Leading school change: How to overcome resistance, increase buy-in, and accomplish your goals* (2nd ed.). Routledge.

Yadusky, K., Kheang, S., & Hoggan, C. (2020). Helping underprepared students succeed: Minimizing threats to identity. *Community College of Research and Practice*, *45*(6), 423–436. 10.1080/10668926.2020.1719939

Zhao, L., Heyman, G. D., Chen, L., & Lee, K. (2017). Praising young children for being smart promotes cheating. *Psychological Science*, *28*(12), 1868–1870. 10.1177/0956797617721529

3 Parents Teach Preschoolers about the Internet

A Message to the Reader

During early adulthood (ages 20–40), people often become parents. This responsibility requires that mothers and fathers meet a broad range of child needs that redefine the adult sense of purpose, enlarge scope of satisfactions and concerns, and expand the criteria used for self-evaluation. This chapter and Chapter 4 will explore parent goals and concerns about how to fulfill the new family obligation of teaching young children. Studies conducted for the Pew Foundation show that parents believe their role is harder today than it was for parents 20 years ago, with many of them citing technologies such as social media or smartphones as a reason (Auxier et al., 2020; Minkin & Horowitz, 2023).

Family Curriculum for Preschoolers

Historically, parents have been expected to get their children ready for kindergarten by learning letters of the alphabet and reciting numbers in progression. Preschoolers cannot read so they have to rely on observation for many lessons. Between ages 3 and 6, children are in a developmental stage called *identification*. During this stage they imitate and adopt the attitudes and actions of others they spend time with including their parents, grandparents, babysitters, preschool staff, and peers (Bouffard, 2017; Done, 2022).

Parents admit uncertainty about the content of lessons they should teach their children. Fortunately, just being together motivates valuable conversations. Visual and audio stimulation encourages children to reveal their feelings, ask questions, interpret images and situations, show curiosity, engage in guessing, detect difficulties, admit and correct mistakes, experience feeling of success, and gain confidence. Corresponding opportunities for adults are to share their opinions, arrange for discoveries, model curiosity, respond to questions, encourage perseverance, correct errors, recognize achievement, convey attitudes necessary for acceptable behavior, foster caring about feelings of others, and contribute to acquisition of social skills. Parents should teach these lessons that collectively support the growth and development of young children.

We offered parents of 3- to 6-year-olds a free online course that focused on *Thinking in Early Childhood*. Before instruction began, the parents were invited to ask questions about their readiness for becoming an Internet teacher. Their most frequent questions along with our responses are described.

DOI: 10.4324/9781003401261-5

What Should Be My Focus to Support Child Learning Online?

Many adults think of the Internet as a huge library that contains infinite knowledge. Easy access to information is a wonderful advance over how learning was gained by prior generations. However, rather than expose children to as much information as possible, greater benefit can come from an emphasis on the mental processes that permit a child to practice creative and critical thinking (Abraham, 2018; Goldberg, 2018). Assigning lower priority to teaching factual information might seem strange at the outset because adults have historically believed that the mission of a teacher is to provide lessons students are expected to memorize. This common expectation should be left behind because it does not yield as much benefit. Greater results are possible by respecting child interest in discovery and identifying Internet search skills everyone needs (Cleese, 2020; Davis, 2023).

The reason for spending time practicing mental processes is because this experience helps children learn how to frame questions for online searches, urges persistence in locating hard to find data, and motivates thinking critically about truthfulness of messages presented online (Levitin, 2016). The main challenge for parents is to model creative thinking processes by demonstrating curiosity and wonder, generate insightful questions, propose hunches, check out guesses, explore possibilities, decide about the credibility of sources, and apply insights for solving problems (Abraham, 2018; Goldberg, 2018; Mayo Clinic, 2023). There is also value in showing that some desired results do not require trial and error but instead call for following directions when a series of progressive steps are already known to complete a particular task. This strategy supports cause and effect thinking, urges memorization only as needed, and enables satisfaction in achieving personal goals.

Previous generations viewed learning mostly in terms of information students needed to know instead of the thinking processes that are necessary for involvement on the Internet. By emphasizing how children learn, ways they think, a different emphasis emerges that assigns priority to practicing search skills, processing new ideas, and adapting to an ever-changing social environment. Teaching about thinking is a responsibility of families and schools so that children become able to adjust to a future that is bound to transcend current ways of looking at events and interpreting situations (Strom & Strom, 2020).

Families are not alone in feeling uncertain regarding ways to provide instruction about the Internet. The nationwide closure of schools during the COVID-19 pandemic challenged most teachers who lacked prior experience in provision of virtual learning. Teachers of every grade level want to know how to maximize the benefits of student reliance on Internet resources. All adults should realize that the Internet allows individual students to learn at their own pace and progress toward becoming a self-directed learner who is able to find wanted information, and gradually decrease dependence on adult direction.

Because some of the knowledge students currently acquire on their own goes beyond lessons provided by classroom teachers, textbooks and software programs, the traditional evaluation practices are no longer sufficient to estimate the scope of student knowledge. The revolutionary shift to reliance on the Internet as the main source of information and discovery enables students to decide some of their own preferred content for learning and supports the motivation of individuals and peers to share what they learn with cooperative teammates. The potential for learning using the Internet is enormous even though uncertainty remains about what families and schools should independently do to enhance this possibility.

How Can I Support Motivation for Online Learning?

Parents should recognize that some of their personal habits can interfere with teaching and therefore should be left behind. First, it is necessary to set aside an assumption that was prevalent when parents grew up about the relationship between pleasure and learning. Many parents incorrectly suppose that the activities students enjoy do not qualify as learning. Instead, educators at home and in school should realize that, besides offering rapid information retrieval, technology tools have great appeal for students, can motivate participation, encourage conversation, increase attention span, and sustain student willingness to persist when faced with difficulties. A common reason dropouts give for their decision to leave school is that classroom experiences did not provide them with any pleasure. All teachers should know motivation for learning throughout life depends on trying to ensure students experience satisfaction that motivates them to continue learning.

Early childhood educators are concerned about lack of parent involvement with child development. They wish that more families would take greater responsibility for instruction. However, encouraging parents to increase participation with teaching presumes grownups are uniformly comfortable with reading, searching the Internet, and guiding discussions. Instead, there are many parents, particularly in low-income families, who feel uncomfortable within the culture of learning. This is because their years in school were mostly disappointing and caused them to gradually withdraw. These parents have to experience the pleasure of learning online before they can convey a sense of enthusiasm to daughters and sons. Carefully selected website visits can enable parent joy of learning with children. Rideout and Katz (2016) conducted a national survey of 1,200 low-income parents of 6- to 13-year-olds. Over 90% of these parents had Internet access and recognized their need to provide child guidance about ways to use this tool for greater learning.

What Are the Optimal Conditions for Child Orientation?

The best way to acquire and apply knowledge is to practice a skill as soon as it is learned, followed by corrective feedback, and further guidance. Situated learning in the family contrasts with how knowledge is gained in the classroom where teachers have many students but not enough time to figure out whether lessons have been learned by everyone in class. Consequently, teachers have accepted memorization as sufficient evidence of student comprehension. A more practical form of assessment is to gain understanding about the context where learning should be applied. Situated learning for children whose observation is a basis for formation of concepts encourages adults to behave as models, the most influential method of instruction.

A goal of early childhood education is exposure to different ways of learning. In the future this goal will require greater exposure to technology tools and careful supervision, the one-to-one arrangement that can best be provided by parents. Daycare and preschool staff have many children to care for so they cannot be expected to provide the individualized instruction necessary for Internet learning (United States Department of Labor Statistics, 2023). Parents should assume leadership for initial online instruction to guide young children (Mayo Clinic, 2023).

How Should I Convey Caution about Credibility of Sources?

Years ago, children were taught they should believe whatever adults told them. This is no longer reasonable and, in some instances, can be dangerous. Indeed, deciding what to believe has become a common problem experienced by people in all age groups. To illustrate, go on the Internet and enter these search words—General Mills Total Mind Games (https://www.youtube.com/watch?v=ZBpMxgRyq48). This comedy skit focuses on Total Blueberry Pomegranate Cereal and presents the dilemmas of familiar obstacles encountered by everyone. Distinguishing the truth from fiction is becoming ever more difficult because people are so frequently exposed to truth distortion (Levitin, 2016). The scale of this challenge can be reduced by checking the origins of a website, background of sources providing information, date of posting, and verification by comparisons with messages on other sites. Searching, verifying, questioning, challenging, and discussing can all contribute to better decision making needed to assess the worth of information presented online (Katz et al., 2021).

How Should I Help with the Search Process?

Knowing how to locate desired information is more important to support child thinking than it is to memorize information. Practice with the search process is needed to find out things a child wants to know. Conner, age 4, and his mother take turns each day choosing a topic to explore on the Internet. Today Conner says that he wants to learn more about *dogs*. Some of the words mother enters for their mutual search are *dogs*, *puppies*, and *what do dogs eat*. In addition, she enters the word *breed*, *veterinarian*, and *kennel*. As Conner's mother generates additional search words, Conner becomes aware of her extensive vocabulary, observes how important key words are to find things you want to know, and provides greater benefit when search words can be further defined for additional descriptors like breed (collies, bulldogs, cocker spaniels) or kennel (place dogs are cared for while owners take a vacation or dogs stay while they wait for someone to adopt them). Helping children search while also building their vocabulary should be goals linked with instruction. The reason that adults should define words they use during a search is because these words are context relevant, making them key words.

Parents vary in the size of their vocabulary, enabling some to draw more connections and appropriate words, especially important for advanced searching. Children discover that knowing words related to any topic they want to learn more about is a way to enable better searching. Later, as children grow older, their ability to locate information, organize it, and summarize results provides credible evidence of problem-solving ability (Strom et al., 2023).

How Will the Internet Impact My Child's Education?

In the past, schools assigned higher priority to memorization than to thinking. One of the reasons was that, until recently, educators believed they knew with a high degree of certainty the knowledge students would need to secure their future. Consequently, results of tests designed to assess learning were considered to be the best predictors of student academic success. Tests revealed the extent to which students were able to recall the lessons they were taught by teachers. Memorization was the main indicator of understanding and considered evidence of comprehension.

New conditions of learning emerged when the Internet enabled students to become more self-directed and less dependent on direct instruction provided by adults. Because some of the knowledge students acquire on their own from Internet searching is bound to go beyond the content of lessons provided by teachers, tests that measure only what is taught in class can no longer be portrayed as an accurate measure of student knowledge. Education cannot continue to be limited to the influence of teachers and curriculum because a greater amount of what students learn will take place outside school. This shift that allows students to govern more of their learning can support individual motivation and enrich the information they can share with cooperative learning teammates. The change implicates revision of the teacher role and expectations so students can view peers as being helpful resources for learning and requires innovative formats that apply to evaluate thinking and performance (Strom et al., 2019). Classroom teachers should regularly make assignments that call on parents to be essential sources for learning. Parents should realize their continuing efforts to establish healthy attitudes and skills about the Internet as the main source of external knowledge and insight can contribute much to child development.

How Much Screen Time Should I Schedule for My Child?

Parents want to protect health of their children. They recognize the necessity to set limitations on child consumption of sugar, salt, soda, and exposure to sunlight. However, it is less common to think about screen time as a form of consumption. *Screen time* is defined as all the activities that happen in front of a screen such as watching television, playing electronic games, and using a computer or mobile device (Auxier et al., 2020; Robertson, 2021). Screen time research has consistently found that, when the amount of time is excessive, this inhibits restorative sleep, contributes to attention deficits, encourages unhealthy snack habits, correlates with increased anxiety, depression, anger, and undermines learning (Heitner, 2023; Lauricella et al., 2015).

The Mayo Clinic (2023) recommends that children younger than 18 months should not be allowed to have any screen time—yes, none. Children from 2 to 5 years old should be limited to one hour each day of high-quality programming, not allowed to be alone on the Internet, and no screens should be located in a child's bedroom. Bear in mind that unstructured playtime is more valuable for a young child's developing brain than is electronic media. Children younger than age 2 are more likely to learn when they interact and play with parents, siblings, and other children and adults.

How well do parents implement these guidelines recommended by pediatricians? Madigan et al. (2019) followed 2,440 mothers and their 2-year-olds to examine prevalence of meeting and exceeding guidelines for screen time. The mothers kept track of how much time their children spent in front of television or a computer screen and reported on developmental measures by answering questions about communication skills, behavior, and social interaction of children. Data were collected at the beginning when the children were age 2 and again at ages 3 and 5. Findings showed that, on average, children spent two to three hours per day in front of a screen. Children exposed to the greatest amount of screen time performed the poorest on measures of development. Researchers concluded parents should be informed that when a child is watching a screen, s/he is missing out on opportunities to be walking, talking, and participating in pretend play with their friends.

A separate study by McArthur et al. (2021) was conducted involving the same 2,440 mothers and preschool children from the Madigan et al. (2019) research. Given the increasing consumption of digital media, the purpose was to determine whether screen use impacts offline enrichment activities such as reading and whether reading offsets screen use. The screen time of children and reading activities were assessed by maternal reports at ages 2, 3, and 5 years old. Results indicated that greater child screen time at 2 years old was associated with lower reading activities at 3 years ($p < .02$). In turn, lower reading at 3 years was associated with more screen time at age 5 ($p < .02$). Early screen use by children was associated with lower print book reading, resulting in greater screen use at later ages. Results of these studies suggested that parents should read to children from books as the basis for literacy (Abrams, 2022).

What Should I Know about Video Games?

Video games appeal to a broad age range, beginning with preschoolers. However, most gamers (70%) are adults (age 18 or older); the average gamer is 34 years old, owns a home, and is a parent (Yanev, 2023). Video games are the biggest form of entertainment in the United States, generating more revenue than Hollywood films and the music industry combined (Mitic, 2023).

Most parents (70%) who play video games with their children believe that this activity has a positive influence (Yanev, 2023). Involvement includes team competition along with a sense of power and control, a place to go to satisfy the need to be in charge. A study to detect stressful conditions experienced by 351 community college students included 210 females (60%) and 141 males (40%). In response to the question of how they reduce stress, 59.6% of the males reported playing video games; only 9.5% of females reduced stress by playing video games (Strom et al., 2021).

Because most video games require that players select violent-type responses to score well, critics have questioned whether assuming the role of game characters might result in emotional desensitization to the effects of aggression in real life. Those who oppose video games worry that they might encourage aggressive behavior in other sectors of life while restricting the development of compassion, empathy, and concern for others (Borba, 2017). The link between exposure to video games and aggressive behavior remains a controversy. Some researchers have reported video game usage is associated with a decrease in prosocial behavior such as congenial relationships, moral judgment, and regard for well-being of others, essential for development of empathy. Such results have relevance for youth because their personality and moral character are being formed.

The good news is that video games designed specifically for preschoolers such as the many LeapFrog products have been around 20 years and do not involve conflict situations, survival, or imitation of aggressive characters. Instead, they present fun tasks to motivate the whole family, provide teaching tools for parents, help children jump ahead in reading readiness activities, select healthy characters to aspire to become like, and practice other important qualities of social and emotional development. The more than 2,000 LeapFrog games are categorized by age, from early childhood (age 3) to age 7 (Robertson, 2021).

Should I Use a Mobile Phone to Distract My Upset Child?

Mobile media provides multiple modalities of videos, games, and education apps with interactive capabilities. When a family goes to a public place like a restaurant, their young child may show disturbing restlessness and perhaps start to cry. In such cases, parents may pull out their smart phone or media tablet and hand it to the preschooler who momentarily becomes focused on the app, game, or video. Parents consider mobile devices to be the most effective tools to quiet children, often referred to as "the shut-up toy." Visual entertainment from media apps such as Daniel Tiger's neighborhood can distract children from what might be causing them to fuss. This strategy is convenient in the short term as a way to settle children down but could it be detrimental later on if this has been the main method to teach children self-control?

Radesky et al. (2015) studied 144 parents of children who were 15–36 months of age to track frequency with which parents used a smart phone or tablet to calm children down and keep them quiet during the day or at bedtime. Results showed that parents of toddlers who displayed the most difficult behavior were nearly three times more likely to hand them a device to get peace and quiet. In a related study, McDaniel and Radesky (2018) followed 183 couples who had newborn children to age 5 over a six-month period. Parents provided information about their child's behavior and reported how often they interrupted parent-child activities by picking up the mobile phone, watching television, or working on a laptop. Results of the study showed that parents whose child was exhibiting bad behavior such as tantrums, hitting or yelling, showed increased stress and were more likely to turn to devices for relief or avoid confrontation with their child.

Technoference is defined as parent use of technological devices that interfere with or interrupt every day normal family relations and interactions including but not limited to face-to-face conversations, mealtimes, and leisure time together (Mackay et al., 2022; Sundqvist et al., 2020). Furthermore, technoference also predicts greater behavior problems at a later age. One alternative strategy is to look a child in the eyes when s/he is upset, try to be soothing and reassuring about being able to solve the problem. This approach can help children develop self-control, extend attention span, and lead to better organization of thinking (McDaniel, 2020; McDaniel & Radesky, 2017; Morris et al., 2022).

Radesky et al. (2023) urge parents to recognize the importance of teaching their child about self-regulation. The results of their study showed that use of mobile devices to calm children is associated with long-term difficulties in executive functioning (skills that implicate self-control) and being able to stay focused despite distractions. A cohort study with 422 parents and 422 children determined that increased parent reliance on mobile devices to calm 3- to 5-year-olds is related to decreased executive functioning and increased emotional reactivity. These findings suggest that parent reliance on devices to distract children should be avoided in favor of instruction about self-regulation of emotions and recognizing that parent overuse of technology that results in ignoring children is poor parenting. Boys and girls who do not learn self-control skills in early childhood are more likely to struggle when they experience added stress in the school environment (Davis, 2023).

How Can I Know My Teaching Is Successful?

Parents often wonder how effective they are as teachers because they cannot get evaluative feedback from young children. There are numerous learning skills that can be identified by parents showing a lesson has been learned, detect deficiencies that should focus further instruction, and identify feedback related to outcomes of instruction. When

Table 3.1 Parent Observations of Child Learning Skills Shown While on the Internet

Child Learning Skills to Learn	*Demonstrates Learning Skill*
Asks questions that reflect curiosity	_____
Shows a willingness to keep on trying	_____
Talks about preferences and concerns	_____
Exhibits a sense of accomplishment	_____
Accepts challenges that are unfamiliar	_____
Listens carefully and follows directions	_____
Likes participation in repetitious activity	_____
Explains the difficulties of certain tasks	_____
Demonstrates the willingness to wait	_____
Makes guesses for experimentation	_____
Attention and concentration to a task	_____
Displays carefulness along with caution	_____
Reflective in making decisions	_____
Manages frustration without getting mad	_____
Views failure as an aspect of learning	_____
Requests help whenever it is needed	_____
Uses vocabulary terms of the Internet	_____
Predicts what is going to happen next	_____
Accepts time limits on the computer	_____
Recalls sequence of steps in a process	_____
Able to accurately interpret symbols	_____
Risks mistakes and accepts correction	_____
Summarizes a lesson that was learned	_____

adults have evidence that their efforts have a favorable effect on child progress, parent motivation increases for teaching with self-confidence.

Table 3.1 includes a parent observation list we devised to evaluate child learning skills. The left-hand column includes learning skills to be assessed. During occasional observations, parents can write notes in the right column beside the learning skills their child has demonstrated. Parents can enlarge the list to include more items they want their child to learn.

Child Internet Safety Practices

Adults generally consider the Internet to be a wonderful resource but also fear that exposure to some messages could endanger children. These fears decline in families where efforts are made to carry out the following practices that collectively contribute to greater child safety (Brooks & Lasser, 2018; Davis, 2023).

Always Sit beside a Child While S/He Does Anything on the Computer

Non-stop supervision is essential for Internet guidance and protection of young children. Most boys and girls age 10 and younger do not possess the critical thinking skills needed to be online alone. Most 7-year-olds and older will disagree with this suggested age restriction; nevertheless, parents should not relent. A good practice is to support child independence but only when adults are present to provide supervision. Generally, by age 10 s/he should be allowed online alone.

Begin Conversations about the Meaning and Importance of Privacy

Children know the frustration they feel when peers intrude on play space or fail to respect their wish to play alone. In contrast, children are inclined to trust adults and rarely challenge authority. Preschoolers should be told and often reminded that an important family rule is we never share information about ourselves with anyone else. If a website parents believe is worthwhile invites children to submit their name(s) to personalize content, create an unrelated nickname instead.

Devise a Menu of a Child's Favorite Websites So They Are Easy to Access

Restrict a child to these websites. Young children are dependent on adult relatives to be able to locate their favorite websites. This practice allows a child to recognize that returning to familiar and safe Internet sites is easier when parents keep a word file on the desktop listing preferred addresses to quickly access for a return to fun experiences.

Recognize Internet-Filter Tools Cannot Substitute for Adult Supervision

Knowing whether certain situations are unsafe might not be evident to children. Tell the child to always share any doubts or worries s/he has about being online. When children are encouraged to share their concerns, adults can provide information needed to assess whether certain conditions pose a risk or require assistance. Respond to child reports by reinforcing positive statements such as, "I am glad that you told me about that situation because I would not have known otherwise." Software enables parents to block some inappropriate content and prevent requests for personal data. Besides being reliant on protective software, adult supervision is always necessary (Kaliebe & Weigle, 2018).

Asking Questions Is a Method to Assess Conditions of Safety

The decision of children to proceed with Internet responses by themselves should be based on certainty that parents would approve of actions they choose. Inviting children to ask questions about the Internet should be continually encouraged as the right thing to do and represents the best procedure to gain greater knowledge that will ensure self-protection.

Caution Is Needed to Avoid Unreasonable Risks on the Internet

One reason children are injured more often than adults is because they lack caution that greater experience will allow them to apply when faced with unfamiliar situations. Making certain children avoid risk-taking until they are more able to foresee possible adverse consequences is an essential condition for safety in the current environment.

Should There Be Social Networking for Preschoolers?

Young children are not ready to engage with the social networks of interest to adolescents, such as Snapchat, Instagram, Facebook, Twitter, and YouTube. Instead, some social networks designed to motivate young children such as Club Penguin, Webkinz, LeapFrog, and ABCmouse compete for this growing market of young consumers (Heitner, 2023).

Guidelines for Teaching Internet Learning Skills

Parents welcome insights about how to enrich child guidance online. The following guidelines can help define aspects of this important and complex responsibility for families.

Situations That Require Waiting Are Opportunities to Model Patience

While you wait for Internet materials to load, explain that the computer is getting things ready for play. Responding in this way conveys a lesson about learning how to wait and being able to manage frustration associated with delay. Adopting such attitudes contributes more to the healthy adjustment of children than blaming the computer for being too slow or complaining about the inconvenience of having to wait. When children demonstrate patience, tell them this shows they are making progress. Children need to know parents and other relatives appreciate their expression of patience as an asset needed to support relationships and time management habits.

Respect Child Desire for Repetition during Exploration on the Internet

Playing a game or repeatedly participating in any satisfying activity is more appealing to children than to adults. These repetitive experiences foster confidence that, in certain situations, children know in advance what is going to happen next. Being able to predict some things will remain the same like a daily schedule for meals and going to bed at the same time at night satisfies a need for order and consistency that is much stronger in early childhood than later stages of development.

Let the Child Navigate the Mouse and Acquire Practice without Criticism

This experience allows a greater sense of control than just watching a parent always be the sole control agent. Certainly, control by adults is easier because they are able to make the pace of events proceed more quickly. Nevertheless, sharing control in most situations is more helpful than constant dominance by an adult. Recognize that being able to move a mouse properly is difficult in the beginning, particularly because young children lack muscle control. Encourage practice. Responses such as "You can do it" and "You did it correctly" are more appropriate to confirm progress than praises like, "You are amazing," "You are awesome," or "You are really smart."

Following Directions Is the Best Way to Carry Out Tasks Already Understood

Parents who read aloud directions that are given online and then follow them present a far more effective method to get things done than resorting to random trial and error owing to impatience. Children should be asked to explain directions in their own words to confirm their understanding about the proper sequence of steps that should be taken.

Asking Questions Should Be Encouraged to Support Self-Directed Learning

When parents reveal uncertainty by asking questions, children tend to adopt this behavior as their way to confront unfamiliar situations. Premature conclusions and impulsive responses can be prevented with questions that motivate reliance on reflective thinking. When a child asks a question the adult is unable to answer, then it is recommended to support curiosity and wonder by sometimes searching together to find out more about a particular topic on the Internet.

Schedule Unhurried and Uninterrupted Time for Internet Exploration

A comfortable pace for learning avoids feeling hurried or rushed and confirms for a child the priority s/he has in the parent's life. In the beginning, 15 minutes seems a good length of time for Internet visits together. Devote complete attention to the child; this means turning off all distractors such as a cell phone or other devices that could intrude and capture your attention.

Allow Time for Children to Reflect about Their Answers to Questions

Parents who develop this strategy support creative and critical thinking. Having enough time to examine possibilities motivates children to realize the importance of deliberation as an essential aspect of the thinking process for reaching decisions about what they will do or say. In contrast, expecting rapid responses without giving time for reflection fosters impulsive behavior (Abraham, 2018).

Listen Carefully to Respond Thoughtfully to Questions, Feelings, and Opinions

This practice recognizes the value of curiosity and confirms for a child that s/he has undivided attention. When adults multi-task, try to do more than one thing at the same time such as texting on the cellphone and talking with a child, it is difficult to remain attentive and distractions can cause grownups to miss comments made by a child. Boys and girls who feel they are repeatedly ignored often seek advice from peers who show greater willingness to listen to them (Levine, 2020).

Identify Failure and Offer Correction as a Way to Motivate Continued Effort

Acknowledging failure is necessary because it helps to identify learning needs and amend goals. Detection of failure should be followed by remedial instruction, urging further effort to increase success and provide feedback about progress. Persistence is needed to become competent and attain personal goals. Giving up when a task becomes difficult can avoid further mistakes but also prevent success that can follow correction of behavior. Willingness to keep on trying while also getting help is essential for achievement in all sectors of life (Duckworth, 2016).

Recognize That All Children Prefer to Control Their Pace of Learning Online

The Internet allows users to return to a task, begin consideration of the task again, and retrace steps required in a sequence to solve some problems. In this way, Internet activities promote the practice needed to build comprehension, problem-solving skills, and self-confidence.

Conclusion

A century ago it was common for parents and children to read books together. As time went by, families were able to listen to the radio, and still later they watched television. Visits to the Internet can also be enjoyable as parents communicate their values during the stage when children are most inclined to adopt them. Getting children ready for expectations of a digital environment means parents should provide a continuous orientation to lessons for learning online and becoming self-directed. Technology encourages children to question, challenge, and disagree, behaviors that can increase potential to become critical thinkers.

Daycare and preschool staff are responsible for ensuring the safety of many immature children. This means the student-to-adult ratio is too high for these caregivers to be able to offer the one-to-one supervision children need to work on the Internet. Parents should take a leadership role for online learning at a time when children are easily directed to discovery tasks, search skills, and formation of attitudes needed to develop healthy social networking. As more children have Internet experiences, they increase their potential for learning. Elementary schools should help families of preschoolers prepare children to meet digital readiness expectations with supervision, corrective feedback, safety and encouragement.

Key Concepts

1 The Internet focus of young children should be on mental processes that provide practice in creative and critical thinking. This might seem strange in the beginning because adults suppose the mission of teachers is to convey lessons students are expected to memorize. However, greater learning can emerge from respecting child interests in the discovery process and search skills.

2 Encouraging a child to navigate the mouse allows for greater control than watching parents always be the sole control agent. Recognize that being able to move a mouse is difficult in the beginning so practice is required. Responses such as "You can do it" and "You did it correctly" are more suitable ways to confirm progress is being made than reliance on praise.

3 When parents demonstrate uncertainty by asking questions, this behavior is usually adopted by children as their method to confront unfamiliar situations on the Internet. If a child asks a question that the grownup cannot answer, support child curiosity and wonder by searching online together to find out some of what is known about the particular topic.

4 Day care workers and preschool staff typically have many children they must supervise so it is unreasonable to expect them to provide one-to-one attention necessary to offer instruction about the Internet. Parents are the teachers who should assume leadership for introducing children to the Internet, and eventually help them to become self-directed learners.

5 Searching the Internet while also learning vocabulary are complementary goals. Adults should define the words they use during the search process because these words are context relevant, making them key words. As children get older, the ability to find information, organize it, and summarize results in a rational way is credible evidence of their problem-solving ability.

6 Video games for preschoolers such as the many Leapfrog products avoid conflict situations, survival strategies, or imitation of aggressive characters. Instead, they present tasks that

motivate family involvement, provide teaching tools, help children with readiness for reading, select healthy characters to imitate, and practice social and emotional attitudes.

7 Young children are self-centered and have few responsibilities but should be expected to stay in contact with their older relatives. This practice should begin with children dictating messages that parents send by e-mail. Family relatives want to learn from children about the activities that are exciting for them, worrisome situations, and opportunities they want to explore.

8 Always sit beside a child while s/he is doing anything on the computer. Before age 10, most children do not have the critical thinking skills needed to be online by themselves. Generally, children will disagree with this assessment but parents should not relent. They can support independence of children best when continual supervision is offered by adults.

9 Children are inclined to trust grownups so they rarely challenge the authority of adults. Young children should be told that an important family rule is to never share information about ourselves with anyone else online. If a website that parents believe is worthwhile invites children to submit their name to personalize content, create an unrelated nickname instead.

10 Playing a game repeatedly can be more appealing to children than for adults. These repetitive experiences provide confidence that, in some situations, children know in advance what will happen next. Being able to predict some things will remain the same like meal time and going to bed satisfies a need for order and consistency that is far stronger during early childhood.

Generational Perspectives Activities

3.1 Team Discussion
3.2 Agenda for Interviews with Parents
3.3 Agenda for Interviews with Young Children
3.4 A Scenario: Reasoning and Problem Solving
3.5 Team Chapter Review
3.6 Criteria for Parent Self-Evaluation

3.1 Team Discussion

1 Why should parents help introduce their preschool children to learning about the Internet?

2 What aspects of a child's social development can be nurtured by instruction about the Internet?

3 How could the Internet teach parents to become more involved as educators of their children?

4 Parents expect much from schools but do schools expect enough collaboration from parents?

5 In what ways should society expect parents of preschool children to provide more instruction?

6 How should schools redefine readiness for kindergarten that includes Internet understanding?

7 How does teaching preschoolers on the Internet differ from traditional methods of instruction?
8 How will Internet learning of preschoolers impact school evaluation of their knowledge?
9 How could school homework for young children include a role for parents as teachers?
10 Speculate about the motivational value of including self-directed learning for young children.

3.2 Agenda for Interviews with Parents

1 What attitudes and skills do you want children to learn while on the Internet?
2 How is the Internet changing expectations for schools, students, and parents?
3 What are your views about social networking experience for young children?
4 How do you suppose involvement with electronic games influences children?
5 What are some potential dangers when children spend too much time online?
6 How do you feel about the amount of screen time experienced by your children?
7 How often do your children contact grandparents by texting? Skype? Email? iPhone?
8 How do you suppose the Internet will have an influence on the patience of children?
9 What challenges do you anticipate when trying to teach children on the Internet?
10 What experiences are satisfying for you while exploring websites on the Internet?

3.3 Agenda for Interviews with Young Children

1 What are some favorite websites you like to visit on the Internet?
2 What rules do parents want you to follow when you are on the Internet?
3 What are the things you like to do most when you are on the Internet?
4 How much time each day do parents spend with you on the Internet?
5 What have parents taught you about how to explore the Internet?
6 How has the Internet been helpful in finding things you want to know?
7 What do parents do when they are on the Internet?
8 How do you stay in contact with friends and relatives on the Internet?
9 What are the hardest things to do while you spend time on the Internet?
10 What dangers on the Internet have parents said that you must avoid?

3.4 A Scenario: Reasoning and Problem Solving

Problem solving scenarios present an opportunity to look at situations that might happen for a family and think about possible solutions. Your task is to look at pros and cons of choices that are stated, think of additional options, identify relevant information that might be missing, find out how teammates view the options, and defend your reasoning on advice you consider best.

Richard is 6 years old and likes to play games on the Internet. When 20 minutes that parents have set for his daily limit have passed, Richard complains that his friends are given more time by their parents. What suggestions do you have for Richard's parents?

a Do not cave in about the sensible time restriction you have established.
b Explain to Richard that you want exercise to also be a priority for him.
c Allow more time for games if Richard agrees he will stop crying about it.

d Remind him about the possible dangers related to child media addiction.
e Other _____

3.5 Team Chapter Review

Efforts to assess participant learning, provide feedback, and improve quality of instruction is enhanced by a group review of each chapter.

1 What ideas in the lesson changed the way I think about this topic?
2 What insights from the lesson will I try to apply in my relationships?
3 What is the most important point for me presented in this lesson?
4 What are some aspects of this lesson I would like to better understand?
5 Which aspects of this lesson do I wish that I had known about earlier?

3.6 Criteria for Parent Self-Evaluation

Directions: For each question, place a check beside statements that describe your feelings. You may want to give several answers on some items. If your feelings are not on choices list, write them on the line marked "other." If a lesson persuaded you to change your mind, make it known by underlining any statements showing these answers reflect a change in feelings.

1 Introducing my child to the Internet

    a is a task I accept and will try to do my best
    b scares me because I do not feel well prepared
    c can be a learning experience for both of us
    d should be expected of schools, not families
    e Other _____

2 The biggest problem I anticipate teaching on the Internet is

    a making sure that my child is safe online
    b being patient and allowing child exploration
    c knowing the attitudes and skills to focus on
    d conveying importance of privacy and safety
    e Other _____

3 I want to schedule time so my child

    a does not spend too long a period on the computer
    b is involved with regular physical exercise outside
    c also has time every day to engage in solitary play
    d dictates email messages to relatives that I send
    e Other _____

4 As a digital teacher of my child, I hope to

    a avoid domination so there can be exploration
    b provide correction and support self-confidence

    c prevent distraction so I listen to child questions
    d illustrate how learning from failure is necessary
    e Other _____

5 My feeling about being a parent Internet teacher is

    a having a one-to-one ratio for tutoring is absolutely necessary
    b that it is basically a family obligation, not daycare or preschool
    c everyone in the family should try to help educate preschoolers
    d healthy attitudes that are established at this age will pay off
    e Other _____

6 Readiness for kindergarten means families should recognize

    a they alone have the teacher-child ratio needed to introduce the Internet
    b there is a need to orient children to the Internet as a source of learning
    c the Internet offers a basis for conversation to support mutual learning
    d teaching about letters and numbers is only part of their responsibility
    e Other _____

7 Families can take advantage of the childhood stage of "identification" to

    a teach attitudes and skills necessary for communication on the Internet
    b serve as mature examples for children about civil treatment of others
    c provide feedback to children about progress in social development
    d illustrate the sense of caution that is necessary for online safety
    e Other _____

8 When I think about the amount of my child's screen time,

    a I feel the family needs to guard against excessive viewing
    b we all need to set a better example of more balanced activities
    c need for physical exercise must become a daily activity
    d being online or watching television keeps them out of trouble
    e Other _____

9 Keeping in touch with grandparents is a responsibility that

    a more parents must make an effort to teach their children
    b has not been well taught to children in our family
    c children should show they care about older relatives
    d I fulfilled more effectively as a child than my children
    e Other _____

10 The importance of having safety rules online is a lesson

    a I intend to reinforce continually to my children
    b that won't matter much with the increase in hacking
    c my children should learn to value safety
    d that schools should encourage for all of the students
    e Other _____

References

Abraham, A. (2018). *The neuroscience of creativity*. Cambridge University Press.

Abrams, Z. (2022, August 25). *Why young brains are especially vulnerable to social media*. American Psychological Association. https://www.apa.org/news/apa/2022/social-media-children-teens

Auxier, B., Anderson, M., Perrin, A., & Turner, E. (2020, July 28). *Parenting children in the age of screens*. Pew Research Center. https://www.pewresearch.org/internet/2020/07/28/parenting-children-in-the-age-of-screens/

Borba, M. (2017). *UnSelfie: Why empathetic kids succeed in our all-about-me-world*. Touchstone.

Bouffard, S. (2017). *The most important year: Prekindergarten and the future of our children*. Avery.

Brooks, M., & Lasser, J. (2018). *Tech generation: Raising balanced kids in a hyper-connected world*. Oxford University Press.

Cleese, J. (2020). *Creativity: A short and cheerful guide*. Crown.

Davis, K. (2023). *Technology's child: Digital media's role in the ages and stages of growing up*. MIT Press.

Done, P. (2022). *The art of teaching children: All I learned from a lifetime in the classroom*. Simon & Schuster.

Duckworth, A. (2016). *Grit: The power of passion and perseverance*. Scribner.

Goldberg, E. (2018). *Creativity: The human brain in the age of innovation*. Oxford University Press.

Heitner, D. (2023). *Screenwise: Helping kids thrive (and survive) in their digital world* (2nd ed.). Routledge.

Kaliebe, K., & Weigle, P. (2018). *Youth Internet habits and mental health, an issue of child and adolescent psychiatric clinics of North America*. Elsevier.

Katz, R., Ogilvie, S., Shaw, J., & Woodhead, L. (2021). *Gen Z, explained: The art of living in a digital world*. University of Chicago Press.

Lauricella, A., Wartella, E., & Rideout, V. (2015, January–February). Young children's screen time: The complex role of parent and child factors. *Journal of Applied Developmental Psychology*, *36*, 11–17. 10.1016/j.appdev.2014.12.001

Levine, M. (2020). *Ready or not: Preparing our kids to thrive in an uncertain and rapidly changing world*. Harper.

Levitin, D. J. (2016). *A field guide to lies: Critical thinking in the information age*. Dutton.

Mackay, L. J., Komanchuk, J., Hayden, K. A., & Letourneau, N. (2022, March). Impacts of parent technoference on parent-child relationships and child health and developmental outcomes: A scoping review protocol. *Systematic Reviews*, *11*(45). 10.1186/s13643-022-01918-3

Madigan, S., Racine, N., & Tough, S. (2019, November 25). Prevalence of preschoolers meeting vs exceeding screen time guidelines. *JAMA Pediatrics*, *174*(1), 93–95. 10.1001/jamapediatrics.2019.4495

Mayo Clinic. (2023). *Screen time and children: How to guide your child*. Children's Health. https://www.mayoclinic.org/healthy-lifestyle/childrens-health/in-depth/screen-time/art-20047952

McArthur, B., Browne, D., McDonald, S., Tough, S., & Madigan, S. (2021, June 1). Longitudinal associations between screen use and reading in preschool-aged children. *Pediatrics*, *147*(6), e2020011429. 10.1542/peds.2020-011429

McDaniel, B. T. (2020, December 5). Technoference: Parent mobile device use and implications for children and parent-child relationships. *Zero to Three*, *41*(2), 30–36. https://www.zerotothree.org/resource/technoference-parent-mobile-device-use-and-implications-for-children-and-parent-child-relationships/

McDaniel, B. T., & Radesky, J. S. (2017, May 10). Technoference: Parent distraction with technology and associations with child behavior problems. *Child Development*, *89*(1), 100–109. 10.1111/cdev.12822

McDaniel, B. T., & Radesky, J. S. (2018, June 13). Technoference: Longitudinal associations between parent technology use, parenting stress, and child behavior problems. *Pediatric Research*, *84*, 210–218. 10.1038/s41390-018-0052-6

Minkin, R., & Horowitz, J. (2023, January 24). *Parenting in America today*. Pew Research Center. https://www.pewresearch.org/social-trends/2023/01/24/parenting-in-america-today/

Mitic, I. (2023, July 4). *Video game industry revenue set for another record-breaking year*. https://fortunly.com/articles/video-game-industry-revenue/

Morris, A. J., Filippetti, M. L., & Rigato, S. (2022, June). The impact of parents' smartphone use on language development in young children. *Child Development Perspectives, 16*(2), 103–109. 10.1111/cdep.12449

Radesky, J., Kaciroti, N., Weeks, H. M., Schaller, A., & Miller, A. L. (2023). Longitudinal associations between use of mobile devices for calming and emotional reactivity and executive functioning in children aged 3 to 5 years. *JAMA Pediatrics, 177*(1), 62–70. 10.1001/jamapediatrics.2022.4793

Radesky, J., Schumacher, J., & Zuckerman, B. (2015, January 1). Mobile and interactive media use by young children: The good, the bad, and the unknown. *Pediatrics, 135*(1), 1–3. 10.1542/peds. 2014-2251

Rideout, V., & Katz, V. (2016). *Opportunity for all? Technology and learning in lower-income families*. Joan Ganz Cooney Center at Sesame Workshop. https://joanganzcooneycenter.org/wp-content/uploads/2016/01/jgcc_opportunityforall.pdf

Robertson, A. (2021). *Taming gaming: Guide your child to healthy video game habits*. Unbound.

Strom, P. S., Hendon, K., Strom, R. D., & Wang, C.-h. (2019). How peers support and inhibit learning in the classroom: Assessment of high school students in collaborative groups. School Community Journal, 29(2), 183–202. http://www.schoolcommunitynetwork.org/SCJ.aspx

Strom, P. S., Hendon, K. L., & Strom, R. D. (2023). Assessment of Internet learning for high school students. *Journal of Educational and Developmental Psychology, 13*(1), 17–28.

Strom, P. S., Strom, R. D., Sindel-Arrington, T., Rude, R., & Wang, C.-h. (2021). Gender differences in stress of community college students. *Community College Journal of Research and Practice, 46*(7), 472–487.

Strom, R. D., & Strom, P. S. (2020). Learning throughout life about the needs of all generations: Recognizing and counteracting generational isolation. In M. London (Ed.), *The Oxford handbook of lifelong learning* (2nd ed., pp. 183–206). Oxford University Press.

Sundqvist, A., Heimann, M., & Koch, F. S. (2020, June). Relationship between family technoference and behavior problems in children aged 4–5 years. *Cyberpsychology, Behavior, and Social Network, 23*(6), 371–376. 10.1089/cyber.2019.0512

United States Department of Labor Statistics. (2023). *Occupational outlook handbook: Preschool teachers*. https://www.bls.gov/ooh/education-training-and-library/preschool-teachers.htm

Yanev, V. (2023, July 26). Video game demographics – Who plays video games in 2023? *Tech Jury*. https://techjury.net/blog/video-game-demographics/#gref

4   Parents Teach Critical and Creative Thinking

Family Challenges of Television

Watching television presents a social context for parents and children to learn from each other Most families spend a greater amount of time watching television together than any other leisure activity. Television presents parents with three major challenges: (1) parents must decide the programs they will allow their children to watch, (2) parents should support critical thinking and creative thinking by helping children interpret the accuracy of some media information, and (3) the willingness of parents to ask questions and listen carefully to child answers increases the likelihood they will continue to be seen as valued sources of advice.

Agenda to Promote Conversations with Preschoolers and Primary Grade Children

Parents choose television programs based on their beliefs and lifestyles. When parents and children watch television together, they see the same pictures and hear the same words. However, because the generations have a dissimilar background of experiences they do not interpret some media messages in the same way. Instead, they may sometimes reach different conclusions. These differences in perceptions mean that there is much to be gained when generations share their observations. One way to learn how a child interprets stories on television is to ask questions that can reveal understanding. Table 4.1 presents an agenda that can guide parent-child interaction. These questions can be used in any sequence with preschoolers and primary grade children; parents should ask a specific question when it seems to fit the events of a story or program the family is watching together. Do not expect that all of the questions must be answered; emphasize only the questions you choose. The following questions are examples and clarified with a purpose and brief explanation.

What Would You Do in This Situation?

Being able to think of choices is a valuable asset to rely on at every age. Individuals who can see many possibilities in a single situation are more able to negotiate, get along with others, and generate alternatives that can become solutions to problems. These strengths are helpful to learn from interpersonal conflict and can preserve mental health. Sharing interpretations allows parents and children to make known limitations of individual thinking. This knowledge helps gauge the comprehension of children and identify learning attitudes and skills that require further instruction and practice.

DOI: 10.4324/9781003401261-6

Table 4.1 Television Questions for Parent-Child Conversations

Question	Purpose
1 What would you do in this situation?	Identify choices
2 What do you suppose will happen next?	Anticipation of events
3 What parts of the program did you like most?	Expression of interest
4 If you were a friend, how could you help?	Responding to needs
5 What does _____ mean?	Vocabulary growth
6 Do you think s/he is making the right decision?	Evaluation of judgment
7 What kind of person does s/he seem to be?	Assessment of character
8 What has happened in the story so far?	Sequence recognition
9 How do you want the story to end?	Identify preferences
10 What was learned from this situation?	Evaluation of learning

What Do You Suppose Will Happen Next?

By asking questions that call on children to guess, to speculate, adults motivate thinking beyond what is directly observed, imagine what is unseen, express a futuristic perspective. This approach encourages children to talk more because there is no single correct answer to discover for questions that are open-ended. The strategy also approves of children expressing differences of opinion from adults. When parents become aware that their child has created ideas the adults were unable to generate, respect for child thinking grows and the level of a relationship is enhanced. In addition, parents who ask guessing-type questions soon become more comfortable admitting uncertainty and showing willingness to discuss topics for which they do not know the correct answers (Harari, 2017; Leski, 2015).

What Parts of the Program Did You like Most?

This question invites expression of personal interest. An important condition for nurturing a close relationship is being aware of what pleases or disappoints the other person and, in turn, make personal choices and preferences understood. A mutual expression of likes and dislikes offers information needed to make sensible decisions about compromise and sacrifice. Sharing enjoyable times is an easy focus for conversation.

If You Were a Friend, How Could You Help?

Children should learn to care about the feelings of others and be motivated to provide assistance as needed. A combination of loyalty, willingness to offer support, and ability to recognize the help a friend needs can be taught by conversation and example. Parents and children benefit from sharing their own friendship difficulties and methods they rely on to maintain satisfying relationships. Primary school children often ask parents for advice about how to preserve friendships with classmates while also trying to maintain their independence. This concern for how to manage conflict begins early and becomes prominent by age 8 or 9 when peer pressure begins to exert a strong influence (Bentley & Jordan, 2017).

Some parents tell children, "If other kids do not treat you right, forget about them and find new friends who will be nice." This advice suggests that withdrawal is the best way to handle insensitivity of peers who at this stage of development are more inclined to mistreat one another. Children want to get along with classmates, even those who treat them poorly. They are eager to figure out how to transform difficult relationships to become satisfying ones. If parents indicate that they do not share the same goal, they inadvertently disqualify themselves as important sources of advice (Minkin & Horowitz, 2023).

What Does _____ Mean? (A Word We Heard on Television)

The development of vocabulary should be a lifelong ambition that contributes to the benefit of conversation with people of other generations. Some words children hear on television may not be understood by them and should become a focus for their questions. Parents are usually amazed at the number of words they could define that otherwise remain unknown to a child. There are also words that children might understand but adults do not and can be shared while watching shows preferred by children. The most effective method to gain new words is in context. Therefore, conversations that occur while watching television can augment the vocabulary lessons taught in school. This strategy calls on whomever is the more informed family viewer to define words and bring meaning for others who are watching.

During a family program, everybody repeats aloud any words they do not understand that are spoken by characters on the screen. At the end of the program it is time to share the meanings of identified words by looking them up and talk about using them. Vocabulary is more easily gained when words are visually defined. For example, what is the meaning of *fairness*? Children learn the importance of this concept early and use it during discussions with parents about equity. Go to YouTube and enter Two Monkeys Paid Unequally—see how obvious the concept of fairness becomes for you.

Do You Think S/He Is Making the Right Decision?

The purpose is to evaluate judgment about actions taken by a character on a program. Parents want children to acquire good judgment so they can be better prepared to avoid serious mistakes. Sometimes disappointing consequences happen before important lessons are learned. This situation is often referred to as learning the hard way. By reacting to televised versions of real-life dilemmas, families simulate predictable problems and can explore the worth of individual judgment without having to personally suffer disappointment or other undesirable consequences (Grant, 2021).

What Kind of Person Does S/He Seem to Be?

The assessment of character is imprecise but considered a valuable skill. Parents want children to have practice in evaluating situations so they can decide on their own whether being with certain people or engaging in particular events is in their best interest. One way to learn to assess character is compare how a parent and child evaluate television characters early during a program and again at the end of an episode. Parents may not always know what is best but children generally conclude mom or dad have lessons of value to teach them about estimating conditions before making decisions.

What Has Happened in the Story So Far?

The need to recognize sequence begins in early childhood, around ages 3–5. The main purpose for learning to read is comprehension, being able to understand what has been read. This skill requires more than memorizing letters of the alphabet and recognizing words. Understanding the progression of events that have been read about is necessary. In the books from which children learn to read, the words are simple and the story line can seem uneventful. In contrast, most television programs have a beginning, middle, and end.. Many television programs are well suited for teaching about sequence of events and can become a valuable medium for improvement of comprehension (Scott, 2016).

Children need to practice accurately summarizing so they can improve their ability to communicate. This can be done at the end of a TV program or reading a children's book aloud with a parent, and asking the child to describe the main events that have happened. Young children should practice summarizing by reporting to the parent about "the big picture." This helps parents learn what was understood, details a child considered most important, and things that were missed. Such child reports can help parents correct when details are misunderstood.

How Do You Want the Story to End?

Expressing preferences is a way to make child values known. Public polls report on adult opinions and priorities. However, the likes and dislikes of children are seldom identified and often overlooked by parents and classroom teachers. This is unfortunate because the future adults hope the young will enjoy depends in part on helping them gain a sense of what is possible, an optimistic outlook on the future, and establish a willingness to express personal values. Adults are able to reinforce these behaviors for children while they watch television together.

What Was Learned from This Situation?

Television offers an opportunity to witness difficulties other people encounter and see how they try to solve problems. Parents and children can identify with some issues portrayed on the screen by describing related events and struggles in their own lives. The most beneficial way to gain moral learning is in the role of an observer. When the misconduct of someone else is the focus of attention instead of our own behavior, we are less defensive and more able to consider applications for changes in our own conduct (Scott, 2016).

Rationale and Guidelines for Watching Television

Moral Lessons and Media

Talking with children about right or wrong decisions made by characters on the screen can support moral learning. There is growing public concern that the moral development of children is not keeping pace with growth of their mental abilities. A powerful method for teaching morals originated with the ancient Greeks who received moral education at the theater. The Greeks recognized that, unlike other forms of instruction, a theatrical production sustained attention and also conveyed a profound influence (Groton & May, 2014).

Accordingly, the most eminent playwrights were commissioned by the Greek government to teach morals to the public by observation of dramatic presentations. All the well-known Greek tragedies consisted of a common format following a predictable succession of events. The leading characters were always people with high social status but whose departure from their admirable characteristics resulted in facing desperate circumstances. Later, as they renewed commitments to their original values, the reputation of the character was restored along with the audience esteem. Whether the plot was Oedipus Rex, Medea, Hippolytus, or other familiar characters, the lesson was always the same—no one, not even those with the greatest status can desert their moral code without suffering tragedy and remorse.

Shakespeare's (ca. 1623/2020) great tragedies, written hundreds of years later, corresponded with the Greek design. Prince Hamlet, King Lear, Macbeth, and Othello are examples of heroes who turned away from their values only to find that the consequence was great personal loss and regret. How does this reliance in the past on theater as a context for moral education relate to the present environment? Children are often exposed to dramatic productions on television. Parents should take advantage of this appealing context by exploring child values and sharing their own values during time spent together in mutual observation.

Table 4.2 provides additional opportunity to practice asking agenda questions in the primary grades (ages 5–9 years old). The purpose of each question is provided along with anticipated benefits.

Table 4.2 Television Questions for Conversations with Children Ages 5–9 Years Old

Questions	*Purposes and Benefits*
1 What did you like about each character?	*Perception of potential*: Realize that children can see added possibilities because they are more optimistic.
2 Why did this person do what s/he did?	*Recognizing motivation*: A common error is attributing untrue motives to young children.
3 How will that person's behavior affect others?	*Influence on others*: Forecasting outcomes of actions is an aspect of decision making.
4 How do you think s/he should be punished?	*Scaling consequences*: Kids can be severe in their judgment.
5 What questions would you like to ask any of the characters?	*Curiosity about uncertainties*: Desire to know motivation for behavior.
6 What choices does s/he have in this situation?	*Thinking of possibilities*: Generating alternatives can be a key to success.
7 How are you like any of these people?	*Personal identification*: Move away from egocentrism toward development of empathy.
8 Why do you think s/he made that decision?	*Evaluating purpose*: Emphasize what is important and possible.
9 What did she or he do wrong?	*Recognizing behavior that is unacceptable*: Reinforce the honest path.
10 What is an important lesson in this story?	*Detection of main events*: Get to the point, see the main message for comprehension.
11 Who were the important people in the story?	*Significance of characters*: Children may see some characters differently than the adults do.

Influence of Curiosity on Creativity

In describing himself Albert Einstein (1879–1955) stated he did not have any special talents beyond a passionate curiosity (Kaku, 2023). This observation suggested that one way to nurture creative thinking was to encourage child curiosity (Duckworth, 2016). Another icon who revealed clues about his creative thinking was Leonardo da Vinci (1452–1519) (Heydenreich, 2023). His broad range of competencies included painting, sculpture, engineering, and anatomy. The core skill and passion da Vinci relied on was observation, as shown by extensive notes and drawings he kept of nature and portraits of people he saw in Rome, Florence, and Milan. These examples of people recognized for their extraordinary abilities reinforced the need for children to retain their sense of curiosity. This is important because the less people are self-absorbed or narcissistic, the more they are able to notice details in their environment. In da Vinci's opinion, "Many people look, but few see – and mindful seeing is a foundation of experience, itself the base of direct knowledge" (Hoque & Baer, 2022).

Parents realize young children look to them as their most important sources of learning. This is why young boys and girls typically ask 100 or more questions every day. A study of more than 1,000 parents in England was conducted by the Institution of Engineering and Technology (Goldberg, 2018). Results determined that most of the parents admitted children had asked them questions for which they did not know the correct answers. Nevertheless, two-thirds of the parents chose to provide incorrect answers instead of acknowledging their own ignorance to children or suggest collaborative efforts to search together for the answers.

The passion to solve problems shows the impact that curiosity has on initial motivation of young children to learn (Duckworth, 2016; Dweck, 2017). Yet, in just a few years, even before the students complete elementary school, many stop asking questions of parents and teachers. What is it that occurs between early childhood and the onset of adolescence that undermines interest in discovery of new knowledge, causes students to give up on exploring how the world works, and eliminates fascination with mysteries of the unknown? There are no answers that completely explain the reasons for common decline of curiosity on such a grand scale. However, it seems clear that when a person ceases to be curious, s/he gives up the opportunity to become a self-directed learner (Abraham, 2018; Cleese, 2020). The concept of self-directed learning should be a prominent goal because of access to the Internet. One premise is that individuals are naturally curious and will search for knowledge of interest to them at the same time they acquire academic skills everyone needs. However, individuals who abandon curiosity are unlikely to continue searching for knowledge. Given this prospect, preservation of child curiosity should be given high priority by families, schools, and communities (Jackson, 2009, 2018).

In this context parents should realize the importance of restricting the time children are allowed to watch television. A longitudinal study of 1,000 children has been conducted by the Department of Medicine at Dunedin University in New Zealand (Landhuis et al., 2007). They found that children who watched more television at ages 5 and 7 were more likely to show signs of attention deficit at ages 13 and 15. Reports of attention deficits in adolescence were compared to amount of time parents reported their children watched television at ages 5, 7, 9, and 11. A group of psychologists rated the attention span and ability of each child to concentrate at ages 3 and 5.

Even after gender, cognitive ability, socioeconomic status, and amount of viewing time during adolescence were factored in, results showed that students who were spectators 3 or more hours a day between ages 5 and 11 had greater attention problems at ages 13 and

15 than peers who watched television two hour or less a day. More than a decade later, at age 26, children in the study were re-examined. The young adults who spent more time watching television during childhood and adolescence were significantly more likely to have a criminal conviction, diagnosis of antisocial disorder, and more aggressive traits compared to peers who saw less television (Robertson et al., 2013). This continuing 50-year study is the longest longitudinal research on human development ever conducted (Poulton et al., 2020).

The following guidelines are suggested for parents during family televiewing.

Strive for a Well-Rounded Selection of Programs

This is a good rule so a father who likes to watch only sports, a mother who watches only reality shows, or a child who sees only cartoons can expand their scope of viewing. A variety of programs should be seen including news, nature, ballet, concerts, sports, comedies, religious programs, and documentaries. This practice can enable all family members to acquire a broader range of interests.

Everyone Should Get to Choose Some Programs

Taking the interests of others into account seldom happens when the program choice of individuals leads them to watch alone. Families have a common need to take part in activities that are chosen by someone else. When children are allowed to participate in decisions about what will be watched together on television, they are motivated to discuss the programs they see with the family and honor compromise about making choices (Hari, 2022).

Share Feelings and Opinions Together during Observation

Allow children time to express their views and then share your impressions. Remember that when child opinion is invited, parent feedback should not center on being right or wrong. By exchanging opinions you share more than personal experiences. Parents also invite children to be open-minded, aware of alternatives, and add to knowledge. Talking about how each of us interpret what we have seen together can be enjoyable and educational. Don't be surprised if you are often the learner.

Encourage Questions While Watching Television

One way people demonstrate their individuality is by the questions they ask. When people no longer express curiosity and stop asking questions, they are destined to become dependent on others for a sense of direction. This means parents should recognize question asking by children is a powerful sign of growth, a necessary key to becoming self-directed. Besides questions children pose for you, invite them to tell what they would like to ask characters on the screen that you have observed together.

Answer Child Questions Honestly

Children may ask some questions you would rather not answer. But remember, good relationships are based on honesty. Provide an honest answer, even if the answer is "I would rather not answer that question." From middle school onward, there is no guarantee that children will seek advice from their parents. However, parents who are willing to share their feelings are more likely to be approached as a source of guidance.

Help Children Increase Their Vocabulary

Choose a weekly program when everyone is expected to identify words they do not understand, immediately repeating unknown words aloud after being spoken on television. Designate someone in the family to write down unknown words. When the program is over, turn off the television. Then help one another by defining words on the list that you know and rely on the Internet or a dictionary as needed. This activity demonstrates willingness to learn together, admit uncertainty, consult written references, and have fun (Auxier et al., 2020).

Valuing Doubt and Critical Thinking

History of Doubt

The most visible evidence someone is no longer curious is their failure to ask questions. Parents are seldom aware of when this behavior begins to decline and therefore might not help their children understand that generating questions is essential for a good education. A common challenge for teachers is enabling students to become comfortable admitting confusion and being willing to seek guidance about the lessons and concerns that they do not understand. Solving problems often requires asking questions and applying rational procedures to discover answers. The French philosopher Voltaire (1694–1778) recommended, "Judge a man by his questions, not his answers" (Pomeau, 2022). This advice implies adults should do all they can to help children retain curiosity by recognizing questions as a form of achievement. By using this strategy children can be credited for their questions as well as answers.

Presenting questions that motivate students to concentrate and reflect was considered by Plato as a basic skill all good teachers should apply. In *The Republic,* Plato (428–348 BCE) described how Socrates would provide a series of probing questions to engage students in critical thinking, and, eventually acquire understanding. Steps referred to as the Socratic method remain a strategy teachers rely on to assess student comprehension and detect lessons that have yet to be understood (Plato, 380 BCE/2016).

Fifteen hundred years after Plato's observations about the high value of questions, Peter Abelard (1079–1142) established the University of Paris in France (Luscombe, 2023). Historical accounts indicate that he was an extraordinary teacher whose students included 20 cardinals, 50 archbishops, and one Pope (Celestin II). Abelard's assertion that reasoning and religious belief could coexist was a departure from the common authority worship of his time. His famous book entitled *Yes and No* examines 158 questions related to Bible verses (Abelard, 1115–1117/2007). For each of the questions conflicting views of theological authorities were described. Abelard explained that, regardless of the elevated status of religious commentators, no one should believe them without examining their logic. Because God is the creator of reason, then reason is the tool He wants mankind to use instead of looking to celebrities for answers. Abelard argued that when authorities disagreed, deciding the source to believe should not favor the person with the highest status but instead the individual whose logic and reasoning appears to be the most persuasive. Abelard thought common people, most of whom could neither read or write, should reach their own decisions and realize their potential to be critical thinkers long before other scholars agreed this was a reasonable expectation.

Abelard contended that truth cannot be at variance with itself. Because the truth of reason and revelation come from the same God, there must be a defect in the reasoning of men or some mistake in theological citations when the views of religious authorities conflict. His *Yes and No* questions were regarded as offensive by authority quoting scholars because it made transparent the confusion and irreconcilable statements regarding most of the 158 biblical questions. This view also bothered conservatives who could not foresee that reasoning would be on the side of revelation.

Abelard was persecuted for his assertion that doubt should be seen as a commendable attribute because it can motivate curiosity, encourage questions, and generate creative thinking. When people ask questions they become more able to find out the truth. Abelard saw curiosity as a key to personal enlightenment. In contrast, a prevailing attitude was that only religious authorities were in possession of the truth. Therefore, to doubt them was evidence of distrust, unacceptable to God and clergymen (no women) representing him in the church hierarchy. At the present time, people are subjected to many conflicting voices that claim authority. The result is often confusion and greater need than ever to rely on critical thinking to check the logic of people who call on us to entrust our sense of direction to them.

Keep Creativity and Critical Thinking Alive

If parents are able to convey the importance of asking questions, their children will adopt an attitude that enables them to retain their curiosity to find solutions for problems throughout life. Children can become self-directed individuals, able to find out things they want to know by framing questions of the sources they locate on the Internet. On the other hand, benefits of the Internet are jeopardized when curiosity is lost, rejected, ignored, ceases to function, or no longer expressed (Torrance, 1994, 2002).

Society should acknowledge the need to supporting creative thinking in schools. Consider an investigation of creative student performance. Kyung Hee Kim (2011) teaches at William and Mary University. She completed a meta-analysis of articles regarding creativity and intelligence published between 1965 and 2005. Kim found a negligible relationship between creative thinking and intelligence. This means these two aspects of ability originate from a different realm of thinking. The same conclusions were reached 40 years earlier by researchers from the National Testing Service and Duke University (Wallach & Kogan, 1965).

Kim hypothesized that if IQ scores are continually rising, referred to as the Flynn Effect, then creativity might not be rising because studies had confirmed their origins were unrelated. To find out, she examined 300,000 student scores recorded on the *Torrance Tests of Creative Thinking* (Torrance, 2002) that identifies original thinking and ability to look at situations and events in new ways. Kim (2016) found that creativity scores had risen steadily in the same way as IQ scores but that progression for creativity ended in 1990. During the following two decades, creativity scores declined across the full age range with students in kindergarten through sixth grade recording the greatest losses.

Kim (2019) maintained that the foundation of creative thinking is expertise. Her review of studies determined that not all Nobel Prize winners and other innovators have measured high IQs. Instead, each had expertise in some particular field. The foundation of creative thinking seems to be expertise that develops by devoting significant amounts of time to deep exploration.

The way to value originality is appreciate imaginative thinking. Individuals are unique in having imagination, a wonderful attribute that enables them to look beyond the moment. Imagination allows us to go back in time, revisit the past, look ahead, and envision ways to create conditions for a more desirable future. No one can predict what will happen tomorrow but actions that are motivated and shaped by imagination can influence what life becomes. Mankind might be evolving biologically at a similar rate to other living organisms. However, in cultural terms, people have to change and make adjustments more rapidly. As far as we can tell the cats and dogs we cherish are not changing socially at a corresponding rate. Left to themselves, they continue doing what has always been their behavior and concern themselves with the same things they did in the past. There is no need to keep checking up on them to find out what is new (de Waal, 2022). But, something will always be new in the thinking of humanity because imagination triggers creativity and innovation.

Parents who educate primary grade children can count on curiosity and imagination as assets that may be less available when children grow older. For example, young students are generally eager to ask questions in school and suppose teachers know almost everything. We do not understand what happens between early childhood and early adolescence (around age 10), but it seems clear that the peer norms established in middle school shut down questioning that was prominent only a few years earlier. Parents should realize middle school students will do almost anything to avoid being seen as different from peers so admitting ignorance by raising questions declines because it could result in being teased, ridiculed, and rejected. These common peer norms inhibit normal development of creative thinking. Such norms should be recognized as dysfunctional and become the target for replacement by supportive cooperative learning teams in class along with parents and teachers (Strom & Strom, 2021).

Family Observation of Play

An important factor that distinguishes creative children from their less creative peers is family support for imagination. Play is the method children prefer to express their imagination. So, parents should watch children play. That boys and girls want adults to observe them is clear from their near constant plea to "See me," "Look at this, watch how I do it." By observing a child pretend, adults are able to communicate approval of imagination and ensure their acceptance of creativity. In this context boys and girls realize they do not have to change their behavior to get parental attention. Children must believe their creative play is worthwhile for parents to bother watching before they can conclude the ability to pretend is important enough to retain. Parents should learn to value the qualities they want children to retain beyond childhood (Auxier et al., 2020; Minkin & Horowitz, 2023).

Parents can be quickly distracted when they watch a four-year-old play. Is this because we do not know what to look for, what to find pleasing, how to identify success, what to say about a form of play that has no rules, no hits, no runs, and so cannot be scored. Why is it that my wife and I could invite friends to see our 10-year-old son participate in a hockey game, but if we asked them to stop by and watch our four-year-old boy play, they would decline and then ask, "Why? Does he have a special trick?" Whatever prevents us from becoming regular observers of little children pretending should be revised if we seek to nurture creative thinking.

It is one thing to lack the power to pretend and quite another to reject that power when shown by someone else. This has been made clear from many observations of 4- and 5-year-olds during play with parents. When Greg wanted to drive his toy truck to Africa and join a safari, his father did not respond with enthusiasm. Instead, he dismissed the venture by reminding Greg that Africa is across the ocean and trucks cannot travel by water unless they are first loaded onto boats.

A similar discount of imagination is likely when children identify relationships between toys that adults do not recognize. Steven did not feel that his account of what was happening had to be plausible. But his explanation that a man in a crash between two toy trucks was not hurt because he was wearing a brick coat was immediately dismissed by the parent, who insisted on using this occasion to point out the value of seat belts.

A parent's preference for realism and unwillingness to accept divergent thinking combine in Maria's case. Her mother felt compelled to remove the policeman from a group of cowboys because "He doesn't fit." Maria saw the matter differently and kept the officer in the group. She pointed out that because the fort was already surrounded by the enemy, cowboys needed all the help they could get and should not exclude this person just because he dressed differently by wearing a blue uniform.

Parent Types of Questions

Young children often introduce news they want to share by asking, "Guess what?" Most parents do not respond as requested. Instead of generating hunches, they generally reply, "What?" In effect, they make it known that guessing is not a way they prefer to learn something new. Instead, they choose to learn by being told. This means that parents are likely to expect children to adopt the same choice for the ways they prefer to learn. The seriousness of this mistake is typically overlooked (Kellerman & Seligman, 2023).

To explore aspects of questioning, we observed 60 parents and preschoolers engaged in pretend play (Strom & Strom, 2010). A family fun jet with colorful wooden passengers and suitcases, served as the focus for play. Time sampling of interaction were audio recorded in each home. The parents collectively asked over 800 separate questions. An examination of questions showed that 57% were classification type. For example, "Which suitcases are square?" "Where is the blue toy in the group?" Another 33% of the questions were descriptive. For example, "How many passengers are children? or "What is going on in the control tower? In combination, the classification and description questions made up 90% of the total parents presented to their children. Even though every parent had expressed the desire to foster creative thinking, less than 2% of questions called on their child to guess, hypothesize, or speculate.

By using hypothesis-type questions, such as "What will happen if the river rises and covers the airport runway?" or "What do you suppose a passenger will do if she loses her cell phone?" These questions motivate children to go beyond what they can see, to imagine what is possible—a futuristic perspective. Hypothetical questions encourage children to talk more because there is no single correct answer. For the same reason such questions allow children to express differences from adult opinion. A greater proportion of questions should legitimize guessing and imagination by children.

Descriptive questions are also important, especially when a teacher and students see things together while on a field trip or in class. Questions can disclose what children see and what escapes their notice. By calling to their attention the details young students do not see, the teacher can provide the benefit of her broader perspective. This is important for preschoolers and some primary students whose perception is limited by centration, being able to focus on only one aspect of a situation at a time, and egocentrism, the inability to take into account the view of someone else.

Critical Thinking and Reflection

Waiting for students to respond is another factor adults should consider when asking children questions. Those who undervalue the importance of reflection for critical thinking often misjudge its silent process as a sign of child misunderstanding. Consequently, an adult may tend to amend questions or provide cues. However well intended, efforts to motivate premature answers disrespects the child pace of thinking or what is called cognitive tempo. Children who have an impulsive tempo are inclined to act on a first impression without pausing to evaluate its merit. So, they respond quickly but also make more errors. Reflective tempo children take more time, and, because they think before acting, make less mistakes. Even though society declares that reflective thinking is valued, children are often expected to respond to questions immediately. In our study we observed mothers waited a minimum of five seconds for their child to answer to a question 60% of the time. Fathers, whose need for closure was higher, waited five seconds in only 40% of cases. In contrast, children were the most respectful of deliberation, waiting five seconds or more in 86% of cases. Teachers in class should avoid calling on students to give an answer just because they are first to raise their hand. Select someone to respond only after everyone has time for reflective thought. A rush-oriented environment cannot support child reflection. Ditch the contradictory practice of calling on students based on who raises hands ahead of others (Davis, 2023).

Conclusion

Parents should monitor content of television programs observed by children. Otherwise children could be exposed to scenes that involve adult intimacy or violence. Some of what children could watch is inappropriate because of their age and unsuitability of subject matter. Parents should forbid watching some programs, even if children plead that their friends are permitted to see them. Parents should feel comfortable recognizing that their role goes beyond acting as censors and includes responsibility for guidance to help children interpret what they see.

By talking about what the family sees together, familiar topics and seldom-considered issues can be shared. A continuing dialogue helps everyone understand opinions of others, and develop a broader outlook. Many parents are disappointed that it is difficult to get their child to share feelings and thinking. This is seldom a problem when watching television together. Asking questions while seeing a program motivates self-disclosure, reveals how people view situations, and elicits feelings, thoughts, and values.

Presenting questions while watching television disturbs some parents in the beginning. They consider this behavior distracting and liken it to the noisy conduct of others who make watching a movie at a theater disappointing. They believe that observers should be quiet to avoid interrupting concentration of others. However, parents and children can easily follow a story and talk at the same time. Adults underestimate the child capacity to manage two concurrent tasks. Adults also show this ability when watching television and reading the message that may appear across the bottom of a screen. Children and parents readily keep up with the flow of content and can talk about changing events as they unfold. You could record a program, push pause to discuss or to repeat something that is misunderstood. When parents make this shift, they experience the satisfaction of having children express themselves more. Adults also recognize that conversation benefits are greater than the entertainment any program can offer. Seeking child opinions influences the amount of attention they pay to comments made by the grownups.

There is much to learn about using television to support creative and critical thinking. Parents should set new expectations for themselves that enable them to contribute to their child's education. Specifically, watch television together—this requires time. Next, ask questions during mutual observations—this takes practice. And, just as children are expected to express personal impressions, parents and grandparents should share their experiences—this requires self-disclosure. Finally, children should select some of the programs that a family watches, showing acceptance of child interests. When adults subject themselves to these expectations they are able to communicate more easily and establish themselves as a lasting source of guidance.

Key Concepts

1 Parents who ask children guessing-type questions approve of speculation, making guesses. They are also more comfortable with uncertainty and willing to discuss issues for which they may not know the full range of possible answers.

2 Children begin asking for parent advice about preserving and building friendships while also trying to establish independence. This topic arises early and is pronounced by age 8 or 9 when pressure from peers begin to build and become a strong force that influences behavior of all group members.

3 By reacting to televised versions of real-life dilemmas, families simulate predictable problems and can explore the merits of individual judgment without having to experience disappointment, embarrassment, or other undesirable consequences.

4 There can be benefit in comparing how a parent and child assess characters at the beginning and end of a program. Parents might not always know best but children usually conclude that the grownups have something of value to teach them about evaluating situations.

5 At the end of a program or when reading a book, ask the child to summarize the main events that happened. You will find out what was understood, the details a child considered important, and elements that were overlooked.

6 The most beneficial way for children to acquire moral learning is as an observer. When someone else's behavior is the focus of children's attention instead of their own conduct, they are less defensive and more able to consider making personal changes that are suitable.

7 Critical thinking should have high priority for education at home and school because students must be well prepared to distinguish between fact and opinion, determine quality of judgment, and evaluate reasons that govern decision-making.

8 During the past two decades creativity scores have declined with the students in kindergarten through 6th grade recording the largest losses. This is worrisome because business executives identify creativity as the most important leadership competence needed for the future.

9 Some of what children might watch on television is inappropriate because of their age and unacceptable subject matter. Parents should forbid children from seeing some programs, even when they plead that the parents of their friends are allowed to watch them.

10 Asking questions at the same time you observe a program with children motivates self-disclosure, reveals how individual family member interpret situations, and elicits sharing of feelings, thoughts, and values.

Generational Perspectives Activities

4.1 Team Discussion
4.2 Agenda for Interviews with Parents
4.3 Agenda for Interviews with Young Children
4.4 A Scenario: Reasoning and Problem Solving
4.5 Team Chapter Review
4.6 Criteria for Parent Self-Evaluation

4.1 Team Discussion

1 How can parents become teachers while they watch television with young children?
2 Why do the young children ask many questions but stop by middle school?
3 What are some consequences if 5-to-8-year olds spend excessive time with television?
4 How can parents increase child vocabulary while they watch television together?
5 How do views of Abelard regarding the value of doubt compare with your own opinions?
6 What should be done by parents and schools to offset a decline in student creativity?
7 How do you suppose peer influence contributes to student decline in creative behavior?
8 How does expecting students to answer without reflection effect cognitive tempo?
9 What are some lessons parents can learn while they watch television with their children?
10 What are some important lessons children can learn as they watch TV with their parents?

4.2 Agenda for Interviews with Parents

1 What are some favorite television shows of children that you also enjoy?
2 What television programs do your children like that you do not want to watch?
3 What changes would you like in television viewing habits of children?
4 What are your impressions about the children's programs on television?
5 How do you feel about television commercials directed to children?
6 What are some benefits your children gain from watching television?
7 What are your favorite programs and why do you like watching them?
8 What programs are on television you do not want children to watch?
9 What strategies have you used to influence the language of children?
10 How is speech of children influenced by attending daycare or preschool?

4.3 Agenda for Interviews with Young Children

1 What are some of the television shows you always want to watch?
2 What kinds of programs do you dislike and do not want to watch?
3 What television programs do you and your parents watch together?
4 While watching television together, what does your family talk about?
5 Who are some favorite characters that you like to watch on television?
6 What are the cartoons that you enjoy seeing more than any of the others?
7 What rules do parents have about the programs you are allowed to watch?
8 How are Mom and Dad different from you in the programs they like most?

4.4 A Scenario: Reasoning and Problem Solving

Problem solving scenarios present an opportunity to look at situations that might happen for a family and think about possible solutions. Your task is to look at pros and cons of choices that are stated, think of additional options, identify relevant information that might be missing, find out how teammates view the alternatives, and defend your reasoning about the advice that you consider best.

Parents can learn and teach while watching television with children. But, a familiar problem is that many adults do not recognize their potential for influence. How can reluctant parents be motivated to apply their creativity?

a Use an agenda of questions while watching television with a child.
b Identify and build skills that are essential for doing well in school.
c Become an interpreter of story events and define vocabulary words.
d Share personal failures like those portrayed by actors in programs.
e Show your values by asking questions about right and wrong behaviors.
f Other _____

4.5 Team Chapter Review

Efforts to assess participant learning, provide feedback, and improve quality of instruction is enhanced by a group review of each chapter.

1 What ideas in the lesson changed the way I think about this topic?
2 What insights from the lesson will I try to apply in my relationships?
3 What is the most important point for me presented in this lesson?
4 What are some aspects of this lesson I would like to better understand?
5 Which aspects of this lesson do I wish that I had known about earlier?

4.6 Criteria for Parent Self-Evaluation

Directions: For each question, place a check beside statements that describe your feelings. You may want to give several answers on some items. If your feelings are not on choices list, write them on the line marked "Other."

1 How could you improve your television watching habits?

   a Spend less time watching just for something to do.
   b Plan better for what programs are worth watching.

   c Concentrate more instead of channel switching.
   d Turn television off when I am doing other things.
   e Other _____

2 In what ways does television contribute to your education?

   a Stimulates new ideas and interests for me.
   b Helps me reduce the stress of everyday life.
   c Keeps me informed about news of the day.
   d Supports my involvement with imagination.
   e Causes me to be curious and ask questions.
   f Other _____

3 What methods can help children improve television viewing habits?

   a Limit the amount of time allowed for watching television.
   b Parental censorship of the child's choice of programs.
   c Observing good spectator behavior by family members.
   d Media courses at school that include television literacy.
   e Other _____

4 When I watch television with my child

   a we mostly talk about other things but watch too
   b we share interpretations of a show as we watch
   c we pay attention but interact during commercials
   d we mostly watch and don't interrupt the program
   e Other _____

5 My views about watching television with a child

   a have changed from being a spectator to learning together
   b recognize that asking questions is a way to inform us both
   c is a context where we each of us can share interpretations
   d allows me a guidance role I did not previously recognize
   e Other _____

6 Asking questions as a method to motivate curiosity

   a is a procedure I will use to support creative thinking
   b encourages my child to be a self-directed learner
   c shows my child that inquiry is basic for learning
   d is a behavior I want to adopt for relating to my child
   e Other _____

7 Helping a child learn how to process failure is an important lesson that

   a I can teach by drawing attention to failure of characters on TV
   b can be conveyed by revealing some of my own failures
   c I feel is overlooked as many families deny failure experiences
   d they learn from setbacks instead of becoming defensive
   e Other _____

8 Waiting for children to respond after I ask a question

    a allows an opportunity to reflect before giving a response
    b is a behavior I should adopt instead of encouraging hurry
    c lets them know I respect processing ideas before answering
    d is a habit I must check myself on to contribute to thinking
    e Other _____

9 Besides watching TV together

    a my child and I read children's books
    b we play games together
    c my child and I talk about bullying
    d I ask my child about friendships
    e Other _____

10 My views of child thinking are

    a I encourage my child to ask questions
    b I like the idea of schools linking creative thinking and mental health
    c I would approve of students being given grades for critical thinking
    d I think creativity should be emphasized in school for problem solving
    e Other _____

References

Abelard, P. (2007). *Yes and no* (P. Throop, Trans.). MedievalMS. (Original work published 1115–1117)

Abraham, A. (2018). *The neuroscience of creativity*. Cambridge University Press.

Auxier, B., Anderson, M., Perrin, A., & Turner, E. (2020, July 28). *Parenting children in the age of screens*. Pew Research Center. https://www.pewresearch.org/internet/2020/07/28/parenting-children-in-the-age-of-screens/

Bentley, R., & Jordan, M. (2017). *The acceleration of cultural change: From ancestors to algorithms*. Massachusetts Institute of Technology.

Cleese, J. (2020). *Creativity: A short and cheerful guide*. Crown.

Davis, K. (2023). *Technology's child: Digital media's role in the ages and stages of growing up*. MIT Press.

de Waal, F. (2022). *Different: Gender through the eyes of a primatologist*. W.W. Norton.

Duckworth, A. (2016). *Grit: The power of passion and perseverance*. Scribner.

Dweck, C. S. (2017, January 30). The journey to children's mindsets – and beyond. *Child Development Perspectives*, *11*(2), 139–144. 10.1111/cdep.12225

Goldberg, E. (2018). *Creativity: The human brain in the age of innovation*. Oxford University Press.

Grant, A. (2021). *Think again: The power of knowing what you don't know*. Viking.

Groton, A. H., & May, J. M. (2014). *Forty-six stories in classical Greek*. Focus.

Harari, Y. N. (2017). *Homo Deus: A brief history of tomorrow*. Harper Collins.

Hari, J. (2022). *Stolen focus: Why you can't pay attention—and how to think deeply again*. Crown.

Heydenreich, L. H. (2023, April 11). Leonardo da Vinci. *Encyclopedia Britannica*. https://www.britannica.com/biography/Leonardo-da-Vinci

Hoque, F., & Baer, D. (2022). *Everything connects: Cultivating mindfulness, creativity, and innovation for long-term value* (2nd ed.). Fast Company Press.

Jackson, M. (2009). *Distracted: The erosion of attention and the coming dark age*. Prometheus.

Jackson, M. (2018). *Distracted: Reclaiming our focus in a world of lost attention*. Prometheus.

Kaku, M. (2023, April 14). Albert Einstein. *Encyclopedia Britannica.* https://www.britannica.com/biography/Albert-Einstein

Kellerman, G., & Seligman, M. E. P. (2023). *Tomorrowmind: Thriving at work with resilience, creativity, and connection – now and in an uncertain future.* Atria.

Kim, K. H. (2011). The creativity crisis: The decrease in creativity thinking scores on the Torrance *Tests of Creative Thinking. Creativity Research Journal, 23*(4), 285–295. 10.1080/10400419.2011.627805

Kim, K. H. (2016). *The creativity challenge: How we can recapture American innovation.* Prometheus.

Kim, K. H. (2019). Demystifying creativity: What creativity isn't and is? *Roeper Review, 41*(2), 119–128. 10.1080/02783193.2019.1585397

Landhuis, E., Poulton, R., Welch, D., & Hancox, R. (2007). Does television viewing lead to attention problems in adolescence? Results from a longitudinal study. *Pediatrics, 120*(3), 532–537. 10.1542/peds.2007-0978

Leski, K. (2015). *The storm of creativity.* MIT Press.

Luscombe, D. E. (2023, April 17). Peter Abelard. *Encyclopedia Britannica.* https://www.britannica.com/biography/Peter-Abelard

Minkin, R., & Horowitz, J. (2023, January 24). *Parenting in America Today.* Pew Research Center. https://www.pewresearch.org/social-trends/2023/01/24/parenting-in-america-today/

Plato. (2016). *The republic* (B. Jowett, Trans.). Digireads.com. (Original work published 380 BCE)

Pomeau, R. H. (2022, November 17). Voltaire. *Encyclopedia Britannica.* https://www.britannica.com/biography/Voltaire

Poulton, R., Guiney, H., Ramrakha, S., & Moffitt, T. (2020). The Dunnedin study after half a century: Reflections on the past and course for the future. *Journal of the Royal Society of New Zealand.* 10.1080/03036758.2022.2114508

Robertson L., McAnally, H., & Hancox, R. (2013). Childhood and adolescent televiewing and anti-social behavior in early adulthood. *Pediatrics, 131*(3), 439–446. 10.1542/peds.2012-1582

Scott, A. O. (2016). *Better living through criticism: How to think about art, pleasure, beauty and truth.* Penguin.

Shakespeare, W. (2020). *Greatest tragedies of Shakespeare.* Fingerprint! (Original work published ca. 1623)

Strom, P. S., & Strom, R. D. (2021). *Adolescents in the Internet age: A team learning and teaching perspective.* Information Age Publishing.

Strom, R. D., & Strom, P. S. (2010). *Parenting young children.* Information Age.

Torrance, E. P. (1994). *Creativity: Just wanting to know.* Benedict Books.

Torrance, E. P. (2002). *Torrance Tests of Creative Thinking®.* Scholastic Testing Service.

Wallach, M., & Kogan, N. (1965). *Modes of Thinking in Young Children.* Holt, Rinehart, & Winston.

Part II
Middle Age (Ages 40–60)

5 Goals and Self-Evaluation

Personal Goals

Psychologists agree that some reassessment of personal direction is necessary during middle age. However, there is little agreement about the particular goals men and women should strive to achieve at this stage of life (Buchinger et al., 2022). This lack of consensus is actually beneficial because it encourages individuals to direct self-evaluation to the issues that require the greatest attention for their own circumstance.

Middle age is a time to assess how we deal with our emerging perspectives on aging. It is important for people to take stock of their situation, especially their long-standing illusions that motivated occupational goals, intimate relationships, and impressions of what someone really wants from life. By age 40, middle-aged men and women are aware of how they stand in relation to achieving plans made during early adulthood and how much more progress can reasonably be expected. When there has been failure in achieving particular aspirations, there is regret and adjustment is necessary to accept that knowledge. Even individuals who are seen by peers as highly successful, those whose career dreams have already been met and surpassed, report they sometimes experience feelings of futility and meaninglessness. In fact, discontent during middle age is so widespread it can be seen as normal personality development (R. D. Strom & Strom, 2021).

What seems to happen is that some of the previously obvious truths, basic beliefs, and support values, suddenly come into question? The sense of disparity between "what I have attained and what I really wanted" motivates a self search for "what I want now." The necessity to amend dreams that have dominated thinking for a long time can be difficult for most people because the inclination is to retain fantasies that should be replaced; uncertainty keeps other people from contemplating their future and making changes (Kellerman & Seligman, 2023). Nevertheless, the necessity to construct a more appropriate dream should be recognized as an important developmental task in midlife. Everyone should restructure some goals formulated at an earlier age so the worthwhile and mature dimensions of their original form are retained while, at the same time, emerging priorities consistent with being middle age are added to govern personal direction (Mintz, 2015).

Sources of Discontent

Anecdotal reports reveal discontent that triggers the desire to amend goals but do not identify the desired direction for change. Four areas typically relate to discontent in middle age. Because individuals differ in the source(s) of discontent, they vary in

DOI: 10.4324/9781003401261-8

questions that are suitable for self-evaluation. First, when marriage is viewed as the main reason for being unhappy, people think about what is missing in the relationship they have with their spouse. Accordingly, persons in this situation typically ask themselves: Do I want to remain with my husband or wife now that our children are old enough to adjust if we decide to divorce? Should I make an effort to recover the passion we enjoyed earlier in life? Should I have an extramarital affair to compensate for the loss of affection or lack of sexual pleasure in my marriage?

Many men and women consider their spouse to be the greatest source of satisfaction, so they do not ask themselves questions about the management of discontent with their marriage. Instead, what bothers some of them most could be coping with unpleasant conditions on the job. This second context of discontent appears to be increasing in scope. Dual career couples are 80% of all households that include parents and children. As they review the commitment to their job, these people may struggle to decide whether the time and effort they have devoted to this aspect of their life has turned out to be as worthwhile as intended. Whether they are subject to boredom or feel pressure-ridden by relationships with colleagues, the questions they ask themselves tend to be similar: Do I want to keep doing the same type of job for the rest of my career? Is it too late to make a change in what I do for a living? Is it reasonable to think about starting over, to begin anew in a different line of work? These questions are most likely to surface at about the same time adolescent sons and daughters are beginning to explore their occupational alternatives. It is unfortunate that, as adolescents struggle with doubts about the choice of a career path, parents who are engaged in intense self-evaluation seldom share the processes that they use to support reflective thinking, decision-making, psychological and emotional adjustment.

A third context of possible discontent involves physical decline that accompanies middle age. In a society that assigns enormous value to looking young, physical aging has become the main cause of discontent for many women and men. In such cases declining efficiency of their body causes people to become anxious and experience worry about potential for heart disease, leads others to consider shifting to a more moderate lifestyle, and still others to be preoccupied by changes in appearance they believe could undermine their relationships. The prominent questions these people present for self-consideration usually include: What habits must I give up or renew to improve my chances to maintain good health? What should I do to keep my body fit, youthful and attractive? An army of middle-aged people who become members of health clubs, exercise programs, diet clinics, and cosmetic services reflect these worries and concerns. Just as puberty signals the onset of adolescence, physical changes inform parents they are experiencing middle age. Usually this awareness comes at about the same time their adolescent daughters and sons are developing mature attractive bodies and appealing physiques (Hagerty, 2017).

Besides marriage, work, and physical decline, a fourth realm of discontent can center on the inconsistency between expressed religious beliefs or philosophical values and less mature personal behavior. Carl Jung was a Swiss psychoanalyst whose fame allowed him to become a sought after provider of treatment for celebrities and affluent patients across the world. In Jung's (1955) book, *Modern Man in Search of a Soul*, he described this insight from his experiences:

> Among all my patients in the second half of their life, there has not been a single individual whose problems in the last resort was not a matter of finding a religious outlook on life. It seems safe to say that every one of them fell ill because s/he had lost

that which living religions from every era have given their followers, and none of them had been really healed who did not regain a religious outlook.

Self-examination for each of the four realms of discontent implicate the consistency of lifestyle. For example, if my children matter so much to me, then why do I spend so little time with them? How can my definition of success expand to go beyond workplace tasks to include achievement in other roles such as husband, father, wife, mother, adult child or friend? Why do I resolve to have a more healthy lifestyle but do not schedule the time needed for exercise or adopt a healthier diet? What changes should be made to reconcile my behavior and beliefs as priorities that can serve as a guide for my behavior?

Intensity of Discontent

Individuals differ not only in the sources that foster their discontent but also in intensity related to discontent. The severity of discontent appears to account for why the process of self-evaluation in middle age can significantly modify future attitudes and behaviors of some people but result in only slight changes for others. Clinical psychologists, whose purpose is to help people find a path to mental health, have been responsible for the main body of literature that describes experiences of middle-aged people. Most of the generalizations they provide in self-help books are based on their conversations and observations of only a small representation of middle-aged people who come to them for advice. Consequently, the public has been misled to believe that a midlife crisis is common, perhaps even normative. Some scenarios suggest that self-evaluation without reliance on professional guidance could be a gateway to depression, alcoholism, sexual disorder, divorce, obesity, and other type of dysfunctional behavior. Certainly, people who feel overwhelmed, helpless, and hopeless about their situation should seek help from a professional counselor.

However, for most people, middle age is not a time of crisis but a period of transition for further development that leads to greater maturity and increased happiness. The thought leader of India, Mahatma Gandhi, urged people to recognize that "Happiness is when what you think, what you say, and what you do are in harmony." The transition needed in middle age is demonstrated by greater intimacy in marriage, increased satisfaction at work, greater attention to mental and physical health and fitness, and stronger commitment to ethical and moral principles.

The way parents view adolescents can prompt favorable change in perception as well. They assign greater importance to the child's emotional growth and take pride in the kind of person a daughter or son is becoming rather than limit approval and encouragement to only academic progress or athletic achievements. Successful parents encourage youth to set some of their own goals and take credit for personal accomplishments. Some parents become more willing to listen and show undivided attention to revelations by teenagers regarding their feelings, hopes, fears, uncertainties, and concerns that are worrisome for them. It is difficult to overstate the relationship gains that can be made when parents make an effort to engage in healthy self-evaluation during middle age (Thompson, 2021).

Limitations of Self-Assessment

Self-evaluation is essential to determine the extent to which personal aspirations have been attained, whether they remain appropriate, or if amendments are needed in certain sectors. However, research has consistently found that self-assessment focused on skills and character is often flawed. The correlation between self-impression and behavior as observed by others is usually meager to moderate. Most individuals who report they consider themselves as 'above average', overestimate their commendable behavior, announce overly optimistic speculation about when they will complete tasks, and reach judgments based on unwarranted self-confidence (Dunning, 2012). Despite our best efforts none of us are able to identify all personal learning needs by just relying on self-evaluation. People can often be their own worst enemies. There is no greater obstacle to achieving goals as much as lack of insight regarding our own limitations and short-comings. For these reasons there is usually benefit in seeking a second opinion from someone who observes us on a regular basis, understands the goals we are trying to pursue, and wants to support us so that we can achieve our purposes. Accordingly, observations by a spouse, adolescent daughters or sons, older relative, friends or co-worker can help improve the accuracy of self-evaluation.

Criteria for Success at Work and Home

There are differences in criteria that should be applied to judge personal success at the workplace and criteria suitable to perform well in the family. Many people assume that being in the fast lane is the best path to travel through life. This is the impression of 40-year-old Jeff Hansen, husband of Ann and father of their three sons. As manager of a prospering insurance agency, Jeff earns a high salary that allows Ann the choice to remain at home and supervise their children. During a typical week, Jeff spends 70 hours at work. The reason for his demanding schedule is that Jeff believes personal contacts that bring in business require devoting considerable time and besides Jeff enjoys his job. Jeff's devotion to the company means sometimes he unintentionally neglects his wife and children. He is proud that the needs of his clients are taken care of immediately. In contrast, family needs often must await a slowdown in activity at the office.

It is not surprising that Jeff acknowledges lack of time to be his greatest limitation. When company demands have been met, there does not seem enough hours or energy left for activities with Ann, to take children places in the community, listen to older relatives or monitor the goals he expresses as a parent. Although insufficiently involved with his family, Jeff finds it possible to schedule time for workouts at the gym, play tennis, golf, and other activities he says help reduce stress and enable him to stay physically fit. He admits his children are the source of greater worry and stress than all other sources including his job (Livingston, 2018).

The attributes Jeff depends on for his responsibilities as a father are not the same ones that he relies to ensure success on the job. At the office, intensity and determination are the key factors that trigger increased sales. Jeff is accustomed to a high level of control at the workplace but this is an inappropriate expectation for relationships with relatives. Teenagers have a need to assert themselves, express their beliefs, and identify expectations for how they wish to be treated. Jeff would not tolerate this behavior by subordinates at the company. Perfectionism and efficiency may contribute to progress at the office but the more worthwhile qualities in raising children are patience, being a good listener, spending time together, and encouraging individual goals.

Jeff often returns home late. One night Ann was already sleeping but 16-year-old Larry was watching television in his bedroom. The room seemed in disarray with clothes, books, and papers scattered around the floor. Jeff took one look and questioned:

"When are you ever going to become responsible?" Larry did not reply. The next morning when Jeff told his wife about it, she listened and then said, "You haven't talked to Larry much in the last few weeks. It should please you to know he has been volunteering for the Sierra Club planting trees. He is concerned about the environment beyond his bedroom including the planet and the future of people he has never met. I believe Larry is developing a broader sense of responsibility than we had at his age; there are better ways to gauge his progress than how he maintains the bedroom." Perhaps it is time for Jeff to re-evaluate his conception of what being a teenager is about (Harrington et al., 2017).

Changes in Parent and Adolescent Experiences

Many parents believe their obligations become more difficult when children transition to adolescence, sometime between 10-to-14 years old (Minkin & Horowitz, 2023). Some of the anxiety and frustration comes from efforts to help daughters and sons handle their interpersonal problems that did not exist or were less prevalent while they were growing up. Parents realize their background is an insufficient basis for providing all of the guidance that adolescents need (Turkle, 2016; Twenge, 2014, 2023). Parenting is further complicated because media-declared experts about family relationships offer conflicting opinions. Adjustments must also be made by adolescents. When they enter middle school, they experience increased peer pressures. Compared to the elementary grades, there are more teachers to satisfy, higher levels of thinking are required, the amount of homework increases, competition from classmates becomes greater, uncertainty about careers emerge, and maintaining friendships can be worrisome. These stresses often combine to trigger conflict within families (Ripley, 2021; Schulte, 2015).

Value the Views of Adolescent Observers

Adolescents can support emotional and social development of their middle-aged parents by helping them more accurately recognize their strengths and learning needs. Such insights can be drawn from *the Parent Success Indicator* (R. D. Strom & Strom, 2009, 2012) that identifies favorable qualities of parents and their behaviors that should be considered for improvement. The inventory evolved from a study of 2,893 subjects including 1,296 parents, 907 students, and 700 teachers representing all grade levels, from kindergarten through high school (R. D. Strom, 1985). Corresponding items appeared on the parent, child, and teacher versions of the open-ended form completed by trained interviewers. The interviewers were university students and parents who interviewed students of their own child's age attending some other school. Concerns regarding parent competence were identified and ranked in order of importance for 13 grade levels. A 96% inter-rater agreement level obtained for coding 33,000 responses. Topics with the highest priority for families of 10- to 14-year-olds were used to shape a two-generational data gathering instrument. Reliability, validity, and structure of the instrument were deter-mined (Beckert et al., 2006, 2007; Collinsworth et al., 1996; Strom et al., 1996). The inventory of 60 items is equally divided into the following six scales:

1 Communication – skills of advising children and learning from them;
2 Use of time – making decisions about how discretionary time is used;
3 Teaching – scope of guidance and instruction expected of the parents;
4 Frustration – adolescent behaviors that are bothersome to their parents;

5 Satisfaction – aspects of being a parent that bring satisfaction; and
6 Information needs – things parents need to know about their child.

This inventory has two versions, one for parents and one for 10- to 14-year-old daughters and sons. Mothers and fathers provide self-assessments while adolescents describe observations about their parents. The reason for inviting both generations to evaluate behavior of parents is because adults can make better decisions regarding self-improvement when they are aware of the perceptions of those they want to influence. Parents care more about how children perceive their success and failure than they do about view of relationship experts who give advice in the media. Perceptions regarding parent satisfaction has a significant influence, more than other aspects of parenting, in promoting the autonomy and identity of adolescents. Parents know some of their assets and limitations but are bound to overlook some deficiencies when they do not seek other sources of observation regarding their behavior. By relying on a two-generational perspective of interaction, a comprehensive portrayal of parent competencies and learning needs comes into view along with a more realistic picture of how mothers and fathers influence their children.

Lessons Parents Should Teach Adolescents

Many middle-aged parents define their success by how well they manage the customary teaching and guidance role for their children. Like educators in the classroom, parents can benefit from feedback about the quality of their instruction. To provide such insights, 1,544 Black, Hispanic, and White mothers and their adolescents were invited to complete the *Parent Success Indicator* (R. D. Strom & Strom, 2009). The results identified four lessons that these and other parents should consider.

Parents Should Teach Time Management Skills

Time management is a goal that should be achieved to support a lifestyle required for mental health. Individuals who schedule time so their priorities receive sufficient attention feel more in control of their lives, experience greater satisfaction, and demonstrate a more productive record at work. Parents whose schedules include too many activities present their children with a poor example of balance and prevent themselves from spending enough time with their family. As a result, many adolescents are as over scheduled as parents, juggling events, and trying to communicate non-stop with friends. Adolescents should gain the balance time management provides allowing them to spend time with the people they say matter the most to them (Burkeman, 2021).

In the study of 1,544 Black, Hispanic and White families, independent variables were examined to assess individual significance for each of 60 item responses for mothers (R. D. Strom et al., 2004, 2008). The amount of time mothers spent with their adolescents had the most influence on perceptions of maternal success (58 items out of 60) as reported by both adult and adolescent generations. In contrast, household income had a relatively small effect (13 items) on perceptions of maternal success. Variables that can be manipulated such as 'mother and adolescent time spent together' should become prominent criteria for the way parents evaluate themselves. Mothers and fathers cannot readily change their income or level of formal education, but they can choose to take advantage of the powerful influence that comes from spending time with an adolescent. Similar findings were determined in a study that focused on 517 Black fathers in the United States and their adolescent daughters and sons (R. D. Strom et al., 1996, 2000).

Parents Should Teach How To Manage Stress

This limitation was identified only by adolescent respondents. Teenagers from all three American racial groups assigned their mothers unfavorable ratings for teaching them to cope with daily stress. Learning to relax is fundamental for mental health, a path that more parents should model so their children observe how to manage stress. Parents commonly overestimate their favorable influence in this realm. To qualify as an advisor regarding stress, a parent must be seen by daughters and sons as able to demonstrate this capacity in their own lives. One reason to occasionally retreat from carrying out daily tasks is because this helps to recover perspective. It is troubling that mothers from all three ethnic group gave themselves low scores for being able to manage their time. The inability to schedule leisure for themselves was ranked lowest among things mothers thought they did well, 60th out of 60 items and 57th of 60 according to adolescents (R. D. Strom et al., 2004; Strom et al., 2008).

This familiar situation should not be interpreted as just an example of maternal sacrifice. The fact is adolescents need their mothers to provide a healthy example of dealing with stress by setting aside time for themselves and showing how to manage time so they can retain a sense of personal control. Ten items on the Information Needs scale of the *Parent Success Indicator* (R. D. Strom & Strom, 2009) included how to help children cope with anxieties, fears and worries, set goals, manage conflict, explore careers, address concerns about sex, and avoid bullies cannot be met unless the parents become listeners to children. Careful listening requires time and avoiding distractions. Mothers who invested over 10 hours a week talking with their adolescents and doing things together were considered more successful by adolescents and themselves. Providing access to parents when it is needed is a condition that must be arranged by more mothers and fathers.

Parents Should Teach About Friendship And Dating

Unwillingness to talk with adolescents about dating was identified by both generations as a serious omission in parent teaching. The fact that adolescents saw this as the most prominent learning need of their parents may seem surprising. After all, most schools provide a curriculum related to sexual relationships and safe sex practices. However, student responses suggest that instruction from parents often lacks guidance on how to build relationships with friends of the opposite gender. Adolescents should have conversations with grownups about expectations for dating and building friendships to develop respect and self-restraint in an evolving relationship with dating partners (Davis, 2023).

Both generations from three racial groups (Black, Hispanic, White) thought that parents should be more involved in discussions about dating. Teenagers are entering puberty earlier than previous generations and often start to date well before they have knowledge about relationships. Curiosity and lack of information increases anxiety and fosters premature sexual activity. Dating involves the complicated process of friendship formation and can be seen as distressing because it implicates status as being emotionally or socially competent. Adolescents can turn to peers for advice, but their lack of maturity can sometimes have unfortunate results. Parents should accept their responsibility to guide adolescents at the same time they listen to concerns and experiences.

Parents Should Listen To Their Children

Adolescents from all three ethnic groups gave parents unfavorable ratings for willingness to learn from daughters and sons. Furthermore, the time that mothers spent with their adolescents made considerable differences in this context. The more time mothers and adolescents from all ethnic groups spent together, the more favorable maternal ratings were reported by both generations. It appears that when mothers and children spend a lot of time together, both parties conclude that mothers learn from their child.

Fathers received higher scores for listening to adolescents than for their willingness to learn from them (Beckert et al., 2006). Because of enormous changes in technology youth possess a considerable amount of valuable information. Since parenting is transactional, the views of adults and teenagers should be more closely related. Fathers must be encouraged to find new ways to access ideas, feelings, and opinions of adolescents as well as techniques to help them monitor their logic, particularly as it relates to risk-taking. Listening is necessary to know how another person sees things, but fathers must go beyond being good listeners to recognize the need for reciprocal learning. These attributes characterize good teaching at home and in school.

Societal Expectations of Parents

When men and women try to judge their success as parents, the criteria should include common expectations that society has for all families. Meeting these requirements is necessary for the nation to keep important promises that citizens have collectively made to themselves.

Teach the Values of Fairness and Equality

Fairness and equality are core values of American society that parents of all backgrounds are expected to help their children adopt as an essential element for the democratic way of life. Neither value is taught when some students are disadvantaged because classmates participate in cheating. When cheating is a common practice, high achieving students are unable to distinguish themselves, deficiencies in student learning remain hidden, a need for tutoring goes undetected, and school progress reports to parents are inaccurate. Scandals in the workplace and government reveal unethical practices have eroded public trust and are fostering a cynical perspective.

Adolescence is the stage in life when students establish their sense of moral direction, define behavior they consider commendable, actions they view as misconduct, and decide on relationships they approve of and consequent ways they want to treat people. For these reasons, adolescents need adult guidance and examples to choose integrity as their path to shape behavior instead of engaging in cheating to get ahead (International Center for Academic Integrity, 2023). There is substantial evidence that moral lessons families and schools are expected to provide are not being learned by a large proportion of youth. Consider some examples of unethical parent and teacher behavior that warrant concern.

Teach Children to be Honest and Avoid Cheating

Rettinger and Gallant (2022) wrote *Cheating and Academic Integrity: Lessons from 30 years of Research*. They reported that, despite evidence that the moral development of students has not kept pace with mental development, 93% of nationally surveyed students expressed satisfaction with their personal standard of ethics and character. Most, 81%, agreed with this statement, "When it comes to doing what is right, I am better than most people I know."

An unexpected poor example by educators has been recognized. Salaries of teachers and school principals and their career opportunities are sometimes connected to test performance of students. Faculty have been fired for giving students answers to academic tests, prompting changes in test responses of students while being evaluated, changing answers following testing and before submission to the district for processing, and allowing students more time than specified by test directions.

A national high profile case involved the Atlanta, Georgia, public schools. The Atlanta Constitution newspaper pursued a trail of wrongdoing by public school educators dating back for a decade. In 2015, former educators, principals, and other administrators were tried and convicted of conspiring to create false reports about student achievement. The scandal involved changing responses of students on the Georgia state academic examinations by erasing incorrect answers and substituting correct answers. By misrepresenting student progress, many educators were able to retain their current positions and receive bonuses for accomplishments by students that never happened. Evidence showed cheating took place in multiple schools and involved many educators (Lowry, 2015).

Cheating is behavior meant to deceive or mislead others to gain a personal advantage. In the past, it was commonly supposed that cheaters were students with marginal abilities, causing them to resort to dishonesty as the only way they could keep up with higher achieving peers. The assumption was that talented people, the ones destined for leadership positions in society, would not behave this way. However, evidence has shown that high achievers are just as likely to cheat as their less capable peers. For example, the Harvard University administrative board forced 70 students to leave the school in a cheating scandal that involved a course entitled Introduction to Congress (Pérez-Peña, 2013).

During the past decade, the public has become more informed about academic fraud by college athletes. Smith and Willingham (2015) described some of the worst instances related to college basketball in their book *Cheated: The UNC Scandal, the Education of Athletes, and the Future of Big-time College Sports*. They elaborated how athletes are not given what they were promised, a college education. Instead, for twenty years, football and basketball players at the University of North Carolina were enrolled in courses they never attended but received passing grades.

Parents Who Disregard Fairness and Equality

Some parents are recognized as poor example of integrity by cheating to provide their children with unfair advantage in the college admissions process. In a nationally reported case, fifty wealthy families were caught paying bribes to admissions personnel in order to enable their sons and daughters to enter elite colleges and universities. Several people were fined and jailed.

Every educational institution should have policies about student cheating so the faculty can respond to incidents they observe or have reported to them without fear of duress from students or their parents. A majority of students admit that they cheat but, parents often express confidence that their children would never cheat (Twenge, 2023). Perhaps they believe teaching the differences between right and wrong is all that is required of them without linking student awareness with their responsibility to behave in an ethical way (R. D. Strom & Strom, 2021).

A common outcome is that educators of all grade levels feel vulnerable about possible threats from parents who threaten lawsuits if their child's integrity is questioned without providing indisputable proof. Teachers worry that they might falsely accuse a student and then suffer dreadful consequences. In fact, 70% of educators agree that concern about adverse parent reactions discourages them from trying to punish cheaters. An unintended result is student awareness that their misconduct rarely results in punishment and therefore presents a low risk of detection (Moody, 2021).

Methods of Detecting Plagiarism

A well-known source of forensics technology is Caveon Test Security (2023). This company monitors assessments of student achievement tests by detection of cheating and enables prevention strategies. Caveon has developed data forensics, a process that searches to find unusual test response patterns such as getting difficult questions correct while missing easy questions, an abnormally high pass rate for a school, tests where incorrect answers have been erased and replaced with correct ones. The services of Caveon include protection of instruments from fraudulent practices and application of statistical and web patrolling tools that track cheaters, holding them accountable by providing evidence to school administrators.

Software that detects cheating in various ways has existed for several years. Recently, with introduction of artificial intelligence, new software, such as CHatGPT, has become a source for both learning and cheating. To combat the use of artificial intelligence generated essays and other responses, companies have developed software to detect cheating by applying artificial intelligence such as Turnitin.com software.

When students lack the ethical commitment that is needed to conduct Internet searching, they may suppose it is acceptable to present the words and ideas of someone else as representing their own thinking. Plagiarism is a major problem in middle school, high school, and college. Cyber law proposals that define offenses and penalties are emerging as agenda that, during the future, could be decided by courts instead of by schools (International Center for Academic Integrity, 2023; Moody, 2021).

Parents share responsibility for helping children realize that searching for a topic on the web is just the first step in research, similar to going to a library. Copying from books, journals or sources on the Internet and portraying these products as one's own invention is dishonest and defined as plagiarism. Deceptive practices by students have been reported as moving downward to earlier grades (Bretag, 2016; Eaton, 2021; Moody, 2021).

Conclusion

The most important questions that deserve consideration in middle age are those people ask themselves. Self-evaluation motivates individuals to focus on conditions that cause feelings of discontent and encourage amendment of goals that are out of sync with their developmental stage. This process motivates detection of learning needs and supports progress to maturity. Access to a second opinion can improve awareness about changes in behavior that may be necessary to develop more durable and closer relationships. A spouse or a friend sometimes offers this benefit. Similarly, adolescent children should become sources of feedback about parent behavior and their learning needs. Parents should be aware of important lessons they fail to provide in the estimate of their children. Raising self-expectations is a goal more parents should consider. Teaching adolescents to manage stress, adopt a healthy balance for how time is spent, discuss how to build friendships and nurture relationships, and be willing to learn from children are social contexts where some parents perform poorly in the estimate of children.

High rates of cheating show that many students have not been taught or are not learning to value fairness and equality, fundamental expectations of society. Plagiarism presents teachers with uncertainty about whether they are grading students on their own work or work of someone else. Educators are reluctant to express doubts about dishonesty of student without absolute truth because they fear retribution from parents and the school administration. To support ethical decisions, schools pay for statistical services that can detect plagiarism. Another way to reduce cheating is to devise more challenging assignments that call on students to defend or oppose particular views and offer chances for reciprocal learning as generational reporters or cultural reporters gathering input from relatives and other sources. Students are able to understand that becoming mature cannot be achieved unless they demonstrate fairness and equality toward others. There is also a need to provide parents with agenda to guide family discussion about the relationship of honesty, trust, and integrity to enable personal success.

The most common strategy to support student development of empathy and concern for others is participation in community service. The increasing length of formal education needed to prepare students for employment could forfeit their progress in gaining maturity unless the student experience goes beyond academics to include active involvement in demonstrating concern for others. Acquiring experiences related to the helping relationships is a powerful way to build character, civic responsibility, and support for the well-being of others.

Key Concepts

1 The need to construct a more appropriate dream and outlook on life is one of the principal developmental tasks of middle age. Some of the aspirations that were chosen as a young adult should shift to match the goals that are more supportive of growth and maturity.
2 Feelings of discontent can trigger a desire to modify goals and plans but do not provide a guide for what behaviors should change because personal direction depends on the source(s) of discontent experienced by the individual set of circumstances.

3 Severity of discontent accounts for why self-evaluation in middle age brings only slight change in the behavior of some individuals while causing others to reflect more and significantly modify personal attitudes and dreams that can favorably impact the future.

4 For most people middle age is not time of psychological crisis but instead a time of personal growth and development, a transition that usually results in greater maturity, increased concern for others, and more happiness.

5 It is difficult to overstate the relationship gains that can accompany healthy self-evaluation by individuals during middle age. This means encouragement from others is appropriate to reinforce the attention that is necessary to participate in self-reflection.

6 Self-evaluation is essential to gauge whether personal goals have been met, if these aspirations continue to be appropriate, or should be amended to provide a more beneficial set of criteria to apply when trying to assess personal progress.

7 There are often differences in the criteria required to be successful at work and the criteria to be seen as a success within the family as a husband, wife, father or mother. Knowing how to achieve chosen goals in both settings is the balance that is most desirable.

8 Adolescent daughters and sons can support development of their middle-aged parents by helping to identify their learning needs as well as their strengths. Getting feedback from younger relatives based on their observations is an important source of improvement.

9 Parents should learn time management, how to deal with stress, be willing to learn from their children, and teach lessons about healthy friendships and dating. The best method for teaching these lessons is by providing a good example.

10 Encourage creative thinking. Children more readily become creative thinkers when this is a common behavior in the family. By striving to become creative you will provide valuable lessons about how to avoid boredom, make decisions, recognize opportunities, resolve conflicts, feel comfortable with uncertainty, and use time wisely.

Generational Perspectives Activities

5.1 Team Discussion
5.2 Agenda for Interviews with Parents
5.3 Agenda for Interviews with Grandparents and Teenagers for Comparison
5.4 A Scenario: Reasoning and Problem Solving
5.5 Team Chapter Review
5.6 Criteria for Self-Evaluation of Parents

5.1 Team Discussion

1 Why do you think that cheating has become such a widespread problem?
2 How do you suppose artificial intelligence will influence self-assessment?
3 How could self-evaluation be acquired more effectively in teams?
4 Why are middle-aged parents reluctant to ask children to help evaluate them?
5 What role does narcissism have in the self-evaluation of college students?

 6 How well are students being trained to process criticism from their peers?

 7 Why do teachers avoid having student self-evaluate their work in class?

 8 How could young adults help parents to gain insight about their behavior?

 9 What punishment would you suggest for students who are caught cheating?

10 Tell about a middle-aged adult who is a model of self-evaluation.

5.2 Agenda for Interviews with Parents

 1 What are some challenges of raising adolescents for which you were poorly prepared?

 2 How did your goals from ages 40–60 differ from your goals as a young adult (20–40)?

 3 What are the major sources of discontent you have experienced during middle age?

 4 Who do you turn to for observations regarding how well you perform as a parent?

 5 Looking back, what are some lessons that you have poorly taught your adolescents?

 6 How do you feel about amount of time you spend with your spouse and children?

 7 How does school inform you about the misconduct or good behavior of your child?

 8 What topics would you suggest for a curriculum to educate parents of adolescents?

 9 What are some ideas and behaviors adolescent daughters and sons have taught you?

10 What things would you most like to change about the nature of your lifestyle?

5.3 Agenda for Interviews with Grandparents and Teenagers for Comparisons

Movies and films that were made in the past have become more accessible with Netflix, ShowTime, Apple, Turner Classics and many other venues. This allows multiple generations to recommend movies to each other. Grandparents, parents, and children can become acquainted with viewing experience of relatives by answering these questions.

1 What are some of your all-time favorite movies? Summarize the story lines.

2 Who are your favorite actors and actresses? What films did they perform in?

3 What kinds of behavior have you observed in movies and then tried to imitate?

4 What films do you remember as being the funniest? The most frightening?

5 What kinds of movies do you wish Hollywood would try to make more often?

6 What movies caused you to change your mind about some particular problem?

7 What kinds of movies do you usually try to avoid and what is your reasoning?

8 What themes in movies are repeated more often that you think is reasonable?

9 What films about cultures have influenced your thinking about other peoples?

5.4 A Scenario: Reasoning and Problem Solving

Scenarios present an opportunity to look at situations that might happen for a family and think about possible solutions. Your task is to look at the pros and cons of stated choices, think of additional options, identify relevant information that might be missing, find out how teammates view alternatives, and defend your reasoning about advice that you consider best.

Tom has been working 10 hour days and often on the weekends for almost a year. This schedule is difficult, but Tom feels the promotions and bonuses are worth it. Tom's wife Jane urges him to spend more time with her and their three elementary school children even though it might mean less income. What would you recommend for Tom to do?

a He should listen to his wife because young children need access to their father.
b Tom should tell Jane she should be grateful that he raises their standard of living.
c He should have a discussion with the family and let everyone express their views.
d Tom should devote Sundays to the family so that they have no reason to complain.
e Other _____

5.5 Team Chapter Review

Efforts to assess participant learning, provide feedback, and improve quality of instruction is enhanced by a group review of each chapter.

1 What ideas in the lesson changed the way I think about this topic?
2 What insights from the lesson will I try to apply in my relationships?
3 What is the most important point for me presented in this lesson?
4 What are some aspects of this lesson I would like to better understand?
5 Which aspects of this lesson do I wish that I had known about earlier?

5.6 Criteria for Self-Evaluation of Parents

Directions: For each question, place a check beside statements that describe your feelings. You may want to give several answers on some items. If your feelings are not on choices list, write them on the line marked 'Other.'

1 The self-directed questions I consider about my personal goals

   a get little attention because I have such a busy schedule
   b help me reflect on replacement of some current priorities
   c help in causing me to change my definition of success
   d are interesting to think about but unlikely to change me
   e Other _____

2 Amending some of the goals I set for myself as a young adult

   a are difficult to give up so I usually try not to think about it.
   b is unnecessary since dreams should always be the guide
   c seems essential for adjustment to my current stage in life
   d is important so that I am not discontent about getting older
   e Other _____

3 Some regrets that I have about my behavior as a parent are

   a showing anger during disagreements with children
   b not trusting my children when it was appropriate
   c not having conversations about important issues
   d not spending enough time doing things with my children
   e Other _____

4 The source(s) I value for feedback about my behavior as a parent are:

   a spouse
   b parents

c friends

d children

e Other _____

5 Some lessons I must learn before teaching my children are

a time management attitudes and skills

b learning methods to respond to stress

c building durable and healthy friendships

d listening while other people are talking

e Other _____

6 My attitude about experience as a parent is

a I think about how I could do a better job

b I cannot change the past so I try to forget

c I see mistakes as lessons for improvement

d I cannot see value in looking back at errors

e Other _____

7 The misbehaviors that bother me most are

a mistreating someone that I have loved

b not spending enough time with family

c not showing gratitude until it was too late

d not forgiving someone for misbehavior

e Other _____

8 The most difficult aspects of personal development for me are

a helping my children to grow up

b having a job that I do not enjoy

c feeling trapped in my marriage

d becoming less physically attractive

e Other _____

9 Discussions with my children about dating

a involve listening to their curiosity and concerns

b emphasize the need to build healthy friendships

c recognize I started dating at a later age than them

d include mentioning fears and worries as a parent

e Other _____

10 Regrets I sometimes have about past behavior

a mostly relate to actions I should have taken but did not

b mostly relate to actions I took but should have avoided

c lead me to wish I could live again to do things differently

d encourage me to act more wisely in the time I have left

e Other _____

References

Beckert, T. E., Strom, R. D., & Strom, P. S. (2006). Black and White fathers of early adolescents: A cross cultural approach to curriculum development for parent education. *North American Journal of Psychology*, 8(3), 455–469.

Beckert, T. E., Strom, R. D., Strom, P. S., Yang, C., & Singh, A. (2007). *Parent Success Indicator*: Cross-cultural development and factorial validation. *Educational and Psychological Measurement*, 67(2), 311–327. 10.1177/0013164406292039

Bretag, T. (Ed.). (2016). *Handbook of academic integrity*. Springer.

Buchinger, L., Richter, D., & Heckhausen, J. (2022, May). The development of life goals across the adult lifespan. *The Journals of Gerontology*, 77(5), 905–915. 10.1093/geronb/gbab154

Burkeman, O. (2021). *Four thousand weeks: Time management for mortals*. Farr, Strauss and Giroux.

Caveon (2023). *Your ultimate guide to monitoring the web for stolen test content*. Caveon. https://www.caveon.com/insights/ultimate-guide-to-monitoring-the-web-for-stolen-test-content/

Collinsworth, P., Strom, R. D., & Strom, S. (1996, June). Parent Success Indicator: Development and factorial validation. *Educational and Psychological Measurement*, 56(3), 504–513. 10.1177/0013164496056003012

Davis, K. (2023). *Technology's child: Digital media's role in the ages and stages of growing up*. MIT Press.

Dunning, D. (2012). *Self-insight: Roadblocks and detours on the path to knowing thyself*. Routledge.

Eaton, S. E. (2021). *Plagiarism in higher education: Tackling tough topics in academic integrity*. Libraries Unlimited.

Hagerty, B. (2017). *Life reimagined: The science, art, and opportunity of midlife*. Riverhead Books.

Harrington, B., Fraone, J., & Lee, J. (2017). *The new dad: The career-caregiving conflict*. Boston College Center for Work & Family. https://www.bc.edu/content/dam/files/centers/cwf/research/publications/researchreports/BCCWF%20The%20New%20Dad%202017.pdf

International Center for Academic Integrity (2023). *Facts and statistics*. https://academicintegrity.org/resources/facts-and-statistics

Jung, C. (1955). *Modern man in search of a soul*. Harcourt.

Kellerman, G., & Seligman, M. E. P. (2023). *Tomorrowmind: Thriving at work with resilience, creativity, and connection -- now and in an uncertain future*. Atria.

Livingston, G. (2018, January 8). *Most dads say they spend too little time with their children: About one quarter live apart from them*. Pew Research Center. http://pewrsr.ch/2m62cXS

Lowry, D. (2015, April 30). Sentence reduced for 3 in Atlantic cheating scandal. *USA Today*. https://www.usatoday.com/story/news/nation/2015/04/30/atlanta-educators-resentenced/26643997/

Minkin, R., & Horowitz, J. (2023). *Parenting in America today*. Pew Research Center. https://www.pewresearch.org/social-trends/2023/01/24/parenting-in-america-today/

Mintz, S. (2015). *The prime of life: A history of modern adulthood*. Belknap Press of Harvard University.

Moody, J. (2021, March 31). How cheating in college hurts students. *U.S. News & World Report*. https://www.usnews.com/education/best-colleges/articles/how-cheating-in-college-hurts-students

Pérez-Peña, R. (2013, February 1). Students disciplined in Harvard scandal. *The New York Times*. https://www.nytimes.com/2013/02/02/education/harvard-forced-dozens-to-leave-in-cheating-scandal.html

Rettinger, D., & Gallant, T. (Eds.). (2022). *Cheating academic integrity: Lessons from 30 years of research*. Jossey-Bass.

Ripley, A. (2021). *High conflict: Why we get trapped and how we get out*. Simon & Schuster.

Schulte, B. (2015). *Overwhelmed: How to work, love and play when no one has the time*. Picador.

Smith, J., & Willingham, M. (2015). *Cheated: The UNC scandal, the education of athletes, and the future of big-time college sports*. Potomac Books.

Strom, R. D. (1985, April). Developing a curriculum for parent education. *Family Relations*, *34*(2), 161–167. https://eric.ed.gov/?id=EJ320754

Strom, R. D., & Strom, P. S. (2009). *Parent Success Indicator*. Scholastic Testing Service.

Strom, R. D., & Strom, P. S. (2012). *Learning throughout life: An intergenerational perspective.* Information Age Publishing.

Strom, R. D., & Strom, P. S. (2021). Learning throughout life about the needs of all generations: Recognizing and counteracting generational isolation (pp. 183–206). In M. London (Ed.), *The Oxford handbook of lifelong learning* (2nd ed.). Oxford University Press.

Strom, R. D., Strom, S., Collinsworth, P., Strom, P., & Griswold, D. (1996). Intergenerational relationships in Black families. *International Journal of Sociology of the Family*, *26*(2), 129–141.

Strom, R. D., Amukamara, H., Strom, S., Beckert, T., Moore, E., Strom, P., & Griswold, D. (2000 August). African-American fathers: Perceptions of two generations. *Journal of Adolescence*, *23*, 513–516. 10.1006/jado.2000.0335

Strom, R. D., Strom, P. S., Strom, S., Shen, Y.-L., & Beckert, T. (2004 Winter). Black, Hispanic and White American mothers of adolescents: Construction of a national standard. *Adolescence*, *39*(156), 669–686. https://pubmed.ncbi.nlm.nih.gov/15727406

Strom, R. D., Strom, P. S., & Beckert, T. E. (2008, Fall). Comparing Black, Hispanic, and White mothers with a national standard of parenting. *Adolescence*, *43*(171), 525–545. https://pubmed.ncbi.nlm.nih.gov/19086668/

Thompson, M. (2021, May 11). *The benefit of self-evaluation and assessment.* https://wethrive.net/blog/self-evaluation-and-assessment/

Turkle, S. (2016). *Reclaiming conversation: The power of talk in a digital age.* Penguin.

Twenge, J. M. (2014). *Generation Me: Why today's young Americans are more confident, assertive, entitled -- and more miserable than ever before.* Atria Books.

Twenge, J. M. (2023). *Generations: The real differences between Gen Z, Millennials, Gen X, Boomers, and Silents -- and what they mean for America's future.* Atria

6 Caregivers and their Aging Parents

Communication about Parent Needs

Caregivers should receive the favorable feedback they deserve. Caring for aging parents should be acknowledged as an achievement by the family, community, and society. Rosalynn Carter (1927–2023), wife of former U.S. President Jimmy Carter, pointed out there are 53 million caregivers who serve as family caregivers to someone who is aging, ill, or disabled (Rosalynn Carter Institute for Caregivers, 2023). Despite a wide array of caregiver support programs scattered across the federal government, caregivers often struggle to navigate a disjointed system, fail to qualify for the types of benefits they need, and find that the resources available to them are not sufficient or timely. Recognizing the need for better systems of support for caregivers, Rosalynn Carter made a bold proposal to establish a new Office of Caregiver Health within the federal government to elevate and center caregivers like never before. Rosalynn Carter's statement summarizes what life is really like: "There are only four kinds of people in the world--those who have been caregivers, those who are currently caregivers, those who will be caregivers, and those who will need caregivers."

In 2021, about 38 million family caregivers in the United States provided an estimated 36 billion hours of care to an adult with limitations in daily activities. The estimated economic value of their unpaid contributions was approximately $600 billion (Reinhard et al., 2023). Most middle-aged people admit they feel uncertain about how they will manage the family role reversal that will be necessary when they become caregivers for their parents. Making personal needs known is necessary to maintain close relationships between aging parents and their adult children. Both generations should know what older relatives need and agree about identification of reasonable expectations for the caregivers. Initially, older adults will likely need assistance with housekeeping tasks and yard maintenance. When they can afford it, older adults should hire someone outside the family to complete these chores instead of expecting younger relatives will assume the responsibility. Older adults have usually saved money but might be reluctant to hire help. Persuasion may be needed to get them to realize that paying for assistance from outside the family can be a wise expenditure.

Later, when aging parents have to give up driving, their needs expand to include transportation to the store, visiting doctors, going to the beauty shop or barber, and attending church. They may also express a desire to have more contact with their grandchildren. Unless these kinds of needs are expressed, they may be overlooked. Middle-aged caregivers cannot anticipate all the needs of their parents without being told. Many families rely on intuition when the more reasonable strategy is to focus on clear communication (Berman, 2016; Kanter, 2023).

DOI: 10.4324/9781003401261-9

Conversations should focus mainly on current events so everyone feels obliged to keep up with the times and share ideas about what is happening in the family, community, state, nation, and the world. Emphasizing the present is also an effective method to discourage excessive reminiscence, tendency to dwell on events of the past. In this context, caregivers may discover that parents are becoming socially isolated because they refuse to take advantage of interaction opportunities outside the family. As this realization occurs, it should be brought to the attention of older relatives. Children should express their views about all aspects of parental needs including expectations of the family for continued learning, volunteering, and adjusting to change. Aging parents who pursue these goals are recognized as less egocentric, less self-centered, and more concerned about the well-being of others (Hayslip & Fruhauf, 2019).

There is benefit in anticipating contexts of disagreement that are likely to develop with elders. More families must become willing to talk about the issues that matter most to them. A common explanation for why this does not happen is neither party wants to worry or upset the other. We arranged for a group of middle-aged caregivers to talk about conflicts they experienced with their aging parents. Consider some common observations they shared with peers.

Encourage Independence and Interdependence

At the time older adults grew up, independence was the basic principle applied to judge personal success. Depending upon others was generally viewed as evidence of personal failure and identified someone as presenting a burden to their family. Mary gave this example: "My dad is 85 and wants to do everything around the house himself even though he can no longer safely manage some tasks that were reasonable at a younger age. I worry that, when he gets on a ladder or tries heavy lifting, it could be dangerous. When I tell him about my willingness to find someone else who can do certain jobs around the house, he gets mad and says that he doesn't need any help. I'm always afraid he'll fall when he gets up on the ladder." In contrast, secondary school students now are learning interdependent teamwork skills to prepare for employment by working in teams to solve problems together and share assets. Families should make a similar transition to support further development of maturity and harmony. People of all age groups should pursue the goals of independence and interdependence.

There can be benefit in looking at independence from the viewpoint of aging parents. They like to believe younger relatives come to visit because of a desire to interact and share feelings instead of only to check up on them. Do they examine the contents of my refrigerator to find out whether any of the products are past the "use by" date? Does my house pass their cleanliness expectations? Some older adults report they feel as if they are being constantly assessed, overprotected, and led to wonder whether they are still in control of their affairs (American Association of Retired Persons, 2020; Berman, 2016). On the other hand, caregivers should keep track of whether the aging parent is showing weight loss, unopened mail is stacking up, or the refrigerator has spoiled food. This could be a sign of confusion or forgetfulness.

Expand the Scope of Social Interaction

Laura commented, "My dad died two years ago. My mom now lives by herself several miles from my husband and I and our two children. Each day I phone to visit her, find out what is going on, and determine whether she needs or wants anything. Mom likes to spend time with me and enjoys coming to our house for meals but does not want to socialize with people outside the family. When I suggest going to the senior center, she explains that being around old people does not appeal to her."

Social isolation is defined as the objective state of having few social relationships or infrequent contacts with others; *loneliness* is defined as the subjective feeling of being isolated. Both of these conditions present significant public health risks (National Academies of Sciences, Engineering, and Medicine, 2020). About 25% of retirees living in the community report feeling socially isolated and 43% feel lonely. Social isolation has been associated with a 29% increased risk for mortality and 25% increased risk for cancer mortality (Holt-Lunstad, 2021). Loneliness is associated with higher rates of depression, anxiety, and suicidal ideation. In addition, poor social relationships, characterized by social isolation and loneliness, have been associated with increased risk of coronary disease and increased risk of stroke (Valtorta et al., 2016). Caregivers should realize the need to encourage and arrange for increased interaction of elder relatives with members of their peer group, and other people in the community.

Support a Sense of Purpose and Meaning

Jenny is a single parent with a busy and demanding schedule. She is disappointed when her phone calls and visits with Harold, her recently retired father, always focus on complaints about his lack of satisfaction with retirement. Having employment is a source of self-esteem for most young and middle-aged adults. The chance to spend time in ways that someone prefers during retirement is expected to replace having a job as the key to favorable self-impression. Nevertheless, many older adults report that retirement is accompanied by a loss of purpose that should be restored. Many elders find involvement with community service satisfying and realize that helping others contributes to mental health.

Explore Assisted Living Care Facilities

Roger is middle-aged, single, and wondering how he can convince his mother Martha to explore what satisfactions can be had in an assisted living facility. Martha does not take good care of herself. During several visits, Roger discovered that Martha left the stove on, she had overlooked her blood pressure medications, the front door was unlocked, and water was running from an outside hose. When Roger mentions the possibility of changing Martha's residence, she tries to make him feel guilty, "You don't care about me, or you would not suggest making me leave the home I love." Visiting an assisted living or long-term care center can demystify stereotypes held by many retirees. Scheduling an orientation to a nearby institution and taking a tour can provide answers to questions, discover advantages and limitations of this lifestyle, and allow Roger and his mother to discuss what they saw during their visit instead of retaining fears of the unknown. They should ask and understand questions about costs (Thompson, 2022).

Reconciliation to Restore Harmony

There may be times when caregivers and those who receive care experience frustration and they say unkind words to one another that can jeopardize further communication. When this happens there can be value in considering the research of Franz de Waal,

Professor of Psychology and Director of the Primate Research Center at Emory University. Before de Waal's studies, primatologists were reluctant to suggest that animals are capable of thinking.

In contrast, Franz de Waal (2022) went to the only place in the world where a colony of chimpanzees were confined and could be observed at all times. Over a six-year period, he took daily notes and photographs to detail the social life of 23 chimps living on two acres of forest surrounded by a moat at Burgers Zoo in the Netherlands. His observations revealed how closely the social organization of chimpanzees with their continual struggle for power resembles the organization patterns of humans. The data de Waal collected on conflict determined that, after frequent and loud disputes, chimps quickly resumed contact for reconciliation. As a rule, this required only a few moments before they would come together again, kiss, embrace, and begin to groom one another. This pattern was universal even when the process was delayed for several hours. Until the combatants reconciled, both parties revealed observable tension. These findings, corroborated by subsequent primate studies, illustrate how reconciliation can fulfill a necessary purpose of repairing valuable relationships between individuals with close ties and a cooperative partnership.

Reflect on this question: Can people learn from chimpanzees some important lessons about rebuilding relationships? Many adults seem uninformed about how they could repair the damage when it comes to their most important associations. On the other hand, adolescents are frequently reminded by grownups that, when they become angry, say hurtful things or mistreat others, they should try to make amends. Grownups who refuse to engage in reconciliation and forgiveness forfeit a valuable chance to teach younger relatives about accepting expression of differences and still retain harmony. Everyone can make progress toward greater maturity by reflecting on the chimpanzee examples of reconciliation, starting over, and building bridges (de Waal, 2022).

Protecting Health of the Caregivers

The average caregiver is a 49-year-old employed woman who devotes nearly 20 hours a week to providing some forms of assistance for elderly parent(s) (American Association of Retired Persons and National Alliance for Caregiving, 2020). Almost half (48%) of caregivers for older adults are 18–49 years old; 34% of caregivers are 65 years or over. Provision of care for aging relatives will have to be shared in a broader way than is typical at the present time. Middle-aged caregivers should decide what is reasonable for them to expect of themselves. There is concern about combining the caregiver role with other obligations such as the care of a spouse, childcare, meeting the expectations of an employer, and management of a home. The emotional toll is often demonstrated by stress, sadness, worry, and loss of sleep.

Given their extensive responsibilities, it is not surprising that caregivers often report they are emotionally exhausted, sustain high blood pressure, and experience depression. Some might resent their situation, being tied down by a daily care schedule and dislike having to give up on the social and recreational lifestyle they had looked forward to and been planning a long time. Another group of caregivers report dissatisfaction because their aging parents never seem to be satisfied, regardless of how much is done to make their life comfortable. Older adults should be reminded by family and friends to regularly express gratitude to caregivers for the sacrifices they make. Ungrateful older people make themselves unpleasant to be around. The great Roman philosopher Lucius Seneca

(4 BCE–65 CE) identified a need for people to recognize importance of thankfulness: "Homicides, tyrants, thieves, adulterers, robbers, sacrilegious men and traitors there will always be, but worse than all of these is the crime of ingratitude" (Leithart, 2006).

Common Responsibilities of Caregivers

Here are 20 common responsibilities of middle-aged caregivers of older adult relatives.

1 Personal Care: Assisting with daily hygiene tasks such as bathing and dressing.
2 Medication management: Keeping track of medications, administering at the correct times, and refilling prescriptions as needed.
3 Meal preparation: Planning and preparing nutritious meals that meet specific dietary needs.
4 Housekeeping: Maintaining a clean living environment, including cleaning, laundry, and acceptable room temperature.
5 Transportation: Driving the elderly person to appointments, errands, and social affairs.
6 Companionship: Spending time with the person, talking together, playing games, and providing emotional support.
7 Managing finances: Assisting with bill payment, budgeting, and financial planning.
8 Religious involvement: Arrange for participation in religious studies, prayer groups and Bible reading at home, away from home, or online.
9 Safety: Ensuring that the living environment is safe and secure, including preventing falls and other accidents.
10 Coordination of care: Coordinating with other family members and healthcare providers to ensure their needs are met.
11 Medical care: Monitoring the elderly person's health, such as taking vital signs and tracking symptoms, and communicating with healthcare providers.
12 Mobility assistance: Helping the person move around the home including providing support with walking, using a wheelchair, or their mobility devices.
13 Home modifications: Making necessary modifications to the home to improve accessibility and safety, such as grab bars or ramps.
14 End of life planning: Helping the elderly person make decisions about end-of-life care, such as hospice or palliative care, and communicating their wishes to health care providers and family members.
15 Socialization: Encouraging the elderly person to participate in social activities such as attending community events or joining a senior center.
16 Cognitive stimulation: Engaging the elderly person in mentally stimulating activities, such as reading, puzzles, memory games, and discussion groups.
17 Emotional Support: Providing emotional support including listening to their concerns and offering reassurance and encouragement.
18 Respite care: Arranging for temporary caregiving services to give the primary caregiver a break.
19 Record keeping: Keeping detailed records of their medical history, medications, and other important information.
20 Self-care: Taking care of oneself as a caregiver, including getting enough rest, exercise, and social support.

Sharing Responsibilities with Siblings

The need caregivers have for periodic relief implicates their siblings. Brothers and sisters who do not regularly provide care for their aging parents should accept some responsibility to periodically act as a substitute for the main caregiver. They should also share expenses incurred by the main caregiver. Siblings from another town or state can visit parents to allow the main caregiver an uninterrupted vacation. Another option is for non-caregiver siblings to buy travel tickets so parents can come to stay with them for a time (Reinhard et al., 2023). In addition, young children can be involved as "helpful little caregivers" while doing small tasks for aging relatives; this experience can be a beneficial way to set examples of learning to care about others as well as support family relationships (McHeffey et al., 2021). Most American adults (55%) live within an hour's drive of at least some of their extended family members who could become caregivers (Hurst, 2022).

Employer and Community Support

A common assumption has been that families in previous generations more often took care of aging parents. The more accurate observation is families now provide 75% of the care for older relatives whose population is larger than ever before because people are living longer. Goldstein (2022) pointed out that caregivers are the fastest growing identity group in the workforce, making up 73% of employees who have to care for elderly relatives, sick or disabled children, siblings or a spouse. Nearly a third of all employees who quit their job before retirement identify elder care or care of an ill or disabled family member as the main reason for leaving.

United States Census Bureau (Vespa, 2019) demographic forecasts show that by 2034 for the first time in U.S. history older adults (ages 65 and older) will outnumber children (under the age of 18). This means businesses will need to create innovative policies that will enable them to link family caregiving with worker productivity and mental health (Varn, 2020). There are good reasons to establish new practices that contribute to retention of female employees who represent 61% of all caregivers (Tyler, 2022).

Businesses may consider the following strategies to further improve support for employees who are family caregivers (Reinhard et al., 2023):

- Flexible work schedules and possibilities to work on some tasks remotely from home
- Referral services that offer advice about potential financial, legal, and housing issues,
- Self-care suggestions to manage stress such as exercise classes and support groups,
- Medical second opinions to make better care choices and promote peace of mind,
- Specialist coordination of elder record keeping to reduce the risk of medical error,
- Help with processing complicated health insurance and medical bills,
- Expand telehealth access to include more employee involvement with elder care, and
- Establish subsidies to cover the costs of in-home backup care as a safety net.

Employers should try to provide separate education programs for middle-aged caregivers and their aging parents to support adjustment of both groups (Miller, 2021; Reinhard et al., 2023). More caregivers should recognize that their obligation goes beyond getting groceries, doing household chores, and transportation. When these demanding tasks are the sole focus, insufficient attention is given to maintaining satisfying relationships. At the time older adults move to assisted living or long-term care, some caregivers may feel a sense of relief that their responsibilities are completed and the facility staff should now assume future caregiving. In effect, these caregivers believe, "I have done my share; it is someone else's turn now." The situation is further complicated by the reports from a majority of residents living in long-term care that their family does not visit them on a regular basis. Staff can provide care but cannot be a substitute for family relationships. Lack of visitation to relatives in long-term care is a form of neglect imposing loneliness and undermining personal importance (Holt-Lunstad, 2021; Varn, 2020).

The *Recognize, Assist, Include, Support, and Engage Family Caregivers Act* (2018) directs the United States Secretary of Health and Human Services to develop a national family caregiving strategy. The strategy will identify actions that community providers, government, and others are planning to recognize and support family caregivers. These actions include:

- Promoting greater adoption of person-and family-centered care in all healthcare and long-term service and support settings, with the person and the family caregiver at the center of care teams,
- Assessment and service planning (including care transitions and coordination) involving care recipients and family caregivers,
- Information, education, training supports, referral, care coordination, and
- Respite options,
- Financial security and workplace issues.

Volunteerism and Loneliness

Some grandparents between 50 and 75 years of age devote excessive time to personal leisure interests. Over this lengthy period of time they seldom help younger relatives, excusing themselves claiming they do not want to interfere with parents. Later, when elders become frail, those who have been selfish with their time and energy expect their adult children to provide care for them. This familiar family situation suggests a need to link aging parent care with grandparent education. Studies of the relationships between aging parents and their adult children rarely mention responsibilities of the grandparents (Hayslip & Fruhauf, 2019). By encouraging grandparents to pitch in while they are still healthy and independent, adjustment to their less viable status later is easier for everyone and less a source of resentment by younger relatives (Reinhard et al., 2023).

The volunteerism of older men and women can contribute to the mental health of families and society. Cho and Xiang (2023) conducted a systematic review to synthesize evidence between older adult's unpaid productive activities and loneliness. The sample included 5,000 individuals aged 60 and older who did not experience loneliness at the outset of the 12-year longitudinal study. Self-reported participation in formal volunteer work were classified into three levels; (0) no volunteering, (1) less than 100 hours of volunteering per year, and (2) more than 100 hours of volunteering per year. Volunteering more than 100 hours a year was statistically significant associated with a lower risk of loneliness compared to the non-volunteers. This protective effect was not observed for those who volunteered less than 100 hours per year. The benefits of volunteering in mitigating loneliness did not differ by gender. These promising effects of volunteering should be made known to middle-aged and older adults as a way to reduce loneliness (Akhter-Khan et al., 2023).

Caregiving for Relatives with Dementia

According to the Alzheimer's Association (2023), this incurable brain disorder and most common dementia afflicts more than 6.7 million in the United States; 70% live at home while the remainder 30% live in long-term care facilities; approximately 65% are women. These victims present problems related to changes in communication, personality and behavior shifts, coping with issues of aggression, sundowning showing restlessness and agitation in late afternoon and early evening, managing problems of sleep, bathing, dressing, and grooming, physical exercise, healthy eating, locating placement, and direct contact by phone for guidance. People in advanced stages of Alzheimer's have difficulty with one or more basic daily living activities like dressing, bathing, and toileting. They are also disadvantaged by their cognitive limitations presenting difficulties in taking medications when scheduled and managing financial affairs. Assisting relatives with Alzheimer's Disease is more time consuming for caregivers than for those who take care of older family members without disabilities (Harrison et al., 2019; National Institute on Aging, 2023).

Demographics of Dementia

Dementia is a general term used to describe cognitive impairment that implicates the ability to remember, think, or make decisions that interfere with daily activities. In 2019, about 5% of older college graduates (ages 70 and older) were living with dementia compared with 18% of their counterparts who had less than 12 years of education (Population Reference Bureau, 2020). Estimates are that dementia may begin 20 years or more before the onset of symptoms, giving time for intervention with best support practices. While dementia mostly affects adults over the age of 65, this disease is not a normal aspect of aging (National Institute on Aging, 2022; Reckrey et al., 2020).

There is evidence that higher educational attainment is associated with lower risk for dementia and means having more years of a cognitive healthy life (Alzheimer's Association, 2023; Health and Retirement Study Survey Research Center, 2017). The common assumption of researchers is that education early in life directly affects brain development by building a cognitive reserve elders can draw on when memory or reasoning begin to decline. The probable rates of dementia differ by ethnicity with Hispanics and other minorities ages 70 and older 17%, Whites non-Hispanic 8.4%, and Black non-Hispanic 12.7% (Population Reference Bureau, 2020).

Demographers have drawn attention to the shifting structure of families as the large Baby Boomers population (ages 60–78 in 2024) approaches an age of increased risk for dementia and Alzheimer's Disease. Declines in marriage, higher rates of divorce, and lower fertility mean more Boomers reach old age without a spouse and fewer children, on average than previous generations, to rely on for care (Alzheimer's Association, 2023).

Complexities of Care

Alzheimer's victims have difficulty remaining still, a condition that makes caring for them more difficult. Healthy adults might devote attention to some program they see on television, read a book, or interact with other people. This is not the case for patients who no longer have the ability to understand the meanings of words and interpret relationship of images. They view their stillness as a prison. Consequently, their inclination is to wander. The victim's desire to walk outside can result in being hit by a car or getting lost in the neighborhood. Global position system devices allow for tracking victims who are permitted to walk alone, revealing their whereabouts and ensuring they do not go beyond the boundaries that have been set by their caregivers.

Nancy Mace and Peter Rabins (1981/2021) are the authors of *The 36-hour day,* a family guide to caring for people who have Alzheimer disease and other dementias. This provocative book title came about from a Seattle man whose wife had Alzheimer's – he commented "Living with my wife is like living a 36-hour day." The excessive demands these caregivers experience often lead to exhaustion, depression, and persistent feelings of anxiety. Marital conflict is common, with many couples separating or divorcing due to the enormous stress.

Mary Mittelman (2021), Professor of Psychiatry at New York University School of Medicine, initiated a guidance program to assist caregivers of relatives suffering from dementia. This model program received financial support for 20 years from the National Institutes of Health before the current funding was assumed by the state of New York. Assistance begins with two individual counseling sessions that permit caregivers to identify special needs they experience in trying to carry out responsibilities including bathing and administering shots. Next, four family counseling sessions are scheduled, followed by weekly support groups, and additional counseling as needed by phone.

Preliminary research compared the caregivers who received counseling support with other caregivers who were not exposed to counseling. Findings showed that those given counseling were significantly less depressed and demonstrated more healthy behaviors. Results also included less conflict with relatives and reduced anxiety. In addition, social support provided by other relatives made it possible for a spouse or partner to keep an individual with dementia home for 18 months longer than those without this care (Gaugler et al., 2018; Sperling et al., 2020).

This educational guidance strategy also reduces financial expense of care. The program has been adopted by 11 states. Minnesota, an early implementer of the program, estimates the state will save millions of dollars over 15 years when the caregivers are provided with counseling intervention. A comparative study involving Great Britain, Australia, and the United States confirmed benefits across the three cultures (Foldes et al., 2018). Sperling et al. (2020) reported the development of online training for social workers, nurses, and psychologists who want to begin a program.

Caregiver Options for Alternative Care

There are many circumstances that occur where full-time institutional care may be the best or only choice for a caregiver. Getting acquainted with senior care and senior living options nearby is helpful; finding out about availability (short time or long time stays), kinds of care provided, and understanding related costs are important concerns. Options to explore include independent living, senior living, memory care, assisted living, nursing home, and in-home care.

Adult Day Care

There are approximately 27,000 certified adult day care centers across the United States. These are intended to give relief to caregivers and service elderly in useful ways. Usually, family caregivers can bring their loved one to a nearby center in the morning before going to work and pick them up later in the day. Some communities arrange van or bus travel to and from the center. The benefits of day care include group exercise and fitness, receiving medications on time, enjoying a healthy meal or special diet, occupational, speech, music or art therapy, support groups, and counseling. The opportunity for stimulating conversations with peers can counteract feelings of loneliness, improve mental health, and perhaps delay cognitive decline (National Adult Day Services Association, 2023).

For the family, adult day care means being able to continue employment knowing that their loved one is in a safe and secure environment. Caregivers have time to do necessary personal errands, experience relief from constant care, and are able to financially afford this option. The cost for full day care differs by state but provides a daytime safe protective service. Regardless of where a family lives, this is a much cheaper choice than home care as an alternative to 24-hour in-home caregiving, having a live-in caregiver, or placement in assisted living.

Federal Assistance Programs to Support Elderly in Need and Their Caregivers

Knowing about federal (and local) programs can enable caregivers to make good decisions and help them manage the long list of required obligations. The following selected sites in Table 6.1 provide information regarding the common sources of

Table 6.1 Sources of Support for Caregivers

Federal Agency	Website	Description
Eldercare Locator	https://eldercare.acl.gov/Public/Index.aspx	Describes and connects to adult day care local services which include counseling, exercise, recreation, meals, evening care, respite care, socialization, transportation, and education.
U.S. Department of Veterans Affairs Caregiver Support	https://www.caregiver.va.gov/	Promotes the health and well-being of family caregivers who care for veterans through education, resources, support, and services.
National Institute on Aging	https://www.nia.nih.gov/health/caregiving	Provides information and resources for caregivers of older adults about health topics, caregiver support and tips for managing caregiving responsibilities.
Administration for Community Living	https://acl.gov/	Aging and disability networks include national, state and local organizations that support community living options for older adults and people with disabilities.
Medicare	https://www.medicare.gov	Medical coverage includes hospital care, skilled nursing, hospice, lab tests, surgery, doctor care and medical equipment, home health care, and preventive services.
Social Security	https://www.ssa.gov	Benefits cover retirement, disability, family survivors, supplemental security income to disabled adults and children, and those age 65 and older in need.
National Family Caregiver Support Program	https://acl.gov/programs/support-caregivers/national-family-caregiver-support-program	Helps caregivers by providing nutritional support, managing disabilities, long-term-care planning, healthcare, respite care, and caregiving training.
Benefits.gov	https://www.benefits.gov	Browse the wide range of federal agencies to support specific needs.

support for caregivers to help them learn about services such as Social Security, Medicare, Veterans benefits, locations of elder care facilities, support programs for caregivers, services for disabled, and caregiving obligations.

Conclusion

Maintaining a satisfying relationship with aging parents is a priority for most middle-aged people. Achieving this goal depends on having mutual knowledge about the needs of each other. Conversations about important issues, as defined by each generation, can identify needs that require mutual adjustment. More of the community should become involved to support the efforts of middle-aged caregivers. Siblings should share obligation for care of their aging parents instead of expecting the main caregiver to assume sole responsibility. Every daughter and son should assume a share of time and care costs, and provide periodic relief to enable the primary caregiver to sustain their difficult task. Grandchildren also have an important emotional contribution. They should learn that growing up requires caring about the needs of others, beginning with older family members. Employers, government agencies, nonprofits, educational and religious institutions should establish additional methods to improve support for caregivers.

Key Concepts

1 Family conversations to identify aging parent needs is an effective way to improve well-being. In addition to each person stating personal opinions and deciding together what older relatives require, both generations should agree on the expectations of middle-aged caregivers. This consensus effort can result in proper care to enable mutual satisfaction and prevent discontent.

2 Caring for aging parents is a developmental task that must be met by a larger proportion of family members than in the past because of a longer lifespan. This task requires greater maturity than is common in a culture that promotes self-centeredness and narcissism. The qualities of successful caregivers implicate concern for others, patience, compassion, and optimism.

3 Middle-aged women carry a disproportionate share of responsibility for elder care. Their combined tasks to help younger and older relatives and obligation to employers means needs of the main caregivers should be recognized by aging parents, spouses, children, employers and community institutions. Sharing the load of domestic tasks, offering comfort and encouragement, siblings arranging for regular relief, flexible work policies, and arranging for elder daycare at the workplace are ways that can enable caregivers to stay strong for all those who depend on them.

4 Families should discuss matters of importance to each of their members. Discussions about issues of health and death should be welcome. Introduce legal concerns such as estate planning, completing a will or trust, power of attorney, burial preferences and choice regarding the medical directive for life support systems.

5 Older adults benefit when they are exposed to peer norms of socialization and fitness. The influence peers provide should include motivation for engaging in regular exercise, learning, social interaction, reliance on friends as listeners, helping monitor quality of thinking, and encouraging assistance for caregivers.

6 Caregivers need education to become aware of community resources. Churches and civic groups should identify volunteer caregivers who can provide caregivers with

periodic relief. Classes for caregivers should include knowledge of how to prevent elder mistreatment, and rehabilitation of abusers.

7　Recognize that conversations with aging relatives should avoid excessive reminiscence. When events of the past are the dominant topics elders talk about, younger people are relegated to a listener role instead of stimulating thought and sharing feelings. Caregivers should engage aging parents in dialogue focused on current events. This can be done by talking about news in the family, community, nation, and the world. A related need is for social engagement outside the family to prevent social isolation from peers. Enroll in mentally stimulating classes that can help sustain mental viability, self-improvement, and family development.

8　Lack of visitation to relatives in assisted living facilities is not usually recognized as a form of neglect that imposes loneliness and undermines individual sense of personal importance. Institutional staff can provide physical care but cannot be a substitute for loving parent-child relationships.

9　Families should recognize that a majority of elder abuse cases implicate self-neglect by persons living alone who lack motivation to care for their own personal needs. Greater emphasis should be placed on nutritious meals, clean clothes, continuous social interaction, and education.

10　Willingness of elders to explore what life is like in assisted living facilities should be encouraged. This helps demystify the institutional experience. If parents living at home forget to take medications, do not cook nutritious meals, leave the stove on, or ignore running water, it is time for families to consider the next steps to preserve safety and sustain a good quality of life.

Generational Perspectives Activities

6.1 Team Discussion
6.2 Agenda for Interviews with Grandparents
6.3 Conversations with Children about Caregiving of Grandparents
6.4 A Scenario: Reasoning and Problem Solving
6.5 Team Chapter Review
6.6 Criteria for Self-Evaluation of Grandparents

6.1 Team Discussion

1　What do you know about caregiving for the older relatives in your family?
2　How informed are you about the financial standing of your grandparents?
3　What have you observed to be the needs of retired individuals in your family?
4　What are some topics of conflict that you have experienced with older relatives?
5　How much social interaction do your grandparents have outside the family?
6　Looking ahead, how do you suppose caregiving will be handled in your family?
7　What has been your experience in visiting assisted living or long-term care facilities?
8　How do you and your siblings plan to share obligations for care of aging parents?
9　How should the workplace support employees who are caregivers?
10　What have your parents shared with you about their last will and testament?

6.2 Agenda for Interviews with Grandparents

1 Which of your needs do your children not know about or tend to underestimate?
2 What needs of yours have middle-aged caregivers detected that require attention?
3 What kinds of care do middle-aged daughters and sons currently provide for you?
4 How suitable are the expectations middle-aged children have established for you?
5 What are the needs of your middle-age children that you consider to be unmet?
6 How do you ease concerns for middle-aged caregivers who serve in your family?
7 How will your care be different from the way that you cared for your parents?
8 What resources should families rely on to ensure aging parents are not abused?
9 What are your questions about Hospice and implications for family caregivers?
10 What plans have you made for completing a living will about your affairs?

6.3 Conversations with Children about Caregiving of Grandparents

1 Who should take care of relatives when they are become old and require help?
2 How do older relatives find out what they should know about your health needs?
3 What kinds of help have you observed that some of your older relatives need?
4 What needs do your grandparents have that could be better met by your family?
5 What things have you seen your grandparents do to help others?
6 Who is the one person who helps your grandparents more than anyone else?
7 What could public schools do to meet social needs of long-term care residents?
8 How do you suppose caregiving will change years from now when you are old?
9 What do you know about the nation's Social Security and Medicare programs?
10 How could churches be more involved with education and caregiving for old people?

6.4 A Scenario: Reasoning and Problem Solving

Problem solving scenarios present an opportunity to consider situations that might occur for a family and think about possible solutions. Your task is to look at pros and cons of choices that are stated, think of additional options, identify relevant information that might be missing, find out how teammates see the options, and defend your reasoning about advice you consider best.

Judy has experienced occasional dizziness for over a week so her doctor is scheduling diagnostic tests. She is a widow whose daughter Shelly lives in another state. Judy should

a inform Shelly about the scheduled tests and share her feelings about being tested
b wait until the test results are known before she lets Shelly know about them
c confide in a friend instead of causing additional stress and worry for her daughter
d avoid telling anyone about her condition and hope for a favorable test outcome
e Other _____

6.5 Team Chapter Review

Efforts to assess participant learning, provide feedback, and improve quality of instruction is enhanced by a group review of each chapter.

1 What ideas in the lesson changed the way I think about this topic?
2 What insights from the lesson will I try to apply in my relationships?

3 What is the most important point for me presented in this lesson?
4 What are some aspects of this lesson I would like to better understand?
5 Which aspects of this lesson do I wish that I had known about earlier?

6.6 Criteria for Self-Evaluation of Grandparents

Directions: For each question, place a check beside statements that describe your feelings. You may want to give several answers on some items. If your feelings are not on choices list, write them on the line marked 'other.'

1 My need to socialize with others are met by

    a attending church and social events there
    b being with my children and grandchildren
    c going to classes designed for grandparents
    d visiting with friends by phone and online
    e going to the senior center for activities
    f Other _____

2 My expectations to remain independent are

    a ambitious and provide satisfaction
    b modest and can easily be attained
    c such that I would not accept help
    d need revision to be more realistic
    e Other _____

3 The qualities middle-aged caregivers need are

    a common among people in their age group
    b uncommon because of self-centeredness
    c possible if relevant training is provided
    d unlikely to be present in many families
    e Other _____

4 My experience with elder abuse is based on

    a reports of friends who were mistreated
    b seeing older adults who I suspect were abused
    c stories told to me by relatives or neighbors
    d being mistreated by people in my family.
    e media reports that document the problem
    f Other _____

5 The ways I favor to ensure older adult safety is

    a for society to provide free long-term care
    b to encourage more savings for retirement
    c urge more families to care for aging parents
    d give government support to retirement towns
    e Other _____

6 My family is informed about

   a status of my health and care
   b my finances and locations
   c my needs to be independent
   d my fears so they can help
   e Other _____

7 I do not want to become a burden to my family so

   a I will make my own arrangements for help
   b I plan to move to a home for retired people
   c they will not have to resent caring for me
   d living by myself appears the best solution
   e Other _____

8 I believe that employers could help families by

   a providing elder care for parents of employees
   b allowing caregivers to have flexible hours
   c offering support groups for the caregivers
   d devising a curriculum about being a caregiver
   e Other _____

9 I believe the problem of caregiver abuse of elders

   a is underestimated by families and communities
   b should be part of caregiver education curriculum
   c at institutions should be monitored more closely
   d will increase as the length of the lifespan grows
   e Other _____

10 Providing middle-aged caregivers with periodic relief should

   a be provided by volunteers from churches
   b involve students as visitors and readers
   c be met with reliance on Medicare or Hospice
   d be organized by AARP or Area Agency on Aging
   e Other _____

References

Akhter-Khan, S. C., Hofmann, V., Warncke, M., Tamimi, N., Mayston, R., & Prina, M. A. (2023). Caregiving, volunteering, and loneliness in middle-aged and older adults: A systematic review. *Aging & Mental Health, 27*(7), 1233–1245. 10.1080/13607863.2022.2144130

Alzheimer's Association. (2023). *2023 Alzheimer's disease facts and figures.* https://www.alz.org/media/Documents/alzheimers-facts-and-figures.pdf

American Association of Retired Persons and National Alliance for Caregiving. (2020). *Caregiving in the United States 2020.* https://www.caregiving.org/research/caregiving-in-the-us/caregiving-in-the-us-2020/

Berman, C. (2016, March 4). What aging parents want from their kids. *The Atlantic.* https://www.theatlantic.com/health/archive/2016/03/when-youre-the-aging-parent/472290/

Cho, J., & Xiang, X. (2023). The relationship between volunteering and the occurrence of loneliness among older adults: A longitudinal study with 12 years of follow-up. *Journal of Gerontological Social Work*, *66*(5), 680–693. 10.1080/01634372.2022.2139322

de Waal, F. (2022). *Different: Gender through the eyes of a primatologist*. W. W. Norton.

Foldes, S., Moriarty, J., Farseth, P., Mittelman, M., & Long, K. (2018). Medicaid savings from the New York University Caregiver Intervention for families with dementia. *The Gerontologist*, *58*(2), e97–e106. 10.1093/geront/gnx077

Gaugler, J., Reese, M., & Mittelman, M. (2018, June). The effects of a comprehensive psychosocial intervention on secondary stressors and social support for adult caregivers of persons with dementia. *Innovation in Aging*, *2*(2). 10.1093/geroni/igy015

Goldstein, K. (2022, November 21). 5 Things employers get wrong about caregivers at work. *Harvard Business Review*. https://hbr.org/2022/11/5-things-employers-get-wrong-about-caregivers-at-work

Harrison, K., Ritchie, C., Patel, K., Hunt, L., Covinsky, K., Yaffe, K., & Smith, A. K. (2019). Care settings and clinical characteristics of older adults with moderately severe dementia. *Journal of the American Geriatrics Society*, *67*(9), 1907–1912. 10.1111/jgs.16054

Hayslip, B., Jr., & Fruhauf, C. A. (Eds.). (2019). *Grandparenting: Influences on the dynamics of family relationships*. Springer.

Health and Retirement Study Survey Research Center. (2017). *Aging in the 21st century: Challenges and opportunities for Americans*. Health and Retirement Study, University of Michigan, Survey Research Center, Institute for Social Research. https://hrs.isr.umich.edu/about/data-book

Holt-Lunstad, J. (2021, May 6). Loneliness and social isolation as risk factors: The power of social connection in prevention. *American Journal of Lifestyle Medicine*, *15*(5), 567–573. 10.1177/15598276211009454

Hurst, K. (2022, May 18). *More than half of Americans live within an hour of extended family*. Pew Research Center. https://www.pewresearch.org/short-reads/2022/05/18/more-than-half-of-americans-live-within-an-hour-of-extended-family/

Kanter, S. (2023). *Positive caregiving: Caring for loved ones using the power of positive emotions*. Collective Book Studio.

Leithart, P. (2006). *On Seneca, de Beneficiis, Books 1–2*. Theopolis Institute. https://theopolisinstitute.com/leithart_post/on-seneca-de-beneficiis-books/

Mace, N., & Rabins, P. (2021). *The 36-hour day: A family guide to caring for people who have Alzheimer disease and other dementias* (7th ed.). Johns Hopkins University Press. (Original work published 1981)

McHeffey, T., Brush, J., Zanzarov, D., Browne, J., & McHeffey, C. (2021). Volunteerism: A means of lifelong learning. In M. London (Ed.), *The Oxford handbook of lifelong learning* (2nd ed., pp. 633–650). Oxford University Press.

Miller, S. (2021, September 10). *Employers benefit by providing elder care support*. Society for Human Resource Management. https://www.shrm.org

Mittelman, M., O'Connor, M., Donley, T., Epstein-Smith, C., Nguyen, A., Nicholson, R., Salant, R., Shirk, S., & Stevenson, E. (2021). Longitudinal Study: Understanding the lived experiences of couples across the trajectory of dementia. *BMC Geriatrics*, *21*, 558. 10.1186/s12877-021-02503-4

National Academies of Sciences, Engineering, and Medicine. (2020). *Social isolation and loneliness in older adults*. The National Academies Press. 10.17226/25663

National Adult Day Services Association. (2023). *Eldercare locator: Adult day care*. https://eldercare.acl.gov/public/resources/factsheets/adult_day_care.aspx

National Institute on Aging. (2022, November 17). *Providing care and comfort at the end of life*. https://www.nia.nih.gov/health/providing-comfort-end-life

National Institute on Aging. (2023). *Tips for caregivers and families of people with dementia*. Alzheimers.gov. https://www.alzheimers.gov/life-with-dementia/tips-caregivers

Population Reference Bureau. (2020). *Fact sheet: U. S. dementia trends*. https://www.prb.org/resources/fact-sheet-u-s-dementia-trends/#:~:text=Estimates%20vary%2C%20but%20experts%20report,nearly%2012%20million%20by%202040.

Reckrey, J., Morrison, R., Boerner, K., Szanton, S., Bollens-Lund, E., Leff, B., & Orstein, K. (2020). Living in the community with dementia: Who receives paid care?. *Journal of the American Geriatric Society*, *68*(1), 186–191. 10.1111/jgs.16215

Recognize, Assist, Include, Support, and Engage Family Caregivers Act of 2018, Pub. L. No. 115–119, 132 Stat. 23 (2018, January 22).

Reinhard, S., Caldera, S., Houser, A., & Choula, R. (2023, March). *Valuing the invaluable: 2023 Update*. AARP Public Policy Institute. https://www.aarp.org/content/dam/aarp/ppi/2023/3/valuing-the-invaluable-2023-update.doi.10.26419-2Fppi.00082.006.pdf

Rosalynn Carter Institute for Caregivers. (2023). *Promoting caregiver health, strength, and resilience*. Rosalynn Carter Institute for Caregivers. https://rosalynncarter.org/about-us/

Sperling, S., Brown, D., Jensen, C., Inker, J., Mittelman, M., & Manning, C. (2020). FAMILIES: An effective healthcare intervention for caregivers of community dwelling people living with dementia. *Aging & Mental Health*, *24*(10), 1700–1708. 10.1080/13607863.2019.1647141

Thompson, D. (2022). *The unexpected journey of caring*. Rowman and Littlefield.

Tyler, K. (2022, March 10). Supporting employees with caregiving responsibilities. *HR Magazine*. SHRM. https://www.shrm.org/hr-today/news/hr-magazine/spring2022/pages/supporting-employees-with-caregiving-responsibilities.aspx

Valtorta, N., Kanaan, M., Gilbody, S., Ronzi, S., & Hanratty, B. (2016). Loneliness and social isolation as risk factors for coronary heart disease and stroke: Systematic review and meta-analysis of longitudinal observation studies. *Heart*, *102*(13), 1009–1016. 10.1136/heartjnl-2015-308790

Varn, M. (October 28, 2020). Employees are stressed caring for aging parents. How can employers help? *Employees Benefits News*. https://www.benefitnews.com/opinion/employees-are-stressed-caring-for-aging-parents-how-can-employers-help

Vespa, J. (2019, October 8). *The graying of America: More older adults than kids by 2035*. U. S. Census Bureau. https://www.census.gov/library/stories/2018/03/graying-america.html#:~:text=Starting%20in%202030%2C%20when%20all,add%20a%20half%20million%20centenarians

7 Influence of Adolescent Peers

The Power of Peer Influence

Judith Harris was excited. She had just been admitted to the psychology doctoral program at Harvard University. One year later she was disappointed when the program committee notified Harris that her "originality and independence were not up to Harvard standards." She moved on, accepting a job as an editor at a publishing company where she was responsible for all the manuscripts focused on developmental psychology. The materials that she reviewed reflected traditional beliefs about the unmatched benefit of parent influence more than was identified by contradictory scientific evidence. Harris developed her own theory of child and adolescent development to challenge the popular impression that parents have the greatest impact on socialization as adolescents are growing up. She documented her assertion that, in a rapidly changing environment, successive generations have different experiences and, as a result, peers emerge as the most influential source of socialization during the teenage years. Her book *The Nurture Assumption: Why children turn out the way they do* (Harris, 2009) compared the relative influence of parents and peers. She concluded that students are bound to impact peers more than during the past because from early adolescence they spend much of their time with age mates. Harris recommended that it would be wise for parents to carefully monitor their child's choice of friends.

The evidence that peer influence is pre-eminent in adolescence was uniformly dismissed by child development specialists who accused Harris of undermining the authority of parents and education that they provide children at home. Then, in 1995, Harris' theory was awarded the American Psychological Association George Miller Award as the outstanding contribution to developmental psychology. Ironically, George Miller was chair of the psychology department at Harvard where years earlier Harris had been dismissed from the doctoral studies program. Harris' seminal text is recognized for persuasive insights demonstrating how peers are able to contribute in unique ways to the development of their classmates. Psychologists are generally agreed that, from around ages 10 or 11 examples and expectations of peers become the dominant source that students rely on to guide their socialization.

Peer Socialization Lessons

The potential of friends to shape development is illustrated by lessons that students learn primarily from classmates. The relevance of these lessons is that they can support or prevent social adjustment and mental health across a broad range of interpersonal situations (P. S. Strom et al., 2019).

DOI: 10.4324/9781003401261-10

1 *Peers provide the first substantial experiences with equality.*

Children want to be with companions and enjoy their attention. Peers are in the best position to satisfy these needs. When members behave in a way that is approved by the group such as dressing according to a fashion norm, the rewards from peers include greater attention, acceptance, and emotional support.

2 *Peers present different standards than expected by adults.*

The standards set by peers are more attainable and offer a reason for collective opposition to directives given by adults. The greater resources of adults make it impossible for students to declare complete autonomy from them. However, peers show a consistent willingness to listen to friends about dilemmas and encourage one another to express their differences of opinion in the presence of adults.

3 *Positive influence of peers is often ignored by adults.*

Peers make a unique contribution to social and emotional well-being. Adolescents must rely on members of their age group as the most reasonable standard to gauge self-comparison, chances to express themselves without having feelings of guilt or fear of punishment, and chances to engage in leadership situations. They encourage one another to strive for independence and offer the prospect to belong to another significant group besides the family or school classroom.

4 *Students learn friendship from peers and getting along with others of the same status.*

Becoming part of a group requires skills motivated by peers. These social skills typically include cooperation, sharing ideas, striving for independence, expressing discontent and anger, and engaging in reconciliation following arguments. These lessons are more easily learned from peers than from parents. Students discover what friends will tolerate and they become aware of conduct the group refuses to condone. Most students gain a sense of belonging and satisfaction when they are accepted by peers. Students discover they must learn from peers how to resolve conflicts peacefully, although aggressive responses can sometimes become prominent.

Belonging and Rejection

Helping students view themselves as successful is a special contribution of peers. Students also mature by being able to see others in positive ways. Before age 10, students less often engage in social rejection. Most activities for young children are non-competitive so their self-concepts are rarely threatened. Students who perform better than their classmates on tasks in the early grades seldom announce superiority and those who fall below average do not yet feel inferior because academic norms have yet to be established. During childhood, status of the parents is the main source of self-esteem. Children accept as their own the value they believe their parents have attained (Burkholder et al., 2020).

The social environment changes dramatically as students transition to middle school and junior high. Then boys and girls can no longer depend on what their parents have achieved as the basis for their self-pride. Another shift is that, instead of continuing to meet expectations of one teacher, students are obligated to satisfy multiple teachers, each of them providing instruction for a different subject in the curriculum. From this age forward, students have to earn their social standing. In the classroom, students begin to face greater competition and failure along with critical and unfriendly remarks from classmates. Peers are quick to detect weaknesses and identify them by using insults that are meant to be hurtful. As a result, students in the middle grades experience a sharpening sense of self and overall decline in their self-esteem. Teachers should arrange for experiences that enable students to perceive themselves favorably without having to find fault with others (Ferrer-Wreder & Kroger, 2020).

As peers replace parents in supplying the norms to imitate and models for identification, students gravitate to classmates for acceptance, information, and emotional support. It becomes so important to belong that peer group methods are rarely challenged. Instead, most students are eager to conform. Group members feel less anxious when they act in the same way as their peers without knowing why. This inclination to adopt values and attitudes without understanding the reasons can lead to acceptance of behaviors that students would otherwise recognize as wrong.

In order for any group to take on special significance, becoming a member has to be somewhat exclusive. Around age 10, students form clique groups where peers from similar backgrounds, mutual interests, and standards hang out and often refuse to accept others who differ from themselves. Although this can be a way to find and develop friendships, there are also negative outcomes. Sometimes peer rejection escalates to verbal intolerance and prejudice. Social prejudice is more common for 10-year-olds than high school students (Jackson, 2019).

While it is gratifying to realize that the negative social prejudice of rejection will likely decline as grade level of students rises, research has determined that the consequences of peer rejection can last for a lifetime. Individuals who become a target of racial, religious, ethnic, and other prejudices have to divert energy from healthy forms of activity to strategies used for self-protection. Acceptance, rejection, and self-concept are inseparable conditions. To suggest that minority students who suffer prejudice should ignore the low estimate members of a dominant group has of them is to presume children are able to avoid being affected by the impressions of peers. On the contrary, the way others feel about us influences the way we are treated and, to an extent, how we view ourselves (Baumeister & Bushman, 2021).

Acceptance of Group Differences

In addition to anti-bully policies, school boards across the nation have amended some of the ways history is presented. Students are more accepting of differences when they become aware of how particular groups targeted for abuse have contributed to the country. In the 1960s, schools began to acquaint students with notable Blacks who previously were denied recognition even though their contributions improved the quality of life for everyone. During the 1970s, Latinos were first portrayed in a way that recognized leaders in this subpopulation. The Fair Accurate Inclusive Respectful Education Act of 2011 mandates that California schools address missing gaps in curriculum textbooks (California Department of Education, 2022). Specifically, advocates for the rights of disabled persons, racial justice organizations, eminent figures in the lesbian, gay, bisexual, and transgender communities and other groups that have shaped history should be a part of curriculum that chronicles evolution of the society.

Students should also be taught that fear can be a valuable emotion when it motivates cautious behavior that can protect us from harm. People are wise to be guided by fear when it comes to consuming illegal drugs, chatting with online predators, or riding as the passenger of a drunk driver. These kinds of dangers warrant consideration because they have the potential to threaten self-preservation. On the other hand, fear of groups whose behaviors differ from norms does not serve a survival purpose, compromise safety, place general welfare at risk or diminish individual freedom to pursue a lifestyle of our own choosing. The reality is that fear of group differences is sustained only by conveying misinformation used to justify the abuse of targeted groups.

School Practices of Inclusion

History of Inclusion

The practice of forming clique groups can provide benefit but also result in exclusion of others, most often classmates with disabilities. Treatment of people with disabilities has varied throughout history. At times they were viewed as enemies to be disliked, imprisoned, and even killed. During the 1960s, they were often segregated from the regular student population. Since then, dramatic positive improvements have been made resulting in general awareness that people with disabilities are neither helpless nor hopeless but require some assistance to build on their talents (Kauffman et al., 2017). This perspective is reinforced by federal government regulations that apply to employment, access to buildings, and education opportunities. The expectation that disabled persons can become productive members of society is championed by teachers, parents, employers, and the disabled. Transforming potential to achievement is facilitated when regular classroom teachers and special educators collaborate, support is forthcoming from classmates, appropriate standards of conduct are applied for everyone, and strategies of instruction enable disabled students to integrate with non-disabled peers (Doubet & Hockett, 2015).

The stimulus for education reform was a revelation in the 1970s that a million students were being excluded from attending the public schools and denied access to education services. Mainstreaming is the term that initially referred to providing schooling for special education students in regular classes, a practice that began when Congress passed the Education for All Handicapped Children Act of 1975 (Public Law 94–142). In this case, the tradition of setting a timeline for implementing school-related laws was waived. Instead, this reform is meant to govern national policies permanently. Since 1975 the law has been amended several times to reflect changing social considerations. The most recent revision, the Individuals with Disabilities Education Improvement Act of 2005 (2023) requires inclusion of special education students in all aspects of education including after school extracurricular activities (Kauffman et al., 2017).

According to the National Center for Education Statistics (2023), the number of American students who received special education in 2021–2022 was 7.3 million, or the equivalent of 15% of all students attending public schools. A higher proportion of males (18%) than females (10%) were enrolled in special education. Most of these students attended inclusion classrooms throughout much of the school day with peers who were not classified as needing special education. Table 7.1 *Students with Disabilities* presents the percentage distribution of students ages 3–21 by selected disability type and school year 2021–2022.

Special Education Requirements for Public Schools

The requirements for public schools that serve this 15% of total student population are (National Center for Education Statistics, 2023):

• Free public education for disabled persons between ages 3 and 21.
• Access to education in a regular classroom is guaranteed unless the handicap is such that services cannot be properly offered there.

Table 7.1 Students with Disabilities

Percentage distribution of students ages 3–21 served under the Individuals with Disabilities Education Act (IDEA), by selected disability type, school year 2021–2022[*]

Disability Type	%
Specific learning disability	32
Speech/language impairment	19
Other health impairment	15
Autism	12
Developmental delay	7
Intellectual disability	6
Emotional disturbance	5
Multiple disabilities	2
Hearing impairment	1

[*] *Source:* National Center for Education Statistics. (2023). Students with disabilities. Condition of Education. U.S. Department of Education Institute for Education Sciences. https://nces.ed.gov/programs/coe/indicator/cgg/students-with-disabilities.

- School placement and other education decisions are made only after consultation with a child's parents. Continuation in a program requires a re-evaluation once every three years based on testing at no cost to the parents.
- Parents can examine and challenge all school records bearing on identification of their child as disabled and the kind of educational setting for placement. The expense of this independent educational evaluation is borne by the school.

Outcomes of Inclusion

Two-thirds of the students with disabilities who receive special education services spend 80% or more of their time in inclusive classrooms (Barshay, 2023). Separation from non-disabled peers is a less common placement than during the past; only one of eight students with disabilities is taught in a special-needs-only environment. Advocates of inclusion claim segregated education placement causes stigma and social isolation that could have detrimental effects on self-concept, social identity, and self-confidence of special needs students. In contrast, those who favor a segregation placement point out that placement in an inclusive classroom could have adverse effects, especially if time and resources are insufficient to support individualized instruction aligned with student needs.

An international committee reviewed studies involving nine countries as commissioned by the Campbell Collaboration, a non-profit organization whose purpose is to provide research evidence to guide public policy (Dalgaard et al., 2022). Studies conducted from 2000–2021 involving 7,000 students ages 6–16 were examined to explore effects of placing students with special needs in inclusive classrooms compared with segregated placement to measure academic achievement and psychosocial adjustment. The results from the meta-analyses were inconclusive, indicating that some students thrive in an inclusion setting while others perform better in a segregated arrangement. Similar inconsistent results were determined by studies published prior to 2000. "The current evidence base suggests that one size does not fit all, and there is only limited contemporary evidence on what works for whom in special education when it comes to comparing inclusion to segregated placement for subgroups of children with special needs" (Dalgaard et al., 2022). The implication is that a single placement strategy may or may not benefit everyone so greater emphasis should be placed on individual students needs instead of assuming inclusion is best for everyone (Barshay, 2023).

Management of Peer Pressures

One cost of developing a strong sense of belonging and loyalty to a group is conformity. This has benefit when the group norm encourages healthy behavior. When it is not the situation, individuals must be capable of withstanding peer pressure because caving in to group demands could jeopardize health, integrity, safety, and goals. All students should be able to access peer pressure protectors provided by teachers and parents.

Teacher Peer Pressure Protectors

1 *Families rely on educators to take initiatives because school is the place where peers are together most often and for the greatest amount of time.*

   Encouraging involvement with extracurricular activities in after school programs is a way to support healthy interaction with others having similar interests and goals that might not become known in a classroom. The benefit for students can be attained when teachers are willing to act as advisors for operating after-school activities and clubs.

2 *Teachers can set peer influence on a healthy course by arranging cooperative learning teams where peers learn to support one another in being able to think critically and creatively.*

3 *By showing acceptance of imagination, teachers can alter peer judgment.*

   John is a creative 6th grader. In the past when John proposed original ideas, his classmates would usually laugh and the teachers felt it was their role to protect John by insisting the laughter stop. However, this year the teacher listened to John's ideas and, when his peers began to jeer, she said, "Let's pursue John's idea." She wrote the idea on the board and challenged the students to explore beyond their already expressed surface reaction. She pointed out that John's idea may have value and should be considered for what implications could be beneficial to us. In this way, the teacher obligated the class to think about John's idea instead of dismissing it without reflection.

   During the ensuing conversation students came to these conclusions: (a) sometimes good ideas are not recognized when first expressed; (b) judging a concept before understanding it is a form of ideational prejudice; and (c) John's ideas are actually very good. These conclusions contribute more to the welfare of John and the class than trying to protect John from classmates choosing to laugh when they do not understand.

4 *Teachers encourage self-reliance and individuality by rewarding questions in the face of peer pressure to prevent questions, beginning during middle school and junior high.*

   The general unwillingness to be seen by peers as curious can inhibit growth and suggests a false impression that students can become self-directed without motivation to explore their own questions. Instead, if we want students to keep learning after they complete formal schooling, asking questions must be part of the attitudes and skills developed by everyone. Support for questioning does more to improve learning than other kinds of responses.

5 *Urge students to ask questions so they will challenge the thinking of their peer group.*

   Students should learn the importance of examining norms carefully and not accepting that all ideas and norms are reasonable, fair, and deserve support. Recognize that this initiative requires reflection and courage.

6 *Students should have opportunities to discuss the nature of clique groups, how they influence others, and what should be done to prevent inappropriate rejection.*

If someone is behaving in unacceptable ways toward others, peer rejection is the natural response.

7 *When teachers help adolescents establish friendships, students become less vulnerable to rejection from cliques.*

Two can stand apart easier than one. While all students should have opportunities to make friends at school, some classes appear more conducive to friendships. These relationships are more apt to flourish when teachers make assignments where students work together as pairs or triads instead of alone or in large groups.

8 *Most students are achievement-oriented and adopt actions leading to recognition.*

Extra credit is sometimes given for competition. Caring about other people is observable and could be seen by students as a form of accomplishment that deserves consideration in status and leadership (e.g., tutoring, volunteering in a hospital, assisted living facility or long-term care home, peer counseling). Similarly, when teachers see how newcomers are treated without directing students to welcome them, recognition can be given to students whose initiatives enable newcomers to feel they belong.

9 *Teachers counter peer dependence by making themselves available for conversation.*

This allows students someone else to turn to than just peers. To fulfill this role, teachers must be perceived as approachable and trustworthy. Students say some teachers are hard to talk to, leaving them without a valuable source of adult assistance.

Parent Peer Pressure Protectors

In addition to teachers, parents should provide peer pressure protectors.

1 *The best way to minimize peer pressures is to recognize the strengths and goals of individual children.*

Parents should avoid making comparisons of achievements or limitations of their children. When one child is used as the standard of behavior for a sibling, the results can include sustained rivalry and jealousy. The more promising conditions should be to support the efforts and achievements of each family member throughout life. There is satisfaction in observing families where each person feels confident about their unique goals and contributions.

2 *Encourage children to value solitude as a time to reflect, self-evaluate, and look at things anew.*

Solitude allows the individuality and creativity students need so that being around age mates for long periods of time does not lead to excessive dependence.

3 *Parents should listen to adolescents about their difficulties of having arguments and maintaining friendships.*

This task requires high priority, takes time, and is inconvenient. Do it anyway. Beginning about the age of 10 (grade 5) and older, problems involving classmates and friends are likely to be continuous and, depending on how parents respond, they may be asked for advice often or not at all. Help children learn to get along without threatening withdrawal to force concession by others. Share your mistakes – this requires self-disclosure.

4 *Allow privacy.*

Let adolescents confide in you when they will, without insisting that they tell everything that is happening in their lives. Trust is essential for building intimate relationships and parents play the most prominent role in helping adolescents acquire this attribute.

5 *Recognize that the status of an adolescent child no longer depends only on the hierarchy of group members.*

Students with low social status are able to satisfy their need for acceptance and belonging as well as enjoy interaction after school when they go online and communicate with cyber friends. The opportunity to build friendships in a broader context has expanded with the Internet and there may be more conversation with friends online than the face- to-face communication that occurs at school. Parents should encourage cyber friendships with peers who live in other communities.

Learning to Develop Friendships and Dating

Building Close Relationships

When children become adolescents, between ages 10 and 13, the focus of parent worries expands. In addition to worries about the potential of unexpected violence, parents also begin to worry about the negative influences of friends, especially boyfriends, girlfriends, and dating (Zaloom, 2019). Adolescents also place friendships and dating high on their own list of priority concerns. Friendships are based on mutual feelings of trust and affection. Building friendships is a fundamental requirement for the development of healthy socialization. Dating, going out with someone as a social partner, enables adolescents to practice building friendships and to explore romantic connections. Most students between age 12 and 18 report having experienced some romantic relationship. By age 16, many adolescents confide more often in romantic partners than with parents, siblings or friends (Levine, 2020; Montemayor, 2018).

Some students do not learn to build healthy friendships because their parents disregard the sequence of attitudes and knowledge needed to achieve this goal. The orientation parents provide about dating should emphasize equality, mutual respect, and always consider a dating partner's goals. Instead, parents who fear early sexual intercourse and pregnancy are motivated to disregard building lessons about friendship formation in favor of issuing warnings against involvement with premature sex and recognizing the protective purpose of condoms.

Sexual Health Epidemic

The Centers for Disease Control and Prevention (2023a) reported the country has a health epidemic reflected by 26 million sexually transmitted infections (for the year 2020–2021) with half of these cases involving adolescents and young adults between ages 15–24. Suffering from these diseases is disproportionate among ethnic groups. Syphilis rates were nearly seven times higher among Black women than White women and Hispanics had twice the rate of Whites (Martin et al., 2022). Gay and bisexual men comprise nearly half of all syphilis cases, and contract gonorrhea at 42 times the rate of heterosexual men. Blacks accounted for 42% of new diagnoses of HIV, a virus causing AIDS that damages the immune system making it easier to become sick. Similarly, chlamydia rates among Black females were five times greater than for White females.

Cases of gonorrhea rose to become nearly eight times greater among Black females than White females (Centers for Disease Control and Prevention, 2020).

Dating Rights and Responsibilities

Dating abuse occurs when someone resorts to violent behavior using verbal, physical or sexual intimidation to gain power and control of a partner. Parents and teachers should teach gender respect that implicates dating abuse. Comprehensive sex education should be taught as early as grade 4 by schools and parents to reduce adolescent sexual risk (Centers for Disease Control and Prevention, 2020, 2023a; Evans et al., 2020). Parents are frustrated when their children watch television, movies or Internet scenes of intimacy, particularly situations where couples become sexually involved soon after they meet. The parent fear is that teenagers will conclude that speeded up transition to sexual intimacy is acceptable and therefore suitable for their dating expectations.

Education about dating should occur in the classroom and at home where students are able to benefit from guided discussions. Students should understand that common roles such as driving a car, going to school, playing on an athletic team, and dating – and sexual activity – are all accompanied by a set of rights and responsibilities. *Table 7.2 Dating Rights and Responsibilities*, presents guidelines for middle school and high school students that were developed by Washington State Attorney General's Office (2021). Schools and parents should post these guidelines on how to behave and encourage students to self-direct these questions: Do I violate rights of my dating partner? Am I fulfilling my responsibilities to my date? Am I respecting my rights and the rights of the person I date?

Table 7.2 Dating Rights and Responsibilities.[*]

Just like driving a car, going to school or playing a sport, dating someone comes with both rights and responsibilities. Print these out and post them as a reminder for yourself and others. Look at them carefully and ask yourself if you are violating someone else's rights – or if someone is violating yours. Are you fulfilling your responsibilities? Are you respecting your rights and the rights of your date?

RIGHTS

I have the right:
 1 To be treated with respect always
 2 To my own body, thoughts, opinions, and property
 3 To choose and keep my friends
 4 To change my mind – at any time
 5 To not be abused – physically, emotionally, or sexually
 6 To leave a relationship
 7 To say no
 8 To be treated as an equal
 9 To disagree
10 To live without fear and confusion from my boyfriend's or girlfriend's anger

RESPONSIBILITIES

I have the responsibility:
 1 To not threaten to harm myself or another
 2 To encourage my girlfriend or boyfriend to pursue their dreams
 3 To support my girlfriend or boyfriend emotionally
 4 To communicate, not manipulate

(Continued)

Table 7.2 (Continued)

 5　To not humiliate or demean my girlfriend or boyfriend
 6　To refuse to abuse – physically, emotionally or sexually
 7　To take care of myself
 8　To allow my boyfriend or girlfriend to maintain their individuality
 9　To respect myself and my girlfriend or boyfriend
10　To be honest with each other

---

* From: Washington State Office of the Attorney General (2021). Dating rights and responsibilities. https://atg.
wa.gov/dating-rights Copyright © 2021.

Family Conversation about Dating

The purpose for dating should be to get to know another person while having fun. No one should have to convey impressions or commitment beyond "getting to know you." Nevertheless, concerns that a daughter and son might rush into a sexual relationship too early in life distracts many parents from their obligation to provide the dating orientation needed. Empathy is defined as the ability to identify with and understand aspects of another person's feelings, hopes and difficulties. Some ways of showing empathy while dating include listening to hurt feelings and considering goals and aspirations of the dating partner. Building trust and respect are basic ingredients to durable and satisfying emotional ties (Montemayor, 2018).

Some parents defer lessons about dating until their child is the same age as the parents were when they were first allowed to date. However, age of puberty in girls has declined over the past several decades. Consequently, conversations about dating should begin earlier, by grade 4 because some girls enter puberty as early as 8 years old. Studies involving 2,000 Black, White, and Mexican-American parents of adolescents and their adolescent children (ages 10–14) were conducted to rate the relevance of parental guidance. Both generations agreed that parents are not engaged to the extent they should be in talking with their teenage children about dating (P. S. Strom & Strom, 2021).

Peer Advice About Health

Well-Being

Adolescents are uniformly concerned about peer perception of their physical appearance so they rely on friends to give them feedback about how they look, clothes they should wear, and ways to improve how they are seen by classmates. In this context, friends have a unique chance to influence favorable habits that can maintain physical health by encouraging good nutrition, maintaining suitable physical exercise, and avoiding smoking. Consider some of the following ways in which peer advice can contribute to well-being.

Nutrition and Diet Knowledge

Sufficient iron is essential during adolescence because of an expanding volume of blood in the body and increase in muscle mass. During growth spurts extra iron is required because it is vital for muscle development and red blood cells. The need for additional iron is especially acute among girls because of loss of iron that occurs during menstruation. When there is a lack of iron in the diet, the resulting iron deficiency anemia is reflected by a tendency to experience fatigue, feel lightheadedness, loss of appetite, and pale appearance. Teenagers should eat iron-containing foods like meat, fish, poultry, eggs, peas, beans, potatoes and rice (Canavan & Fawzi, 2019).

Another often overlooked health requirement is calcium. Strong bones and teeth depend on calcium. Lack of calcium increases the risk for osteoporosis, a bone-thinning disease viewed as a major public health threat for an estimated 54 million adults. One in two women and one in four men over age 50 will break a bone because of osteoporosis. Only 14% of adolescent girls and 35% of boys meet the government calcium recommendations of 1,300 milligrams a day. One glass of milk contains about 300 milligrams of calcium. Teenage girls should be informed that they are in their biggest and most important growth spurt and this is the time for learning to eat right and treat the body with proper nutrition (Mayo Clinic, 2021).

Students at public high schools have often been surveyed about their food perceptions. Findings have shown that many girls report not eating breakfast in the past week, an unhealthy effort to attain weight management. Excessive diet practices such as fasting, diet pills or laxatives and vomiting to lose weight are reported by one in four students. A healthy form of guidance is to follow government diet guidelines for 2020–2025. This resource describes a healthy diet, by age level, with a focus on fruits, vegetables, whole grains, and low-fat milk and milk products. The diet of lean meats, poultry, fish, beans, eggs, and nuts is low in saturated fats, trans fats, cholesterol, salt (sodium), and added sugars. As Americans experience epidemic rates of overweight and obesity, the United States Department of Agriculture (2020) website can empower young people to make healthy food choices.

Consequences of Obesity

The incidence of obesity among American adolescents has tripled over the past several decades and is now considered to be at epidemic levels. Obesity is a result of caloric imbalance (too few calories that are expended for amount of calories consumed) and mediated by genetic, behavioral, and environmental factors. Physicians acknowledge that obesity is the greatest public health threat, accounting for more fatalities than cancers and accidents combined. The problem begins in childhood with the number of fat cells becoming fixed by age 10. Parents require education to understand that child obesity merits serious concern. Studies have found only 7% of children with normal weight parents grow up to become obese while 80% of children with two obese parents will be obese adults. The medical community is agreed that programs for weight-loss typically do not work; a 1% success rate is the norm. Physical activity must become part of a prevention strategy that can be encouraged by peers (Sanyaolu et al., 2019).

What concerns health care professionals is the cost in lives. Obese youth are three times more likely than peers of healthy weight to develop high blood pressure and twice as likely to suffer heart disease. The assertion that 'you are as old as your arteries' implies that the condition of your arteries can be more important than chronological age in evolution of heart disease and stroke. A sample of 70 obese boys and girls, average age 13, were examined using ultrasound imaging to measure thickness of the inner walls of their carotid arteries in the neck that supply the brain with blood. The purpose was to gauge their vascular age, referring to the age at which the level of arterial thickening would be normal. For these teenagers, their vascular age generally was three decades older than their chronological age. The thickness of their arteries was typical of persons who are

45 years old. The consequences of accelerated vascular aging among adolescents with obesity and diabetes has become a major concern (Ryder et al., 2020).

A related dire prediction is that one of two children will develop Type 2 diabetes because of excess weight, raising their probability of death at a younger age than their parents. Diabetes is the sixth leading cause of death and a major cause of kidney failure, blindness, and non-traumatic leg amputation. An obese adolescent can expect to live a shorter life by 12–14 years less than a peer of desirable weight. The cost of medical treatment for children with obesity is three times greater than treating the average child. Reflection is needed because it is easier to prevent obesity than treat it (Wadden & Bray, 2019).

Physical Exercise

Moderate to intense physical activity is recommended at least 30 minutes per day. An expert panel reviewed the research about effects of physical activity on young people's health and well-being. Over 850 articles and 1,120 abstracts were examined (Pangrazi & Beighle, 2020). The conclusion was that children who participate in moderate to vigorous physical activity one hour or more a day gained significant physiological, health and psychological benefits. Less than half of adolescents are physically active on a regular basis. Instead, many maintain a lazy lifestyle that includes sitting at a desk or computer through the school day and watching television or spending time on the Internet while at home.

Avoid Smoking and Drinking

According to the Centers for Disease Control and Prevention (2022a, 2023b), cigarette smoking remains the leading cause of preventable disease, disability, and death in the United States. Among high school students, 23.6% smoke cigarettes. Each day an estimated 2,000 youth younger than age 18 start to smoke. Adolescents who smoke underestimate the health risks and overestimate their ability to quit once they have established the habit. The reality is that, among high school seniors who smoke several cigarettes a day, 70% of them will still be smokers in five years. The younger a person begins to smoke, the greater the odds they will be a heavy smoker as adults. On average, smokers will die 12–14 years earlier than non-smokers. Smoking is related to level of education. The proportion of people without a high school diploma who smoke is 26.5%; with an associate degree 14%; with an undergraduate degree 7%; and with a graduate degree 4%. Similarly annual household income is implicated.

According to the Centers for Disease Control and Prevention (2022b) underage drinking (younger than age 21) is a significant public health problem in the United States. Youth who drink alcohol are more likely to experience some of these problems.

- Academic issues, such as higher rates of absences or lower grades
- Social difficulties, such as fighting or lack of participation in youth activities
- Arrest for driving or physically hurting someone while drunk
- Physical problems, such as hangovers or illnesses
- Unwanted, unplanned, and unprotected sexual activity
- Increased risk of suicide and homicide
- Alcohol-related motor vehicle crashes

- Substance abuse and addiction, such as opioids
- Alcohol poisoning
- Underage drinking is associated with adult drinking

Excessive drinking is responsible for more than 3,900 deaths among people under age 21 each year. Fortunately, rehabilitation programs can help adolescents recover their well-being.

Conclusion

Peers have a powerful influence on social development of others in their age group. They provide the first substantial experience with equality and often present more attainable standards than those imposed by grownups. Children consider peer norms as suitable criteria to apply for self-evaluation. They find out about friendships mostly from age mates who also encourage the acquisition of cooperation, empathy, compromise, and pursuit of independence.

These lessons are taught more effectively by peers than by adults. Students find out what friends will tolerate and identify the conduct they will not accept. Most early adolescents join a clique that allows them to feel they are accepted and belong. However, some students experience racial, religious, or ethnic discrimination. Prejudice is more prevalent during middle school than high school and the people targeted suffer more than may be supposed by the public. The way others feel about us motivates how we are treated and, as a result, impact how we see ourselves. Middle school should include experiences that help students see themselves favorably without finding fault with peers.

Being able to build friendships is a fundamental asset. Dating offers a social context in which to practice friendship skills and exploration of romantic connections. In many homes, parent worries about adolescent early sexual involvement causes them to overlook basic lessons that they should teach about healthy relationships. One result is teenage dating violence, a greater health and social problem than estimated by parents. Teenagers express frustration that, even during school, opportunities are lacking for friendly conversations with classmates of the other gender. Some education about dating should take place the classroom with teacher monitored discussions. All students should know their dating rights and responsibilities and know where to turn if they are being abused or know about someone else who is mistreated.

Teenagers like being decision makers about what they eat but often choose foods that are not good for them. Many adolescents who want to conform to the idealized thin body image tend to skip meals and experiment with dieting plans that cut calories but ignore needs for nutrients like iron and calcium. A related health danger is a sedentary lifestyle that includes being seated most of the time at school and at home. Obesity and diabetes are related to this choice. Friends can be helpful in reminding peers to eat a healthy diet, get ample exercise. and discourage smoking.

Key Concepts

1 Peers provide the first experience with equality. Everyone seeks companionship and attention from others. Peers are the most able to satisfy these needs. When students behave in keeping with group norms, they are rewarded by attention, acceptance, and emotional support.
2 Peers learn friendship mainly from classmates and how to get along with others of the same status. Becoming part of a group requires exhibiting skills expected by peers like

cooperation, sharing feelings, striving for independence, and making up following arguments. Such lessons are more easily learned from peers than from parents.

3 Before age 10, students demonstrate less social rejection of peers. Activities for young children are non-competitive so self-concepts are not threatened by strengths of others. Better performers in the early grades rarely announce superiority and the below average do not yet report feelings of inferiority since performance norms are not yet established.

4 From the middle grades onward, students can no longer depend on what their parents have accomplished as the basis for self-pride. They must earn their own social standing. In classes they face more competition and failure along with unfriendly remarks of others. Some peers detect limitations and express negative views as insults or hurtful statements.

5 Becoming part of a group requires gaining skills motivated by peers. These skills usually include cooperation, sharing, striving for independence, expressing discontent and anger, and reconciliation after disagreement. Such lessons are more easily learned from peers than parents.

6 Adolescents place friendship and dating high on their list of concerns. Friendships are based on mutual feelings of trust and affection. Dating, to go out with someone as a social partner, allows practice in building friendships and exploring romantic connections. By age 16, many teenagers interact with a romantic partner more than they do with parents, siblings, or friends.

7 The proportion of overweight adolescents tripled in the past generation. Obesity is the greatest public health threat, accounting for more fatalities than drugs, cancers, and accidents combined. The problem begins during childhood with the number of fat cells becoming fixed by age ten.

8 Less than half of all adolescents are physically active on a regular basis. Most of them have a sedentary lifestyle that includes sitting at a desk or computer during the day and watching television or spending time on the Internet at home.

9 Tobacco use is the most preventable cause of death, causing half a million fatalities a year, more than alcohol, accidents, murders, suicides, and substance abuse combined. Adolescents should be aware that regular smokers live an average of 14 years less than nonsmokers.

10 The need for additional iron is especially acute for adolescent girls because of the loss of iron that occurs during menstruation. When there is a lack of iron, the resulting iron deficiency anemia is reflected by tendency to fatigue, light-headedness, appetite loss, and pale appearance.

Generational Perspectives Activities

> **7.1 Team Discussion**
> **7.2 Interview Adolescents about Dating**
> **7.3 Interview Parents about Dating**
> **7.4 A Scenario: Reasoning and Problem Solving**
> **7.5 Team Chapter Review**
> **7.6 Criteria for Self-Evaluation of Team Members**

7.1. Team Discussion

1 What kinds of peer pressure do you have to deal with on a regular basis?
2 What are the biggest problems you sometimes have with your friends?
3 What things are most important in trying to build a lasting friendship?
4 In what ways do friends influence some of your choices and decisions?
5 What things do you like to talk to friends about but not to other people?
6 What happened that ended a friendship you enjoyed at an earlier time?
7 How do you solve a problem when there is a conflict with your friends?
8 What situations have you seen where individuals were rejected by peers?
9 What prejudices were parents taught compared to ones you are taught?
10 What have you done to support inclusion practices at your school?

7.2. Interview Adolescents about Dating

1 How do your parents feel about the dating partners you have chosen so far?
2 What lessons about dating do you wish your parents would share with you?
3 What are advantages and disadvantages of involvement with cyberdating?
4 How could social network platforms contribute more to social development?
5 What are some important lessons that you have learned so far about dating?
6 What has been your experience in breaking up with someone that you dated?
7 How does peer pressure shape how you behave while going out on a date?
8 What are some ways that dating has changed since parents were your age?
9 What concerns your parents most when you go out with someone on a date?
10 How would you handle unfair demands that are made by a dating partner?
11 What are some qualities that you look for in a person that you want to date?

7.3. Interview Parents about Dating

1 How did you meet your spouse and how old were you at the time?
2 What qualities do you suppose caused you to fall in love with your spouse?
3 How long did you date each other before you were engaged? married?
4 What discoveries have you made about getting along with a spouse?
5 How does religious faith influence your lifestyle and relationships?
6 What have you enjoyed most about family life and being a parent?
7 What friends have you tried to keep in contact with for the longest time?
8 Did you ever breakup a relationship with a dating partner?

7.4. A Scenario: Reasoning and Problem Solving

Problem solving scenarios present an opportunity to look at situations that might happen for a family and think of possible solutions. Your task is to look at pros and cons of choices stated, think of additional options, identify relevant information that might be missing, find out how teammates view alternatives, and defend your reasoning about advice that you consider best.

Belief in equality is shown by how adolescents treat dating partners. Success is fostered when relatives share experiences on the importance of friendship building and mutual respect as the basis for satisfying and durable intimate relationships. What are your recommendations?

a acquaint secondary students with their dating rights and dating responsibilities
b encourage empathy by conversations that make known feelings of each individual
c parents and grandparents should share views about the role of trust in relationships
d orient daughters and sons about how to respond to exploitation attempts by others
e suggest involvement in after school programs to meet people with mutual interests
f go on dating websites to meet new people

7.5. Team Chapter Review

Efforts to assess participant learning, provide feedback, and improve quality of instruction is enhanced by a group review of each chapter.

1 What ideas in the lesson changed the way I think about this topic?
2 What insights from the lesson will I try to apply in my relationships?
3 What is the most important point for me presented in this lesson?
4 What are some aspects of this lesson I would like to better understand?
5 Which aspects of this lesson do I wish that I had known about earlier?

7.6. Criteria for Self-Evaluation of the Team

Directions: For each question, place a check beside statements that describe your feelings. You may want to give several answers on some items. If your feelings are not on choices list, write them on the line marked 'other.'

1 The most important lessons I learned from peers while growing up were

    a comparing their behavior to mine as a method to gauge my progress
    b having them listen to me express differences from adults in my life
    c their encouragement for me to strive for independence from adults
    d the need to reconcile after arguments to maintain relationships
    e Other _____

2 When the groups I belonged to rejected others from joining us, I

    a did not object so they would not decide to exclude me as well
    b argued it would be a good to accept differences in our group
    c didn't think about it because empathy was not an asset of mine
    d decided to leave the group because the practice seemed unfair
    e Other _____

3 The way(s) my parents tried to help me with unfair peer pressures included

    a I did not tell so they did not know about peer pressures
    b they felt adults should always step in to stop unfairness
    c they felt I should learn how to manage my own affairs
    d to report such incidents to the teacher or school principal
    e Other _____

4 When I was growing up I took part in teasing some students

    a because they were different from people in my group
    b since they showed difficulties in class with learning

c about their appearance or the clothing that they wore

d regarding conditions that were known about their family

e I never teased anyone

5 Having lots of social network friends can be worthwhile if

a face-to-face relationships do not get sacrificed

b most are seen as being superficial relationships

c not much time is devoted to maintaining them

d friends listen and give advice that is corrective

e Other _____

6 I think dating is more difficult for adolescents now because

a there is a lot of pressure to speed up a relationship

b they are less inclined to seek advice from adults

c having sex is more common at an earlier age

d parents fail to teach lessons about friendships

e Other _____

7 Given the influence that peers have on adolescent mental health

a peer relationships should be part of curriculum

b there should be more counselors on the faculty

c schools should assign topics for family sharing

d peer counseling should have a prominent place

e Other _____

8 Cooperative learning teams can improve their relationships by

a regarding other students as potential sources of learning

b practicing reconciliation about differences of opinion

c recognizing contributions that are made by everyone

d counteracting the exclusion that cliques engage in

e Other _____

9 Orientation to the rights and responsibilities of dating

a is a worthwhile focus for adolescent discussions

b helps teach adolescents to exercise self-control

c could reduce harassment some teenagers suffer

d should include structured discussions with parents

e Other _____

10 I am hopeful the future of social networks will include

a more opportunities to communicate with older generations

b greater exposure to points of view that differ from our own

c sites where new ideas or policies can receive an audience

d discussion of ways to improve school and family practices

e Other _____

References

Barshay, J. (2023, January 9). *Proof points: New research review questions the evidence for special education inclusion.* The Hechinger Report. https://hechingerreport.org/proof-ponts-new-research-review-questions-the-evidence-for-special-education-inclusion/

Baumeister, R. F., & Bushman, B. J. (2021). *Social psychology and human nature* (5th ed.). Cengage.

Burkholder, A. R., Elenbaas, L., & Killen, M. (2020). Children's and adolescents' evaluations of intergroup exclusion in interracial and interwealth peer contexts. *Child Development, 91*(2), e512–e527. 10.1111/cdev.13249

California Department of Education. (2022). *Frequently asked questions: Senate Bill 48*, California Fair Accurate Inclusive Respectful Education Act. https://www.cde.ca.gov/ci/cr/cf/senatebill48faq.asp

Canavan, C. R., & Fawzi, W. W. (2019, July). Addressing knowledge gaps in adolescent nutrition: Toward advancing public health and sustainable development. *Current Developments in Nutrition, 3*(7). 10.1093/cdn/nzz062

Centers for Disease Control and Prevention. (2020). *Health disparities in HIV, viral hepatitis, STDs, and TB.* https://www.cdc.gov/nchhstp/healthdisparities/africanamericans.html

Centers for Disease Control and Prevention. (2022a, April 12). *Trends in tobacco use among youth.* https://www.cdc.gov/tobacco/data_statistics/fact_sheets/fast_facts/trends-in-tobacco-use-among-youth.html

Centers for Disease Control and Prevention. (2022b, October 26). *Underage drinking.* Alcohol and Public Health. https://www.cdc.gov/alcohol/fact-sheets/underage-drinking.htm

Centers for Disease Control and Prevention. (2023a, April 11). *U.S. STI epidemic showed no signs of slowing in 2021 -- Cases continued to escalate.* https://www.cdc.gov/media/releases/2023/s0411-sti.html#:~:text=CDC

Centers for Disease Control and Prevention. (2023b, May 4). *Smoking and tobacco use.* https://www.cdc.gov/tobacco/data_statistics/fact_sheets/fast_facts/index.htm#:~:text=Cigarette%20smoking%20remains%20the%20leading,death%20in%20the%20United%20States

Dalgaard, N., Bondebjerg, A., Viinholt, B., & Filges, T. (2022, December). The effects of inclusion on academic achievement, socioemotional development and wellbeing of children with special educational needs. *Campbell Systematic Reviews, 18*(4), e1291. 10.1002/cl2.1291

Doubet, K., & Hockett, J. (2015). *Differentiation in middle & high school: Strategies to engage all learners.* Association for Supervision and Curriculum Development.

Education for All Handicapped Children Act. (1975). H.R.7217. https://www.congress.gov/bill/94th-congress/house-bill/7217

Evans, R., Widman, L., & Goldey, K. (2020, May). The role of adolescent sex education in sexual satisfaction among LGB+ heterosexual young adults. *American Journal of Sexuality Education, 15*(3), 310–335. https://www.tandfonline.com/doi/full/10.1080/15546128.2020.1763883

Ferrer-Wreder, L., & Kroger, J. (2020). *Identity in adolescence: The balance between self and other* (4th ed.). Routledge.

Harris, J. R. (2009). *The nurture assumption: Why children turn out the way they do.* Free Press.

Individuals with Disabilities Education Improvement Act. (2023, January 11). *A history of the Individuals with Disabilities Education Act.* https://sites.ed.gov/idea/IDEA-History#:~:text=On%20November%2029%2C%201975%2C%20President,and%20locality%20across%20the%20country

Jackson, L. M. (2019). *The psychology of prejudice: From attitudes to social action* (2nd ed.). American Psychological Association.

Kauffman, J. M., Hallahan, D. P., & Pullen, P. C. (Eds.). (2017). *Handbook of special education* (2nd ed.). Routledge.

Levine, M. (2020). *Ready or not: Preparing our kids to thrive in an uncertain and rapidly changing world.* Harper.

Martin, E. G., Ansari, B., Rosenberg, E. S., Hart-Malloy, R., Smith, D., Bernstein, K. T., Chesson, H. W., Delaney, K., Trigg, M., & Gift, T. L. (2022, May 1). Variation in patterns of racial and ethnic disparities in primary and secondary syphilis diagnosis rates among heterosexually active women by region and age group in the United States. *Sexually Transmitted Diseases*, *49*(5), 330–337. 10.1097/OLQ.0000000000001607

Mayo Clinic. (2021). *Osteoporosis*. https://www.mayoclinic.org/diseases-conditions/osteoporosis/symptoms-causes/syc-20351968

Montemayor, R. (2018). *Sexuality in adolescence and emerging adulthood*. Guilford Press.

National Center for Education Statistics. (2023). Students with disabilities. *Condition of Education*. U.S. Department of Education, Institute of Education Sciences. https://nces.ed.gov/programs/coe/indicator/cgg/students-with-disabilities

Pangrazi, R., & Beighle, A. (2020). *Dynamic physical education for elementary school children* (19th ed.). Human Kinetics.

Ryder, J. R., Northrup, E., Rudser, K., Kelly, A., Gao, Z., Khoury, P., Kimball, T., Dolan, L., & Urbina, E. (2020, May). Accelerated early vascular aging among adolescents with obesity and/or type 2 diabetes mellitus. *Journal of the American Heart Association*, *9*, e014891 10.1161/JAHA.119.014891

Sanyaolu, A., Okorie, C., Qi, X., Locke, J. & Rehman, S. (2019). Childhood and adolescent obesity in the United States: A public health concern. *Global Pediatric Health*. 10.1177/2333794X19891305

Strom, P. S., Hendon, K., Strom, R. D., & Wang, C. (2019). Assessment of high school students in the social context: How peers support and inhibit learning in the classroom. *School Community Journal*, *29*(2), 183–202. https://files.eric.ed.gov/fulltext/EJ1236590.pdf

Strom, P. S., & Strom, R. D. (2021) *Adolescents in the Internet Age: A team learning and teaching perspective*. Information Age.

United States Department of Agriculture. (2020 December). *Dietary guidelines for Americans 2020–2025* (9th ed.). https://www.dietaryguidelines.gov/sites/default/files/2021-03/Dietary_Guidelines_for_Americans-2020-2025.pdf

Wadden, T. A., & Bray, G. A. (Eds.). (2019). *Handbook of obesity treatment* (2nd ed.). Guilford Press.

Washington State Office of the Attorney General. (2021). *Dating rights and responsibilities*. https://atg.wa.gov/dating-rights

Zaloom, S. (2019). *Sex, teens and everything in between: The new and necessary conversation today's teenagers need to have about consent, sexual harassment, health relationships, love and more*. Source Books.

8 Family Differences in a Conflict Culture

Guidelines to Manage Family Disputes

Close Family Relationships Require Fairness

Parents and their adolescent children should state personal views so they receive fair consideration. Fairness is a value that has high priority among youth. They reference fairness as their most effective approach to let parents know that the positions they take about some things are unacceptable. In response, parents may acknowledge being strict but are disappointed when they are seen as unfair. Parents should understand how adolescents see a situation before they can determine advice that is relevant. In turn, adolescents should feel an obligation to support worthy advice from parents by revealing continuous insight about their own feelings. Most disagreements can be resolved. The resulting dialogues ensure that disagreements will occur but can be resolved by striving to meet the conditions of fairness and honesty (Ripley, 2022).

Set Rules to Guide How Arguments Proceed

Shouting, put-downs, and sarcasm should not be allowed by families because they contradict the goal to exhibit greater self-control, one sign of maturity. The speaker and listener role should be applied so that while one person speaks, others listen and do not interrupt. Listeners should try to restate what the other person meant to confirm that their message was understood (Branje, 2018). Adolescents should avoid statements such as, "Everybody else's parents let them do it," and parents should avoid saying, "When I was your age …". Attitudes used to guide conflicts should not be limited to determining who is right or wrong, or who concedes. Instead, the desired outcome for both parties should be to capture the most opportune way to solve problems together while making yourself a better person.

Clarify Issues to Ensure a Common Focus

It is frustrating to find out at the end of a lengthy talk that both parties are still unaware of the main concerns felt by the other person. For a daughter, an argument about curfew may be seen as a challenge to her maturity while her parents view it as a matter of safety. There is a difference between telling an adolescent, "I don't trust you" and saying "I am afraid for you because most car accidents happen late at night." Parent concerns about teenagers being out late at night should always be made known and taken seriously by adolescents.

DOI: 10.4324/9781003401261-11

Parents who do not spend enough time with adolescents are often inclined to make concessions to avoid more arguments. A denial of disagreements overlooks the benefit parents can provide their children by allowing them opportunities to practice emerging debate skills in the context of a safe and supportive environment. The family should be the ideal setting for learning to disagree with others because parents love their children and, in most cases, can demonstrate more tolerance. This should motivate adults to rely on restraint rather than anger. The greater maturity of adults also enables them to depend more on prosocial skills like listening, empathy, negotiation, compromise, and independent thinking. Parent and adolescent disputes also confirm that people who disagree can still love each another.

Plan Time to Discuss Bothersome Concerns

Most disputes arise in response to particular events but certain disagreements are continuous. These issues require attention when no one is distracted by mobile devices and are willing to devote time for a serious talk. Recognize parent inattention can fuel further conflict. Parent inattention is increasing because of preoccupation with cell phones and other distractions that undermine the quality of listening that is needed for family members to understand one another (Carter, 2020).

An Example of Parent Inattention

Lack of parental attention is more common but not a new phenomenon. Many years ago, in 1944, Tennessee Williams (1944/2011) presented his play *The Glass Menagerie* that revealed why parent time is well spent listening to the feelings, concerns, and questions of their children. In the play, Tom's mother Amanda never has time to listen to him or tries to understand his views. Consequently, Tom's motives, opinions, dreams, and concerns tend to be consistently misinterpreted. At the end of one of her anger episodes, Amanda shouts a foolish recommendation that Tom should "go to the moon." This remark caused him to run away from home. Years later, as he reflected back on that incident, Tom tells the audience, "I didn't go to the moon. I went much further, for time is the greatest distance between two places." A reminder is that if anger rises, either person should call time-out and return to the topic later when cooler heads prevail. At every age, anger prevents access to logic, consideration for needs and feelings of others, and generation for creative alternatives for problems.

The Talking Circle

In terms of cultural diversity, consider the traditions of the 2.7 million American Indians and Alaskan Natives. The two largest tribes are Navajo (nearly 400,000 members of the tribe), and Cherokee (392,000 members of the tribe) (Romero, 2021). When trying to resolve a conflict situation that involves several people, everyone's views are expected to be heard without interruption. This suggestion would seem to be an easy guideline to fulfill but common experiences demonstrate that it is usually difficult.

The tribes of Native Americans have unique methods to ensure that individual opinions are considered. The Navajo tribe uses a *talking circle* to resolve certain problems. At a hospital in Phoenix, Arizona, a Navajo family allowed our research team to observe their talking circle. In the hospital room, the leader of the circle began by holding an arrowhead over his head while he said, "Sometimes older people in our tribe have to come to the city for medical care. This is a time of worry for him and his family, and he is without spiritual support of the traditional medicine man. How can we help at this time of difficulty?"

The leader then passed the arrowhead to the individual on his right who was part of the talking circle of eight people surrounding the bed. That person had the opportunity to speak and make suggestions. In turn, each person in the circle was given an opportunity to comment. The order of speakers was determined by holding the arrowhead, passing it on only when s/he had finished talking. The talking circle speakers sometimes expressed agreement with views of people who spoke before them. Some speakers supported a suggestion or elaborated an idea that had already been expressed. There were also speakers who presented novel solutions.

At the end, the leader summarized what the talking circle had proposed. Some of the suggestions included having the medicine man to come visit, conduct ceremonies on the reservation in absentia, bring artifacts that were blessed by the medicine man, play messages recorded by the medicine man, and communicate with loved ones and friends on the reservation.

Rural areas of Indian reservations have had less access to high-speed Internet than the general United States population. The U.S. Department of Commerce has approved funding to boost the broadband installation directly to support work, education, housing and health, while protecting local customs and traditions for 157 Tribal entities. This modernization will also bring new opportunities for global engagement and growth (National Telecommunications and Information Administration, 2023; Silversmith, 2022).

Learn the Common Benefits of Conflicts

Parents can become more motivated to be seen as an example when they realize that disagreements can bring benefits for all parties. Adolescents are acquiring the ability to monitor logic so they are inclined to carefully check the reasoning of others. They like to practice this newfound ability by debates in disagreements with parents. These continual challenges are reported by parents as an exhausting experience. Many mothers and fathers who do not recognize that these daily conflicts are opportunities to engage in reciprocal learning instead attribute turmoil to undesirable influences of their child's peer group. A more accurate appraisal is that youth are motivated to initiate some conflicts so parents can teach them how differences should be expressed and given consideration in a civil way (Branje, 2018; Carter, 2020).

Living in a Conflict Culture

Identification of Goals

Adolescents should know more than most of them do about living with conflict. When this goal is stated in general terms, it seems vague and overwhelming. However, when the goal is divided into a number of manageable tasks, a more complete picture of conflict learning can emerge. In addition, it becomes clear that certain lessons should be dealt with at school while others may be better acquired at home. In both environments, parents, grandparents, and teachers can begin by choosing goals they are willing to pursue. Consider some conflict goals that are presented here and identify ones you are trying to reach. Share this information with relatives so they know your goals and can give feedback based on observations of your behavior. Invite them to identify their conflict goals so that you can help them assess their progress.

1 Recognizing people who love each other may still have disagreements.
2 Helping other people may require becoming involved in their conflict.
3 Deciding to talk things over instead of trying to settle issues by fighting.
4 Accepting new goals that are expressed by people we care about.
5 Knowing that self-conflict (conscience) is essential for moral behavior.
6 Developing the ability to respect others by willingness to compromise.
7 Being able to accept defeat when this is the outcome of a competition.
8 Having will power to stand alone in situations when necessary.
9 Understanding that living with a certain amount of uncertainty is inevitable.
10 Finding ways to disagree on things without a loss in status or affection.
11 Being willing to apologize after making hurtful comments about anyone.
12 Realizing that there might be certain differences that are irreconcilable.
13 Learning to share possessions as well as take turns with other people.
14 Respecting personal property of others is a way to reduce conflict.
15 Listening to others when they express contrary feelings or opinions.
16 Analyzing conditions that are needed to result in mutual reconciliation.
17 Sharing dominance and demonstrating an ability to be cooperative.
18 Coping with complex situations that present unfamiliarity and anxiety.
19 Learning to assert personal opinion without having feelings of guilt.
20 Viewing differences as possible opportunities for reciprocal learning.

Family Configuration and Conflict

In the United States, nearly 24 million (34%) children under age 18 live with a single parent (approximately 10 million households) (Annie E. Casey Foundation, 2023a; Chamie, 2023). This is the highest rate in the world; globally the average rate of single parents is 7% (United States Census Bureau, 2023). Mothers maintain 80% of single-parent family groups. About half (51%) of all single mothers have never been married, and 29% are divorced, separated, or widowed (United States Census Bureau, 2022). The likelihood of a child living in a single parent family indicates that, in terms of race, 64% are Black, 49% American Indian, 42% Hispanic, 24% White, and 16% are Asian (Annie E. Casey Foundation, 2023b).

Families headed by single mothers are among the poorest households. Almost a third are considered "food insecure" with two-thirds of their children getting free meals at school that are provided by the government. As these children reach adolescence, they are more likely than their peers from two-parent families to have a poor academic record, engage in sexual intercourse at a younger age, and become involved early with a pregnancy. As grownups they have sustain higher rates of unemployment, lower occupational status, and more troubled marriages and divorces than peers with married parents (Chamie, 2023; Guttmacher Institute, 2023).

Fortunately, family structure is not destiny. Even though students from single parent homes are, on average, more likely to participate in at-risk behavior, such problems are not inevitable. The assumption that all families of any particular configuration have the same experiences and future ignores wide variations in single, blended, and nuclear families (Annie E. Casey Foundation, 2023c). What matters most is the behavior of parents and their access to sources of assistance. Grandparents, teachers, social workers, religious leaders and organizations that serve youth can offer greater support if they are aware of more prevalent problems in certain marital structures and take steps to help build more resilient families (Kearney, 2023).

Causes of Divorce and Survival of Marriages

More than half of marriages in the United States end in divorce. The *Forbes Advisor* commissioned a national online survey to assess the leading causes of divorce (Bieber, 2023). Respondents were 1,000 people divorced or in the process of getting a divorce. Between 35% and 50% of first time marriages had not survived. The figure rose to 67% for second marriages and 73% in subsequent marriages. Only 4% of the divorces took place after 10 years of marriage. Most divorces were initiated by one party; only 27% stated the decision to end their marriage was mutual. Divorces happened most often between year three and year seven of a marriage. Divorce rates among White couples was 15%; Hispanic rates were 18%, and Black rates were 31%.

Participants were initially asked to make known their reasons for getting married. Self reported motivations were financial security 42%, companionship 39%, love 36%, formal act of making a commitment 34%, and to start a family 34%. The common causes indicated for divorce were lack of family support 43%, infidelity or extra marital affairs 34%, lack of compatibility 31%, lack of intimacy 31%, too much conflict or arguing 31%, financial stress 24%, lack of commitment 23%, parenting differences 20%, marrying too young 10%, opposing values or morals 6%, substance abuse 3%, domestic violence 3%, and pursuing different lifestyles 1%.

Survey outcomes also revealed that less than 5% of couples felt that their marriages could not have been saved. Instead, 63% believed that a better understanding of commitment before getting married could have saved the union, and 54% reported that they may not have gotten a divorce if they understood their spouse's morals and values. Over 40% thought their marriage could have been saved by waiting longer to get married and waiting longer to start a family.

Grandparents as Caregivers of Grandchildren

Scope of the Grandparent Challenge

Grandparents have always assumed responsibility for raising their grandchildren whenever there is a family tragedy such as death of a parent, divorce, separation or abandonment. Other conditions that motivate fulltime care of grandchildren include helping unmarried adolescent mothers, parent loss of employment, or need for free childcare and supervision. Some parents become addicted to drugs, particularly opioids (National Institute of Drug Abuse, 2023). Others abuse their children, are deployed overseas by the military, placed in jail because of a crime or demonstrate signs of mental illness. In addition, there are single parent families who acknowledge they are unable to provide all the care their children need (Showalter & McEntyre, 2022).

Nearly 3 million grandparents are responsible for raising their grandchildren. Two-thirds of them are grandmothers without presence of a grandfather (Smith & Segal, 2023). Most grandparents who raise grandchildren believe their responsibility for care will be permanent. This demographic minority group is poorly understood by the public. Generations United (2023), a family research and advocacy group, explained 70% of grandparent caregivers are under 60 years old and 26% have some disability. Estimates are that child care provided by the grandparents saves taxpayers over $4 billion a year. Generally, grandparents do not apply for legal custody because this would mean they would have to take parents of the grandchildren to court. Few grandparents become licensed foster care parents or legal guardians (Saisan et al., 2023). Those who do not attain custody are ineligible for certain services and financial support that states provide for licensed foster care parents.

People of all ethnic and income groups face unexpected demands but the incidence is much higher among racial minorities. A greater percentage of Black (26%) and Hispanic (62%) than Asian (24%), or White (13%) children are living with their grandparents (Cohn et al., 2022). Regardless of the reason younger relatives reside with them, these grandparents share a common resolve to do whatever they can to provide a stable and supportive environment for grandchild growth and development (Showalter & McEntyre, 2022).

In 2018 Congress passed the Supporting Grandparents Raising Grandchildren Act of 2018 (Senate Bill 1091, 115th Congress Public Law 196). This legislation established a federal advisory council to support grandparents and other non-parent relatives raising children. The United States Department of Health and Human Services disseminates data about available resources and best practices to assist relative caregivers in meeting mental health and nutritional basics and other concerns for children in their care as well as maintain their own physical and emotional well-being.

Setting New Goals for New Conditions

Some grandparents believe that taking care of a grandchild means losing freedom. They waited a long time for their children to grow up, supposing it would then become possible to pursue personal ambitions. Perhaps they had planned to travel, begin some hobbies, and participate in leisure activities with their spouse and friends. They may have imagined visiting grandchildren once in a while, taking on occasional babysitting, and indulging younger relatives. However, these dreams never materialized because a child could not manage their personal affairs. Even the future might appear uncertain when grandparents are unable to reasonably predict how long they may have to raise someone else's child. Extraordinary demands on their time, energy, and finances can produce sustained stress (Smith & Segal, 2023).

Sometimes grandparents are angry for being placed in a position of having so many things they are expected to do. There are feelings of resentment toward the relatives who created this situation, remorse, guilt about things they may have done wrong as parents, and doubts about their ability to manage their daunting set of responsibilities. Grandma Rose shared her feelings of ambivalence with a grandparent class: "I don't know whether God thought I did a poor job and wanted to give me a second chance or He thought that I did well enough to be given the job one more time. My daughter told me that she could not handle her children anymore and maybe I won't be able to either."

Grandparents experience mixed emotions. On the one hand, they feel sadness for their grandchildren and their personal isolation from friends who do not understand the priority they must assign to their new mission. Some become depressed about having to give up on previous aspirations to become relatively free of continued responsibilities to others. Despite misgivings, surrogate grandparents generally affirm they would follow the same path again to rescue grandchildren and educate them for a successful future (Dolbin-MacNab & Stucki, 2023).

Grandparents who raise their grandchildren should adopt goals to match their new responsibilities. Otherwise, they remain locked in a state of regret and disappointment over being denied the attainment of earlier dreams that are no longer appropriate. A related danger is that grandchildren could feel unwanted and consider themselves an obstacle to grandparent happiness. These youngsters could be better off living with someone else who can make them feel wanted and provide the sense of belonging they need. Foster care can be a more healthy option than being recipients of care that is grudgingly provided by older relatives (McGowen et al., 2006).

Grandchildren exposed to sustained pessimism are at greater risk for feelings of depression and loss of creative capacity to see possibilities, including their own happiness. A sense of optimism is needed to sustain resilience and should be continually reinforced by grandparents who exhibit this positive outlook about life. Grandchildren should be told on a continual basis that helping them grow up is a priority goal and a source of satisfaction (Hayslip & Fruhauf, 2019).

Grandparent and Parent Agreement

Some reports about grandparents raising children are misleading when they imply most of them lack resources. In two-thirds of families where grandparents are the main caregiver, one of the grandchild's parents also live in the same household. This situation commonly arises when unwed teenagers have a baby. Each year about 750,000 adolescent females get pregnant; about 70% of them give birth, and 95% decide to keep their baby (Centers for Disease Control and Prevention, 2022). Most pregnancies (75%) among 15- to 19-year-olds are unplanned (Guttmacher Institute, 2023). Maternal grandmothers most frequently assume obligation for childcare while the young mother continues to attend school or has a job. This situation often produces disputes between the two women as each of them separately attempt to build a close and satisfying relationship with the child.

An example of mother-daughter conflict involves Carmen who got pregnant at 16. Her mother, Esther, agreed to take care of Juan, Carmen's son, so Carmen could study to earn a general education certificate, GED. That was five years ago but Carmen still lives at home. Grandma Esther and grandson Juan spend most of their day together and get along well. When Carmen comes home after work in the evening she is often tired, routinely denies Juan's request to play with him, and sometimes yells at him for behaving in ways she does not approve. This reaction causes Juan to seek comfort from Grandma Esther. Carmen admits this pattern or behavior causes her to feel jealous and guilty for impatience. Sometimes Carmen tries to regain Juan's favor by suspending Esther's rule about no snacks after dinner.

Carmen's behavior resembles non-custodial grandparents who spend too little time with grandchildren. They seldom have obligations to teach or apply discipline. Therefore, they spoil grandchildren instead of encouraging them to grow by reinforcing the rules of parents for good behavior. However, in this family, roles have been reversed. Esther, Juan's grandparent, is the one who is distraught by permissive behavior of her daughter Carmen. Esther believes that since she is the one who takes care of Juan most of the time, Carmen should support the rules Ester has set instead of contradicting them.

Both women should agree on well-defined responsibilities. Such complimentary roles are essential so Juan can benefit from a stable environment, knowing both women love him and have the same expectations of him. One way to increase continuity is by establishing support groups for young parents living in households where grandparents are the main caregivers. Efforts to unite the adult generations are uncommon but have potential to bring greater benefit for everyone than supposing grandparents are the only ones who require a support group.

Grandparents typically have a more mature outlook than young parents:

"My daughter Lisa lives with us. Her 5-year-old son, Bobby, is a good boy who I take care of while Lisa attends college. Bobby's father has not paid support that he was ordered to by the court. Yet, he comes around when it is birthday and holiday time to give Bobby a piñata or other gifts. My daughter becomes angry because Bobby likes his Dad; on the other hand, she wants to tell him, 'Your dad is a jerk.' When Lisa brought this up again last week, my advice to her was, "I realize you feel bad that Bobby is impressed by his Dad even though he is an irresponsible man. In time, Bobby will consider who does the laundry, feeds him, provides daily care, and is available whenever needed – his Mother and Grandma. So, try not to be overly disappointed with Bobby's early conclusions. The time Bobby's father invests in him compared to your own will be evaluated more fairly later on. Remember too, Bobby can use all of the affection he can get right now. Both of us should not say anything hurtful about his dad. Some day Bobby will make up his own mind about the support base he has and realize who can be counted on."

Protection of Children from Parent Abuse

There are times when it is necessary to protect grandchildren from their parents. Children have historically suffered at the hands of parents dependent on alcohol. Currently drugs are a danger in many families. In fact, drug and alcohol abuse along with the related problems of child abuse and neglect are the two most common reasons why grandparents have to bring up grandchildren (Doblin-MacNab & Stucki, 2023). Drug addicts lose their capacity to provide care for children and themselves. The number of parents consuming illegal drugs is unknown but related dangers for children will continue in the future.

When Denise became addicted to cocaine, she left her 8-year-old son Jason with Edith, his grandmother. At the time Edith took charge of Jason she believed that it would be temporary until Denise completed a rehabilitation program. Three years went by without any phone calls or letters. Then, one day Denise unexpectedly showed up at the front door and requested money so she could pursue job training. At first Edith said no because her intuition was the money would be used for drugs. However, after Denise threatened to take Jason with her, Edith relented and withdrew $800 from the bank. Ever since Edith has worried that some day Denise will return to blackmail her again or abduct Jason. It seems the only way to protect Jason's safety and security is to petition the court for legal custody. This will be the most emotionally difficult thing Edith has ever done because she will have to prove to a judge that Denise is an unfit parent. If Edith wins custody she can also lose any possibility of ever restoring a favorable relationship with her daughter. A battle in court will be expensive and likely to deplete funds Edith has been setting aside for retirement.

Grandparent Views About Raising Grandchildren

An online study of 124 primarily White grandmothers consisted of three groups: (a) custodial grandmothers with legal custody of grandchildren, (b) co-resident grandmothers living with grandchildren and one of the parents, and (c) non-resident grandmothers who provided daycare while the parents were employed (McGowen et al., 2006). Two questions included in the survey were: How is raising grandchildren the same and different from bringing up your own children? Have there been changes in the way you behave as a parent now than you did when raising your own children? Only 25% of the grandmothers reported that having been a parent adequately prepared them for what they needed to know about raising grandchildren because growing up and being a parent had changed so much in one generation.

Most reported they were more patient and relaxed with grandchildren than when raising their own children. They felt less anger and frustration and more concern about the needs of the child. A majority spent more time with grandchildren and participating in their activities. While bringing up their own children, different priorities were in place. At that time, they did not do as many things together or listen as much to the children. Now, grandparents agreed, housework can wait because being with children has greater priority.

To understand more about the motivation of grandmothers assuming their role, they were asked: What happened in your child's family that caused you to become the main caretaker of grandchildren? The women expressed 11 reasons for having to become a substitute parent: substance abuse, abandonment/neglect, working parents, immaturity, mental health, domestic violence, divorce, incarceration, financial problems, death, and military service. When neither parent was capable or willing to carry out their role, grandmothers took over. Substance abuse was the most frequent reason followed by abandonment and neglect as a motivation for those who became custodial caretakers. Working parents were the major reason for co-resident and non-resident surrogates to provide daily assistance.

Another survey item asked: How has parenting your grandchild affected quality of life for you? More custodial (49%) than co-resident (29%) participants felt that the task of caring for grandchildren had enriched their life; they were happier because of assuming the obligation. They had a renewed sense of purpose, more joy, and grandchildren helped them remain more active and feeling as though they were younger. In contrast, grandmothers at both levels of care disliked the fact they had less private time, had lost some freedom, and were obliged to sacrifice opportunities to do preferred activities with a spouse or friends. Many had been looking forward to an empty nest and retirement dreams that had to be set aside. There was a common sense of disappointment about isolation and from being able to do things with their friends because of role demands (McGowen et al., 2006).

Grandparents are often exhausted by all the tasks they have to perform. Sometimes, instead of pacing themselves wisely and accepting that certain chores may have to wait, people overlook their health and psychological needs. They fail to realize that their mental fitness and physical stamina must be preserved in order to remain a source of support for grandchildren. It is essential to schedule rest, hobbies, and opportunities to learn. Regular exercise is never enough to counteract depression and build a necessary positive outlook. Learning to handle continuous stress and feeling a sense of control can prevent giving up or becoming abusive (R. D. Strom & Strom, 2018).

Spending time alone while other trusted adults take over to supervise grandchildren can allow reprieve to recover perspective and renew motivation. These goals to gain relief are modest to be able to do errands, attend religious service, see the hairdresser and visit friends. Nevertheless, some grandparents feel that they must forego relief because there are no relatives to help or the ones willing to be care givers are unreliable and cannot be trusted. Free respite care is a service that more religious institutions should provide as part of their outreach mission to meet community needs.

Conclusion

A fundamental value of democracies is permitting everyone to express personal opinion without fear of rejection. Teaching this value becomes important during adolescence when conflicts with adults, especially parents, accelerate as the students struggle to become independent. The emerging ability to monitor logic motivates adolescents to frequently engage adults in disputes. These confrontations can have value because they offer opportunities to practice debating skills needed for constructive conflict. Parents should know that arguments present opportunities to demonstrate problem solving and to show tolerance for opposing views. There is also benefit in modeling self-conflict, allowing daughters and sons to witness how adults examine and judge themselves. The capacity to introspect emerges in adolescence so youth benefit from adoption of healthy criteria for self-evaluation. They also benefit from recognizing this form of assessment is often a key to conflict resolution because reflection can produce changes in personal behavior.

Most parents recognize arguments with adolescents are normal and help to enable their transition to adulthood. Reliance on practical and respectful guidelines to conduct civil conflict can enable everyone in the family to feel comfortable expressing differences while they gain a less narcissistic perspective. Recognizing that disagreement can result in learning and tolerance can motivate mothers and fathers to wisely use this context for teaching lessons youth cannot acquire in other ways. Learning how to disagree is best taught by parents and grandparents.

More grandparents are bringing up grandchildren than ever before. Their success depends on optimism and willingness to adjust by developing appropriate and attainable goals. They should learn how expectations of parents have changed, become a listener to find out grandchild feelings, encourage creativity and reflective thinking, and emphasize self-evaluation for youth. There is a need for parents to understand what teachers expect of parents at home, recognize how to arrange assistance if a child falls behind at school, cooperate with a parent who shares child care responsibilities, know about available community services to access, and get periodic relief from their stress.

Key Concepts

1 Interpreting all disagreements as a competition in which the goal is to defend personal views prevents reflective processing of another person's perspective. Adults should urge adolescents to take time to reflect on opinions that differ from their own and see it as an aspect of appreciating diversity, causing us to change our minds, and adopt new paradigms to guide behavior.

2 Helping teenagers live with disagreement should include adoption of conflict goals, a desire to strive toward their attainment, and willingness to accept feedback on progress from trusted others who observe them often. Giving attention to this aspect of personal development is more important when adults make known conflict goals they want to reach on a more consistent basis.

3 Grandparents should be a source of help during separation and divorce. They may choose to avoid being involved when a relative goes through a divorce.

However, withdrawal denies the parent and grandchildren a source of comfort, encouragement, and continuity when it is needed most. The willingness to listen when relatives are vulnerable to feelings of despair can help to get them through a difficult experience.

4 Know the benefits of expressing differences. Move away from portraying the differences expressed by children as a sign of disrespect toward adults in the family. Listening carefully and expressing differences allows relatives to better understand and learn from one another.

5 Parents and grandparents should be willing to apologize to daughters, sons or others offended. Making amends, asking for forgiveness, and seeking methods of reconciliation to restore harmony in a relationship is a sign of humility and evidence of maturity.

6 Holding on to feelings of resentment and grudges related to conflict is a common obstacle to mental health. By making an effort to restore positive relationships, even if the other party does not reciprocate allows personal growth to continue and can provide a valuable lesson about having a healthy perspective.

7 Grandparents who bring up grandchildren should choose goals that accord with their obligations. Otherwise, they could remain locked in a state of regret and disappointment about being denied a chance to attain earlier chosen dreams that are no longer appropriate.

8 Instead of pacing themselves and accepting that some chores could to be delayed, some grandparents ignore their own health and psychological needs. They should maintain their physical stamina so they can remain a vital source of support for children.

9 Studies of grandparents raising grandchildren have found that, despite the demands of this role, most believe grandchildren have enriched their lives, given them renewed sense of purpose and meaning, provided more joy, kept them more active and feeling younger.

10 Support groups for grandparents should be led by volunteer professionals who help them move through progressive stages of self-disclosure, constructive self-evaluation, and healthy adjustment instead of continual discontent and seeing themselves as victims.

Generational Perspectives Activities

8.1 Team Discussion
8.2 Agenda for Interviews with Parents
8.3 Conversations with Grandchildren about Conflict
8.4 A Scenario: Reasoning and Problem Solving
8.5 Team Chapter Review
8.6 Criteria for Self-Evaluation of Team Members

8.1 Team Discussion

1 Identify the guidelines to manage disputes that would be most helpful for your family.
2 How have peers from separate or divorced families explained the effects it had on them?

3 What topics of conflict have been a continuing focus between you and your parents?
4 What are three goals for living with conflict you are currently trying to pursue?
5 What are your fears about being able to manage conflicts with an intimate partner?
6 Recount your observations of grandparents who had a prominent family influence?
7 What have parents taught you about how to benefit from interpersonal conflicts?
8 How important are apologies following arguments between parents and adolescents?
9 What advice could you suggest for grandparents who become main child caregivers?
10 What lessons about parenting do grandparents seem to learn over time?

8.2 Agenda for Interviews with Parents

1 What topics do you usually disagree about with your children?
2 Why are you afraid of getting involved with family arguments?
3 How did your parents handle disagreements in your presence?
4 What are controversial topics that families should talk about?
5 What advice would you give relatives on managing conflict?
6 Tell a story about a family argument resolved in a poor way.
7 What topics does your family avoid to prevent disagreement?

8.3 Conversations with Grandchildren about Conflict

1 What are some topics that cause you to disagree with your friends?
2 What issues have caused you to break a friendship with someone?
3 What are the most common conflicts that seem to occur at school?
4 Tell a story about how a disagreement that was handled in a good way.
5 How long does it take for you to get over being angry with someone?
6 How do you feel about apologizing after you make a hurtful comment?
7 What are the common disagreements between you and your parents?
8 What conflicts does your family have regarding the use of cell phones?
9 What topics does your age group disagree about with the older people?

8.4 A Scenario: Reasoning and Problem Solving

Problem solving scenarios present an opportunity to look at situations that might happen for a family and think about possible solutions. Your task is to look at pros and cons of choices that are stated, think of additional options, identify relevant information that might be missing, find out how teammates view the alternatives, and defend your reasoning about the advice that you consider best. Joan is a single parent with a son named Troy. She believes that it would be good if third grade Troy could have the benefit of having a male adult to look up for guidance. However, Joan does not want to find a boyfriend so Troy can have his needs met. What should she do?

a ask her father or other male friend to spend time on a regular basis with Troy
b have Troy join a sports team where he will be able to receive male guidance
c consider getting married again so that Troy benefits from having a real father
d ask the principal if Troy can be reassigned to a third grade taught by a man
e other _____

8.5 Team Chapter Review

Efforts to assess participant learning, provide feedback, and improve quality of instruction is enhanced by a group review of each chapter.

1 What ideas in the lesson changed the way I think about this topic?
2 What insights from the lesson will I try to apply in my relationships?
3 What is the most important point for me presented in this lesson?
4 What are some aspects of this lesson I would like to better understand?
5 Which aspects of this lesson do I wish that I had known about earlier?

8.6 Criteria for Self-Evaluation of Team Members

Directions: For each question, place a check beside statements that describe your feelings. You may want to give several answers on some items. If your feelings are not on choices list, write them on the line marked "other."

1 When I disagree with my father or mother

    a we rely on helpful guidelines to conduct conflict
    b I lose my temper and feel bad afterwards
    c I don't want any trouble so probably I say nothing
    d I listen patiently and attempt to be open-minded
    e Other _____

2 My view about learning from conflict situations is

    a I believe that avoiding arguments is the best practice
    b Making my views known is necessary to help others
    c I always want to stay calm even when others do not
    d Getting over effects of an argument are hard on me
    e Other _____

3 Following a disagreement with family members, I usually

    a apologize for any hurt that I may have caused
    b wait for someone to tell me that they are sorry
    c move on and try to put the matter behind me
    d withdraw from a conversation so I can reflect

4 My feeling about single parent families is that

    a community services should be offered to them
    b their relatives should give the help they need
    c they are too dependent upon the government
    d churches should know and meet their needs
    e Other _____

5 I believe that when parents separate or divorce

    a child support groups should be provided at school
    b teachers should modify some of their expectations
    c children usually adjust without negative effects

    d communities should be ready to help as needed

    e Other _____

6 When I observe conflict between my siblings and my parents

    a I wish children would demonstrate respect as they did in the past

    b it is good to see they show willingness to listen to each another

    c I don't like that they have no ground rules for conducting conflict

    d I wonder whether they recognize how to learn from their disputes

    e Other _____

7 The goals for living with conflict that are most important to me are

    a analyzing conditions that are needed to result in mutual reconciliation

    b learning to assert personal opinion without having feelings of guilt

    c apologizing after making any comments that could be seen as hurtful

    d realizing that there might be some differences that are irreconcilable

    e Other _____

8 Couples who are trying to achieve success in a blended family should

    a determine the rules of equity and avoid favoritism of some children

    b inform siblings with different parents they must resolve differences

    c show patience over a long period without expecting appreciation

    d understand developmental stages for each of their stepchildren

    e Other _____

9 I recognize that family conflict can lead to valuable learning because

    a children get to practice emerging debate skills in a safe setting

    b parents find out how to renegotiate relationships with children

    c denial of disagreements cannot result in resolution of problems

    d parents have an opportunity to model patience and maturity

    e Other _____

10 I believe that many parents of adolescent children

    a do not realize how daily hassles can lead to reciprocal learning

    b overlook the importance of youth learning to assert themselves

    c over rate obedience as a quality they should nurture in children

    d tend to blame peers for motivating challenges to family authority

    e Other _____

References

Annie E. Casey Foundation. (2023a, January). *Children in single-parent families by race and ethnicity in United States*. Kids Count Data Center. https://datacenter.aecf.org/data/tables/107-children-in-single-parent-families-by-race-and-ethnicity#detailed/1/any/false/2048/10,11,9,12,1,13/432,431

Annie E. Casey Foundation. (2023b, June 23). *Child well-being in single-parent families*. https://www.aecf.org/blog/child-well-being-in-single-parent-families

Annie E. Casey Foundation. (2023c, June 14). *2023 Kids Count Data Book: State trends in child well-being* (34th ed.). Kids Count Data Center. https://www.aecf.org/resources/2023-kids-count-data-book#State%20Trends%20in%20Overall%20Child%20Well-Being

Bieber, C. (2023, August 9). Leading causes of divorce: 43% report lack of family support. *Forbes Advisor.* https://www.forbes.com/advisor/legal/divorce/common-causes-divorce/

Branje, S. (2018, January). Development of parent-adolescent relationships: Conflict interactions as a mechanism of change. *Child Development Perspectives, 12*(3), 171–176. 10.1111/cdep.12278

Carter, C. (2020). *The new adolescence: Raising happy and successful teens in an age of anxiety and distraction.* Benbella Books.

Centers for Disease Control and Prevention. (2022). *About teenage pregnancy.* https://www.cdc.gov/teenpregnancy/about/index.htm

Chamie, J. (2023). America's single parent families. In J. Chamie, *Population levels, trends, and differentials* (pp. 197–199). Springer. 10.1007/978-3-031-22479-9_42

Cohn, D., Horowitz, J., Minkin, R., Fry, R., & Hurst, K. (2022, March 24). *The demographics of multigenerational households.* Pew Research Center. https://www.pewresearch.org/social-trends/2022/03/24/the-demographics-of-multigenerational-households/

Dolbin-MacNab, M., & Stucki, B. D. (2023). *Grandparents raising grandchildren.* American Association for Marriage and Family Therapy. https://www.aamft.org/Consumer_Updates/grandparents.aspx#:~:text=Being%20raised%20by%20a%20grandparent,cultural%20identity%20community%20ties

Generations United (2023). *Generations United 2023 Conference.* https://www.gu.org/projects/global-intergenerational-conference/

Guttmacher Institute. (2023). *Teen pregnancy.* https://www.guttmacher.org/united-states/teens/teen-pregnancy?gad=1&gclid=EAIaIQobChMI9Je7_qX__gIVuTLUAR3r3g7GEAAYAiAAEgKsgfD_BwE

Hayslip, Jr., B., & Fruhauf, C. (Eds.). (2019). *Grandparenting: Influences on the dynamics of family relationships* (pp. 159–178). Springer.

Kearney, M. S. (2023). *The two-parent privilege.* University of Chicago Press.

McGowen, M., Ladd, L., & Strom, R. D. (2006). On-line assessment of grandmother experience in raising grandchildren. *Educational Gerontology, 32*(8), 669–684. 10.1080/03601270500494048

National Institute of Drug Abuse. (2023, February 9). *Drug overdose death rates.* https://nida.nih.gov/research-topics/trends-statistics/overdose-death-rates

National Telecommunications and Information Administration. (2023, May 17). Biden-Harris administration announces nearly $5 million in Internet for all grants to tribal lands. Broadband USA. https://broadbandusa.ntia.doc.gov/news/latest-news/biden-harris-administration-announces-nearly-5-million-internet-all-grants-tribal#:~:text=WASHINGTON%20%E2%80%93%20The%20Department%20of%20Commerce's,Broadband%20Connectivity%20Program%20(TBCP)

Ripley, A. (2022). *High conflict: Why we get trapped and how we get out.* Simon & Schuster.

Romero, S. (2021, May 21). Navajo Nation becomes the largest tribe in the U.S. after the pandemic enrollment surge. *The New York Times.* https://www.nytimes.com/2021/05/21/us/navajo-cherokee-population.html#:~:text=the%20main%20story-,Navajo%20Nation%20Becomes%20Largest%20Tribe%20in%20U.S.%20After%20Pandemic%20Enrollment,Cherokee%20Nation's%20to%20nearly%20400%2C000

Saisan, J., Segal, J., & Reid, S. (2023). *Legal and custody help for grandparents raising grandkids.* Helpguide. https://helpguide.org/articles/aging-issues/legal-and-custody-help-for-grandparents-raising-grandkids.htm

Showalter, S., & McEntyre, M. (2022). *The mindful grandmother: The art of loving our children's children.* Broadway Books.

Silversmith, S. (2022, September 8). *Arizona tribes will get $106 million to boost broadband access.* AZMIRROR. https://www.azmirror.com/2022/09/08/arizona-tribes-will-get-106-million-to-boost-broadband-access/

Smith, M., & Segal, J. (2023, April 10). *Grandparents raising grandchildren*. Helpguide. https://www.helpguide.org/articles/parenting-family/grandparents-raising-grandchildren.htm

Strom, R. D., & Strom, P. S. (2018). Education for grandparents in longevity societies. *Journal of Adult and Continuing Education, 24*(2), 208–228. 10.1177/1477971418810652

Supporting Grandparents Raising Grandchildren Act of 2018, Pub. L. No. 115–196, 1511 Stat. (2018). https://www.congress.gov/bill/115th-congress/senate-bill/1091/text

United States Census Bureau. (2022, November 22). *Mothers maintain 80% of single-parent family groups*. https://www.census.gov/newsroom/press-releases/2022/americas-families-and-living-arrangements.html

United States Census Bureau. (2023). *National single parent day: March 21, 2023*. https://www.census.gov/newsroom/stories/single-parent-day.html

Williams, T. (2011). *The collective plays of Tennessee Williams*. Library of America. (Original work published 1944)

Part III

Retirement Age (Ages 60–80)

9 Peer Norms and Productive Aging

Demographic Change and Maturity

Population Increase of Older Adults

Motivating mature behavior in retirement is a goal of the International Longevity Centre Global Alliance (2023). This consortium made up of research centers in 17 countries carry out independent studies to support physical and mental health opportunities of aging adults. The first Longevity Center was established in 1990 by Robert Butler (2008). He was the founder of the National Institute on Aging in 1975 and the first physician to organize a Department of Geriatrics in an American Medical School at Columbia University in 1982.

When the Population Reference Bureau of the United States forecast that the population of retirees would soon increase on an unprecedented scale, Butler (2008) recognized the need to modify prevailing expectations for retirement so a mature lifestyle could become the new norm. He observed that maturity is shown when someone demonstrates a concern for the well-being of others. If, instead retirees are concerned only about their age group, this is self-centeredness or narcissism. Butler posed these questions: "How might older persons be awakened and become engaged responsibly in the present, building a worthy epitaph to the future? How might they be mobilized to found a movement dedicated to various forms of social engagement? This is the true challenge" (Butler, 2008, p. 398).

Fast forward to 2024. We could wish happy birthday to 10,000 Americans born in 1959 who become 65 years old today. The same birthday wish will be appropriate tomorrow and each day thereafter until the year 2030. By then all baby boomers (born between 1946 and 1964) will be older than age 65. A short time later, in 2035, the population of older adults will outnumber children for the first time in the nation's history (Vespa et al., 2020).

Identity Status During Retirement

Most people experience a change in identity when they retire. What matters most is how individuals evaluate themselves and the importance they assign to their family and community status. Two factors can prevent conditions that are needed for a sense of purpose and self-esteem. The first factor implicates disability, possibly becoming a burden for relatives. This could mean being assigned a social status lacking role reciprocity and having nothing to trade with younger family members in return for care provided by them. If retirees, because of age, are defined as having nothing of value to exchange, then

DOI: 10.4324/9781003401261-13

any claims they make for assistance may be seen by them as evidence of dependency and motivate feelings of guilt (R. D. Strom & Strom, 2020).

The second factor to detract from self-worth is a retreat from responsibility. Older people in primitive cultures are expected to continue making a contribution to society. Whether they are collectively seen as having something of value to trade is a matter of cultural definition. Unless they are disabled, older adults have reasonable tasks they are expected to perform and, as a result, by definition, are perceived as possessing something of worth to trade. It is essential that all the generations agree this arrangement provides benefits for the entire society (Bentley & O'Brien, 2017).

Generational Reciprocity in Modern Society

The concept of role reciprocity has long been applied in non-industrialized environments. But, can technological societies establish expectations that incorporate talents of older adults? The answer depends on how deeply committed the American public is to a youth-oriented, anti-aging perspective. When older adults find themselves ignored by younger generations, some of them move to age-segregated communities where peers support the feeling of being appreciated and understood. If society wants young people to value their heritage, aspire to become mature individuals, and prepare for their own aging, then communication with older relatives and friends would seem to be essential. Adolescents and young adults can benefit from the advice of older relatives to maximize emotional growth for building relationships that are durable and satisfying (R. D. Strom & Strom, 2021).

If Americans look at longevity as requiring long-term adaptability, later life can be seen as concluding with a sense of integrity, wisdom, and maturity that should be shared with younger generations. Looking at life through this lens, as a whole, makes it possible to transition from an anti-aging quest to a society where older adults are valued for mature behavior. Men and women should go beyond retirement expectations set by previous generations who had a shorter lifespan.

Maturity in Later Life

The need for everyone to pursue maturity in retirement was described by Aldous Huxley (1932/2017) in his science fiction novel *Brave New World*. The future society Huxley envisioned had created a scientific breakthrough that delayed many physical signs which come with growing old. In this anti-aging environment, wanting to appear younger and constantly pursing personal pleasure had become universal goals. When older adults could no longer hide the effects of their aging, they experienced humiliation and were taken to special hospitals established to supervise their death.

Huxley's frightening forecast was intended as a warning about the possible consequences that could occur if the development of technology was to become the highest priority for society without an equivalent emphasis on the development of human potential for maturity. As Huxley looked ahead, he anticipated people would come to adore technologies that undo their capacity to think. He recognized that a humane and equitable society would enable older adults to retain a sense of purpose, knowing that feeling useless is the most severe shock the human system can endure.

Fulfilling a desire to be needed during retirement depends on attitudes and behaviors that generate respect from younger people. A challenge for longevity societies is to convince retirees that members of other generations need them. They should manage time wisely so their schedule focuses on helping younger generations as well as satisfying their personal interests. Adopting this orientation is a proven way to prevent the otherwise predictable tragedy of feeling useless.

Education and Productive Aging

Content for Adult Education

A longer period of retirement than ever before in history presents a need to motivate people to sustain personal growth, avoid the danger of becoming self-centered, and believing that because their years of employment have been completed, they no longer have the same responsibilities as is the case for younger relatives. Education for maturity is a lifelong process, different from the formal learning of shorter duration focused on preparation for work or upgrading employment skills. A key concept guiding the helping professions is called *productive aging* (Butler, 2008). This concept recognizes older adults are still physically and mentally capable of contributing to society, the time between beginning of retirement and onset of frailty is being extended, and most individuals want an active life that provides them a sense of purpose and satisfaction.

There is substantial evidence that older adults remain capable of learning. However, the literature describing aging does not identify the content of learning to expect of older men and women in societies experiencing rapid social change and transformation of family roles. The strategy relied on to design education for children, adolescents, and young adults begins with the formation of a curriculum to equip them with competencies they will need for employment. In a similar way adult education should orient older relatives with the lives of younger generations. Retirees generally suppose lifelong learning means each individual should decide the curriculum best for them. This avoidance of relevant education focused on their own family prevents older adults from understanding how they might help younger relatives grow, achieve their potential, and adjust to the demands of changing times.

Younger family members are the most credible sources of judgment about the strengths and learning needs of older adults. Asking parents and grandchildren to identify knowledge they think older relatives should learn remains a missing and essential element in the wise design for adult education. Older adults are aware of some of their personal assets and limitations but some of their other deficiencies are bound to be overlooked when education is strictly self-determined. A more accurate way to assess strengths and learning needs of older adults is to compare observations of their behavior as perceived by three generations (grandparents, parents, and grandchildren). When such data is used to shape their education older adults learn about younger relatives and make changes that improve personal influence. Studies by Robert Strom and Strom (2016, 2017, 2021) of multiple generations across cultures have led to the conclusion that the scope of lifelong learning should reflect a common need to understand, strengthen, and protect families. Grandparents recognize many families are fragile, require more support from within, and need greater assistance to become more resilient. Mothers and fathers often need relief from an overload of responsibilities, breakdown of marital relationships, and the erosion of mature guidance to support child and adolescent development. Expectations for grandparents should shift to match contemporary conditions. Their revised role should be clearly defined, include a sense of purpose, and engage their talents to support the mental health of younger relatives.

Mission of Community Volunteers

Retirees should consider themselves as a work in progress, talented individuals with time to help improve the quality of life for relatives, community, and nation. Consider the example of Bill Conrad. One day Bill saw the American flag flying upside down at Arrowhead Elementary School across the street from his home in Phoenix, Arizona. As a retired policeman Bill knew that flying a flag upside down is meant to be a distress signal. Bill decided he would meet with the school principal to find out what was wrong. After the principal was made aware of Bill's observation, he asked Bill to teach the 6th graders how to carry out their flag raising protocol. A few days later Bill returned to the principal's office, this time wanting to know whether there was anything else he and his wife Margaret could do to serve the school. Soon Margaret was tutoring 1st graders in reading, and Bill helped 5th graders in mathematics.

Before long the faculty invited Margaret to become the coordinator of senior volunteers, a new, unpaid but important position. Together Bill and Margaret went house to house around the neighborhood seeking to recruit potential older adult volunteers. They visited churches, senior centers, and fraternal organizations to invite participation in the education of children. The recruitment effort paid off when all 40 of the Arrowhead school classrooms had at least one volunteer scheduled for every day. When asked to discuss the motivation of retired men and women whose efforts she coordinated, Margaret said, "There are great rewards for volunteers. The more people invest in this activity, the more they receive. As they help and encourage children, it is not long until they receive affection in return. This gives a reason to get up in the morning, knowing that I am going to spend time with children. And you feel useful, an important self-impression for those of us who are old."

When retirees decide to become classroom volunteers, most are uncertain about what to expect. This is the reason why, in the beginning, each volunteer should be engaged with several optional placements to try out before being asked to decide the particular task they would like to continue doing. Some of the tasks include listening to children read, checking and correcting homework, tutoring students with deficiencies in reading and mathematics, leading discussion groups, shelving books in the library, and supervising the playground before school and at recess. What matters most is that volunteers feel comfortable, receive positive feedback, decide the amount of time they want to devote to volunteering, and know they can request a change in assignment whenever they wish (R. D. Strom & Strom, 2020).

Projected Changes for Older Adult Housing

The Joint Center for Housing Studies of Harvard University (2019) projects that by 2038, households age 80 and over (the fastest-growing age group) will number 17.5 million and account for 12% of all households. The number of residents in nursing homes and assisted living are expected to decline because of the high costs, and also because residential real estate developers will become more responsive to a growing older-age market, building homes better designed to accommodate their limitations. Older people will require zero-step entrances, single floor homes, wide hallways and doorways to allow for wheelchairs, lever-style handles, robotic assistance, and electronic controls. These future norms represent only 1% of the housing presently available.

Another option for older adult housing that reflects one in five American families is a multigenerational household. This configuration most often serves low-income, minority, and immigrant families. Most older adults living in this arrangement say it is a positive experience because it is convenient and rewarding. About 25% admit it can be stressful, especially among adult children living with a parent. The source of appeal varies but generally involves saving money by sharing expenses, access to supervision for young children, division of household chores, greater awareness of perceptions held by other generations, and providing emotional support and security during times of trouble like divorce, separation, unemployment, and incarceration (Cohn et al., 2022a, 2022b; Henig, 2018).

Attitudes about Independence and Interdependence

Older adults were taught from an early age to equate self-respect with independence and to think of dependence, except among young children and the disabled, as evidence of personal weakness. Consequently, many older people experience conflict within themselves. Yet, even the most steadfast advocates of independence, if they live long enough, will experience disability and require help that should not be interpreted as proof of personal failure or encourage shame of becoming a burden. Merging independence and interdependence is an attitude shift that implicates all of the generations in a longevity society. This essential outlook that is currently being taught in schools should also become a vital element of adult education.

Influence of Peer Norms

Age Expectations

Adolescents and young adults may suppose life in a retirement community would be uniform, dull, and depressing. People age 50 and over generally have a favorable impression about living in a community populated mostly by their peers (Senior Lifestyle, 2023a, 2023b). To account for differences in perceptions about how older and younger people view age-segregated living, it is necessary to take into account the loss in roles, norms, and reference groups that accompany aging.

Children are often reminded to "act your age." This advice implies that, at least during the formative years, there are common expectations from which departure will be disapproved. In early adulthood people generally substitute their occupational expectations as a guide. Later, in retirement, many find themselves for the first time lacking a peer reference group. As a result, to be without norms is to be alone in the worst sense because people are unaware of suitable criteria to use for self-evaluation. This is especially important in retirement when the meager knowledge people have about aging supports fear. To be old and lack norms is to wonder: Do others my age experience the same physical problems? Am I different or average for my age group? Reliance on physicians as a source of information about peer norms is shown by a high frequency of visits by older patients who lack evidence of organic disease (Segal et al., 2018).

Loss of Roles and Norms

For some people the loss of roles and norms can be fatal. This danger was first identified by Emile Durkheim (1897/2018), founder of the sociology department at University of Paris in France. He wanted to find out why individuals commit suicide. Durkheim concluded the most plausible reasons for self-destruction were intense loneliness, combined with the lack of clear expectations that resulted from having marginal social status. Many of the 50,000 suicides that occur in the United States each year are attributed to loss of roles, norms, and reference groups. It is more than coincidence that suicide rate increases significantly after the age of 75, especially among white males (De Leo, 2022; Kautzman-East & Joseph, 2020). Risk factors for suicide in older adults include depression due to bereavement or loss of physical health and independence.

If normlessness contributes to self-destructive behavior, what can be done to compensate for the inevitable loss in roles that people experience at the time of retirement? Gerontologists contend that age-segregated housing can be an effective solution. Older adults living in typical neighborhoods, referred to as "aging in place", are relatively disadvantaged because of a lack of roles, peer interactions, and access to normative expectations. Because older adults have fewer norms to guide their behavior, one way to increase norms is deliberately create an age reference group through residential concentration. By bringing older adults together, a retirement community becomes valuable for socialization, especially for determining individual expectations that are age-appropriate (Aronson, 2019).

Appeal of Retirement Communities

The public is poorly informed about the benefits of retirement communities. One-third of people over age 55 live in age-segregated housing. In this context, one of our research projects began by offering free courses on topics such as aging, health, and relationships to residents of Sun City and Sun City West, retirement communities just outside Phoenix, Arizona (R. D. Strom & Strom, 2017). Graduate students from education, psychology, nursing, and social work accompanied us each week in a university van to monitor the dynamics of classes that we provided in community centers, churches, and synagogues. The student task was to record small group discussions of the retirees and conduct structured interviews with them. These collaborative experiences led to valuable insights about life in an age-segregated community. For example, everyone who is able-bodied is expected to participate in a range of social interaction and physical fitness opportunities. The amenities include golf, swimming, walking tracks, bowling, bike paths, and exercise alternatives. Residents feel responsible to continually motivate and remind one another to avoid the dangers associated with a sedentary schedule. This constructive peer pressure reinforces healthy habits and supports a wellness orientation. The community maintains a sheriff's posse composed of volunteer residents who daily patrol the streets and report observations of potentially dangerous activities to the police department. This surveillance initiative to support safety means there is less criminal activity than other towns in the area. When residents experience illness, they go to nearby outstanding health care institutions, such as the Banner Del Webb Medical Center and Banner Boswell Hospital staffed by geriatric specialists who have extensive experience in the treatment of older adult patients. When residents require other assistance, they know neighborhood volunteers can be counted on. If individuals became ill or frail, assisted living and long-term care facilities are available in the same community.

The high priority assigned to health and wellness is complemented by community efforts to develop a social network of peers. Mental stimulation classes are commonly recognized as a form of protection against dementia and cognitive decline. Fashion remains a concern in old age reflected by local clothing stores that feature styles preferred by older adults. The cost of housing is appealing because a single developer can build many homes in one location for a lower cost. Younger relatives are allowed to visit for up to two weeks. Retirement community residents have less often been divorced and are more financially advantaged.

Friendship and Emotional Ties

Having friendships and strong emotional ties forecast increased longevity. In 2018, the United Kingdom created a new government cabinet position, Minister for Loneliness (John, 2018). Later, Japan established a similar cabinet role as Minister of Loneliness (Tokyo, 2021). These appointments were not intended as a solution but instead to increase public awareness about risks associated with a seldom recognized major health problem (Holt-Lunstad, 2021; Holt-Lunstad, et al., 2015). People who retire in place, stay in their own home, are less likely to experience a high level of social engagement common among retirement community residents (National Academies of Sciences, Engineering, and Medicine, 2020; National Institute on Aging, 2019).

The National Social Life, Health, and Aging Project is a longitudinal study intended to identify crucial social aspects that could postpone mortality (American Sociological Association, 2016). More than 3,000 people born between 1920 and 1947 were interviewed in 2006 when they were ages 57–85 and again in 2011, at ages 62–90. A third wave was completed in 2016 when participants were ages 67–95. Subjects were asked to identify up to five close confidants, describe each relationship in detail, and tell how close they felt to each confidant. Excluding spouses, participants averaged three confidants and reported benefits. At the start of the study, most were married, in good health, and not lonely.

Iveniuk and Schumm reported results of the longitudinal study that close family relations were more important than friendships in extending lifespan (American Sociological Association, 2016). Persons extremely close to family, other than their spouses, had a 6% risk of dying over the next five years compared with 14% among peers who reported not being close to their relatives. The factors most consistently associated with reduced mortality that mattered about the same extent were (a) being married, (b) having a larger size network, (c) greater involvement with social organizations, and (d) feeling closer to confidants. People are more likely to move in and out of someone's social network, especially if a person is difficult to be around. However, family seems more important because the members are expected to take care of us when it is necessary. Everyone can choose their friends but it is the people we cannot choose and have no option about choosing us that seem to provide the greatest contribution to a lengthy lifespan. Family relationships can sometimes be troublesome. However, forgiveness is possible and so is the recognition that maturity is shown by repeated efforts to engage in reconciliation.

Remembering Regrets

Regrets – "I've had a few … ."

Frank Sinatra (1915–1998) recorded a song that became well-known "I Did It My Way." The lyrics declare, "Regrets, I've had a few, but then again too few to mention." This impression does not match the experience of most people who often recall personal failures of the past and consequences that continue to disappoint them, motivate feelings of remorse, and can be painful to review (Stanley, 2020). Regrets are negative self-judgments that cause us to blame ourselves for bad decisions that we made or choices we should have made but chose not to.

Regret is a powerful but seldom acknowledged source of motivation to benefit from past mistakes and failures instead of taking the easier pathway of attempting to deny or ignore them. Actor John Barrymore (1882–1942) commented, "A man is not old until regrets take the place of dreams" (n.d.). When older people review their personal history, their poor choices and missed opportunities are a focus of regret that can undermine the pursuit of further maturity. Everyone can remember actions that they wish had not been taken such as disappointing love affairs, poor financial investments, or loss of relationships because another person was mistreated. These are regrets of commission, feeling bad about certain things that we have done.

Actions people wish they had taken but, at the time, chose not to are regrets of omission. Such regrets include not pursuing opportunities to get more education, failing to show compassion for someone known to be in need, failing to show appreciative feedback to a spouse about behavior or not trying hard enough to preserve a marriage. When older adults have been asked to talk about their greatest regrets, it is the actions that they failed to take, regrets of omission, that are most often mentioned. In his poem "Maud Muller", John Greenleaf Whittier (1854/1912) summarized this familiar experience stating, "Of all sad words of tongue and pen, the saddest are these: "It might have been!" (Line 105).

Short and Long-Term Effects of Regrets

Differences have been found in short-term and long-term impressions of regret. Initially, regrets about inappropriate actions that were taken appear more painful. But, regrets of inaction persist over a longer period and ultimately are judged to be the greater source of disappointment. This pattern is confirmed as people identify what they would do differently if it were possible to go through life again. A greater proportion of responses involved the things people wished they had done than actions they wished had not been taken. Regrets that are reported most often are consequences of inaction such as not spending enough time with relatives, not showing greater assertion in intimate relationships, and not taking risks to enable greater personal development.

Researchers Morrison and Roese (2011) at Northwestern University surveyed 370 retired men and women. The most commonly reported source of regret focused on romance. About 44% of the women surveyed expressed romantic regrets, compared to 19% of the men. This difference might reflect a greater inclination by men to replace lost relationships more quickly with new partners.

Does the observation that greater regret is experienced for things people failed to do than for actions they took apply only to ordinary folks or to the most capable people as well? To find out, researchers examined regrets for a population of geniuses. These 381 men and 331 women, identified in childhood as in the top 2% of the population by having IQs above 140, looked back from an average age of 74. They were asked to explain things they would have done differently if given another chance. Their answers resembled those of less talented peers. Their regrets most often focused on failure to persist in pursuing more formal education, even though 70% were college graduates compared to 8% of peers in their age cohort, and work harder to attain goals, even though 85% of men had professional or managerial positions (Gilovich & Medvec, 1995).

By a ratio of 4 to 1, the older genius's reported regrets focused mostly about their failure to engage in particular actions, avoid taking certain risks. On reflection, they would have been more assertive, paid more attention to preserving and building social relationships, spent more time with their family, been a better parent, taken up a hobby, engaged more often in community affairs, and married after being divorced or suffering death of a spouse. As for the regrets about actions taken, some felt they should not have married at such a young age, not been a smoker, not given such high priority to their job, not made poor financial decisions, not had extramarital affairs, and not been divorced. Some regretted growing old instead of viewing their extended lifespan as a great privilege that many people are denied (Gilovich & Ross, 2016).

Regrets about Parent Behavior

Many regrets vividly recalled by older adults originated during middle age in their role as parents. Some common and foolish actions of parents include showing anger and using poor judgment during conflicts with adolescent daughters and sons, showing lack of trust in relatives, and expressing a pessimistic outlook about situations and the future. There are also regrets that stem from inaction, things parents failed to do but later wished they had done. These risks included allowing daughters and sons to set more of their own goals, being available to listen to children about their experiences, playing with the whole family, having conversations about matters of importance, apologizing to their children after personal misbehavior, showing patience and flexibility in relationships, and carrying through on priorities that we said matter most to us. Most parents should expect that they too will experience regrets but can minimize them by investing greater time and attention to the development of durable, authentic, and satisfying relationships with relatives (Stanley, 2020).

Processing Regrets

People should not allow regrets to define them, permit disappointments to be the only outcomes that are associated with unpleasant memories. Instead, regrets should be seen as lessons that can generate a resolve to currently take particular risks while also avoiding others. Expressing feelings and opinions to younger relatives, asking them for advice, attending classes on family relationships, volunteering in schools, teaching religious beliefs by example, supporting gender equity in domestic tasks, and sharing financial assets with relatives are among many risks worth taking. There are also risks to avoid such as refusing to forgive someone, discounting the value of methods parents rely on to raise children in the current environment, and spending excessive time on personal leisure while ignoring chances to become a more supportive family member.

Memories are one of the greatest gifts mankind has been given; they enable us to relive a particular moment over and over. Some benefits of memories are forming a relationship with a loved one, inspiring others, increasing productivity, and becoming happier because of having positive memories. To review, regret is a negative emotion that could be beneficial if it causes someone to learn from their mistakes and act in a more wise and beneficial way. Continually focusing on regrets when nothing can be done to modify bygone situations or events can undermine health (Greenberg, 2012, 2017). (See Table 9.1.)

Table 9.1 My Regrets – Can I Learn From My Mistakes?

Remember situations you would hope to avoid repeating if similar circumstances arose again and events where you took no action but would do so now if given another chance. These are regrets of *commission*, feeling bad about certain things that you have done. Actions you wish had been taken but at the time chose not to are regrets of *omission*. Reflecting on your regrets can be helpful to improve behavior now and in the future.

1 I would have stayed in school longer.
2 I would have chosen a different career.
3 I would have worked harder at my job.
4 I would have nurtured more friendships.
5 I would have traveled to more places.
6 I would have married someone else.
7 I would have worried less about things.
8 I would have saved more for retirement.
9 I would have helped my parents more.
10 I would have engaged more in fitness.
11 I would have tried to be a better parent.
12 I would have valued my spouse more.
13 I would have spent more time with family.
14 I would have improved my personality.
15 I would have known my relatives better.
16 I would have been more religious.
17 I would have used time more wisely.
18 I would have been more forgiving.
19 I would have been more optimistic.
20 I would have helped others more often.

A Conversation on Processing Regrets

Scene: Howard and John are having a conversation in the lounge of their long-term care center.

Howard: You know, in some ways I envy George.

John: Why would you say something so ridiculous?

Howard: Of course, I recognize his dementia interferes with being able to remember and that is a tragedy. On the other hand, George's situation also means he is not troubled in the way I am by memories of past situations I still regret.

John: But, you are still capable of recognizing opportunities that can support morale of other people. Everyone is guilty of some things they chose not to do and behaviors they wish had never happened. What if we were only able to remember our pleasant experiences? How would that be helpful? Wouldn't it keep us from thinking about behaviors we can still improve?

Howard: I guess you're right. However, my conversations with other residents here have led me to conclude that while disappointments based on past behavior are long lasting, this does not necessarily motivate personal improvement. I wish there was a way to help older people process their regrets in a manner that could stimulate greater advance in maturity.

John: When I look at certain people in this facility, like Mary, who spent her whole life helping others and continues to model compassion, I feel like telling her, "Mary, I wish I had your memories."

Howard: Maybe we should think of ways that would help people re-process their personal information in a non-traditional manner with the goal of supporting greater wellness. Let's try to imagine a creative protocol that could help make processing regrets a more health-enhancing experience.

Conclusion

Relatives, friends, educators, clergy, cultural icons, social media, and civic leaders should collectively encourage older adults to adopt the concept of productive aging as a guide for living. Retirees should be expected to respond to the needs of others while they are viable in exchange for care most are likely to need when they become frail or disabled. A related shift is to persuade men and women to link their commitment to independence with interdependence. This practical outlook can enable older adults to realize that the care others provide them is not evidence of their failure but the natural reciprocal exchange with an older generation that has served society as long as possible.

Educators at all levels of schooling should implement curriculum that fits a well-defined societal vision of lifelong learning. This instruction should begin during adolescence when the emergence of ideals is common and students become capable of looking ahead to their longevity. The scope of adult education should include learning ways to strengthen and protect families, productive aging, role reciprocity, importance of social interaction, and volunteerism. These activities can motivate maturity guided by a schedule that includes time for self-interest activities and time to help younger generations attain their goals. Success in a longevity society requires that every age group becomes aware of and responsive to the priority goals and concerns of five generations. Continuous development of maturity should become a major purpose for life-long learning to foster reciprocal caring, motivate collaboration, and establish satisfying relationships across age groups.

Key Concepts

1 The population growth of older adults (age 60+) is greater than for the younger age groups. A longer retirement presents unprecedented challenges for individuals, families, health care providers, assisted living and long-term care facilities, adult educators, policy makers, employers, schools, and religious institutions.
2 Two factors combine to diminish a sense of purpose and meaning during retirement. One factor is anticipation of losing independence; the other is ignoring continuing responsibility to support well-being of others in the community. Everyone benefits when retirees volunteer in hospitals, schools, community agencies, and non-profit organizations.
3 If Americans are willing to view human development as some cultures do, life can be seen as concluding with a sense of integrity, wisdom, and maturity. When all stages from birth to death are valued instead of only the years of youth and employment, a more favorable view of society can emerge that allows everyone to be treated with respect and kindness.
4 The mental stimulation that accompanies conversations with students at school can promote new ideas, encourage sustained optimism, and counteract loneliness and social isolation. Volunteering at school also supports learning how a grandchild's peer group sees things.
5 The advantages provided by older volunteers should be widely understood and appreciated. Because more than 80% of mothers of school age children are employed,

retired persons have become the main source of an estimated three million volunteers in classrooms.

6 Peer norms remain influential in later life. Healthy norms help continue growth of maturity expressed by responding to the needs of others rather than being self-absorbed and disconnected from continued responsibilities toward relatives, the community, and nation.

7 Middle age adults recognize their obligation to ensure daughters and sons receive the education they need to prepare for employer expectations. In turn, parents should be advocates for suitable education of grandparents so they can adjust to their transforming family role and be a model for younger relatives.

8 Allow your memories of regrets to become a source of motivation so you recognize and take advantage of opportunities for self-improvement. Much can be gained from mistakes that have been made and poor judgment that turned out to be expensive. When such failures are seen as lessons, the focus shifts from wishing actions could be undone or not taken to planning ways to manage related situations in the present and future.

9 Adolescents invited to share observations can help parents and grandparents detect their learning deficiencies and provide insights that can guide reflection about self-evaluation. When teenagers are respected observers whose views can contribute to adult development, this relationship motivates youth to accept reciprocal observations and criticism about their behavior.

10 Retirement communities provide unique benefits to residents. Peer influence places high priority on maintaining health by regular exercise, development of social networks, access to continued learning, reciprocal caring for neighbors, age-appropriate norms of behavior, access to geriatric care, and sense of community.

Generational Perspectives Activities

9.1 Team Discussion
9.2 Interview Parents or Grandparents About Their Regrets
9.3 Agenda for Interview with Grandparents
9.4 A Scenario: Reasoning and Problem Solving
9.5 Team Chapter Review
9.6 Criteria for Self-Evaluation of Older Adults

9.1 Team Discussion

1 How do you suppose the quality of life will change when you retire?
2 What should families expect of their older relatives after they retire?
3 What do you suppose will happen to the social security system in the future?
4 How could schools and churches better connect older and younger people?
5 Why do you suppose some older adults volunteer for their community?
6 Why do you think people find living in a retirement community appealing?
7 What things could people your age do to improve education of older adults?
8 What should older adults learn to help them better adjust to social change?

9 What personal qualities do you want to retain when you are an old person?

10 What are some lessons that you would like retired people to teach you?

9.2 Interview Parents or Grandparents About Their Regrets

Remember situations you would hope to avoid repeating if similar circumstances arose again and events where you took no action but would do so now if given another chance. These are regrets of *commission*, feeling bad about certain things that you have done. Actions you wish had been taken but at the time chose not to are regrets of *omission*. Reflecting on your regrets can be helpful to improve behavior now and in the future.

1 I would have stayed in school longer.
2 I would have chosen a different career.
3 I would have worked harder at my job.
4 I would have nurtured more friendships.
5 I would have traveled to more places.
6 I would have married someone else.
7 I would have worried less about things.
8 I would have saved more for retirement.
9 I would have helped my parents more.
10 I would have engaged more in fitness.
11 I would have tried to be a better parent.
12 I would have valued my spouse more.
13 I would have spent more time with family.
14 I would have improved my personality.
15 I would have known my relatives better.
16 I would have been more religious.
17 I would have used time more wisely.
18 I would have been more forgiving.
19 I would have been more optimistic.
20 I would have helped others more often.

9.3 Agenda for Interview with Grandparents

1 What expectations do you think society should have for people who are retired?
2 What are some regrets that you continue to have looking back on your lifetime?
3 What are some advantages and disadvantages of living in a retirement community?
4 How could being a classroom volunteer become more popular for older adults?
5 What regrets do you have about your performance as a parent or a grandparent?
6 How could religious institutions stimulate more intergenerational conversation?
7 What efforts have you made to spend some time with widowed women or men?
8 Who do you turn to when loneliness and social isolation seem difficult to bear?
9 What could be done to help assisted living residents cope with their loneliness?
10 How could life in retirement become a more mentally healthy experience?

9.4 A Scenario: Reasoning and Problem Solving

Problem solving scenarios present an opportunity to look at situations that might happen for a family and think about possible solutions. Your task is to think about the pros and cons of stated choices, generate additional options, identify relevant information that might be missing, find out how teammates view alternatives, and defend reasoning about advice you consider best.

Marilyn's husband died, her children live in another state, and she is unable to care for the house and property by herself. She wonders whether to consider an assisted living facility. What is your advice for Marilyn?

a Tour the facility with a friend and then consider the advantages and disadvantages.
b Tell your children about visiting the facility and ask them if they have any advice.
c Hire a lawn service and home cleaning service so that she can remain at home.
d Talk to your minister or church group to learn their experience with this facility.
e Other _____

9.5 Team Chapter Review

Efforts to assess participant learning, provide feedback, and improve quality of instruction is enhanced by a group review of each chapter.

1 What ideas in the lesson changed the way I think about this topic?
2 What insights from the lesson will I try to apply in my relationships?
3 What is the most important point for me presented in this lesson?
4 What are some aspects of this lesson I would like to better understand?
5 Which aspects of this lesson do I wish that I had known about earlier?

9.6 Criteria for Self-Evaluation of Older Adults

Directions: For each question, place a check beside statements that describe your feelings. You may want to give several answers on some items.

1 When I see someone who is a burden for their relatives, my reaction is to

  a help my family in all ways possible while I am still healthy and energetic
  b feel depressed and hope my death occurs without a need for lengthy care
  c expect that my family will care for me in the way I took care of my folks
  d hope my savings are enough for a nursing facility and not bother my family
  e Other _____

2 If my spouse died, I would have to learn how to

  a manage finances, pay the bills, and handle investments
  b cook, clean, wash clothes and other household chores
  c become involved with a variety of new social activities
  d adjust to identity change and realize my life is not over
  e Other _____

3 Some older adults move to retirement communities. In my view

  a such places would be boring because residents are the same age
  b this could be appealing because of more involvement with peers

c I would become aware of the peer norms to guide my behavior.
d I would not leave friends to start over in an unfamiliar location
e Other _____

4 My greatest fear regarding the future is

a falling down and getting hurt
b having a heart attack or a stroke
c developing a terminal disease
d acquiring Alzheimer's Disease
e Other _____

5 Socialization support groups for older adults might

a delay the onset of mental dysfunction
b help diminish feelings of loneliness
c produce friendship and satisfaction
d do little to improve mental health
e Other _____

6 I think relatives, friends, and co-workers should

a allow widowed persons enough time for grieving
b help widowed persons to speed up their grieving
c visit widowed persons to reinforce their importance
d encourage widowed persons to volunteer in schools
e Other _____

7 My experience with classroom volunteering is that

a the kids increase my sense of optimism
b helping the students provides satisfaction
c children are grateful when they get help
d I do not have experience in this context
e Other _____

8 If I could choose my ideal place to live it would be

a a retirement community in a warm climate
b to stay in the community where I live now
c living with relatives in an extended family
d somewhere where I could view the ocean
e Other _____

9 For me retirement is

a more pleasant than I had imagined
b just as busy as when I was working
c great because I decide what to do
d allows for a less hurried schedule
e Other _____

10 My stress level during retirement is

    a less than when I was employed
    b greater than when I worked
    c about the same as when at work
    d healthier for me
    e Other _____

References

American Sociological Association. (2016, August 21). Relationships with family members, but not friends, decrease likelihood of death. *ScienceDaily*, https://www.sciencedaily.com/releases/2016/08/160821093058.htm

Aronson, L. (2019). *Elderhood: Redefining aging, transforming medicine, reimagining life*. Bloomsbury.

Barrymore, J. (n.d.). *John Barrymore quotes*. https://quotefancy.com/john-barrymore-quotes

Bentley, R. A., & O'Brien, M. J. (2017). *The acceleration of cultural change: From ancestors to algorithms*. Massachusetts Institute of Technology Press.

Butler, R. N. (2008). *The longevity revolution: The benefits and challenges of living a long life* (p. 398). PublicAffairs.

Cohn, D., Horowitz, J. M., Minkin, R., Fry, R., & Hurst, K. (2022a, March 24). *1. The demographics of multigenerational households*. Pew Research Center. https://www.pewresearch.org/social-trends/2022/03/24/the-demographics-of-multigenerational-households/

Cohn, D., Horowitz, J. M., Minkin, R., Fry, R., & Hurst, K. (2022b, March 24). *2. The experiences of adults in multigenerational households*. https://pewresearch.org/social-trends/2022/03/24/the-experiences-of-adults-in-multigenerational-households/

De Leo, D. (2022, January 20). Late-life suicide in an aging world. *Nature Aging* (2), 7–12. 10.1038/s43587-021-00160-1

Durkheim, E. (2018). *Suicide, a study in sociology*. Franklin Classics Trade Press. (Original work published 1897)

Gilovich, T., & Medvec, V. H. (1995, April). The experience of regret: What, when, and why. *Psychological Review*, *102*(2), 379–395. 10.1037/0033-295X.102.2.379

Gilovich, T., & Ross, L. (2016). *The wisest one in the room: How you can benefit from social psychology's most powerful insights*. Free Press.

Greenberg, M. (2012, May 16). The psychology of regret: Should we really aim to live our lives with no regrets? *Psychology Today*. http://www.psychologytoday.com/blog/the-mindful-self-express/201205/the-psychology-regret

Greenberg, M. (2017). *The stress-proof brain: Master your emotional response to stress using mindfulness and neuroplasticity*. New Harbinger.

Henig, R. M. (2018, June 1). The age of grandparents is made of many tragedies. *The Atlantic*. https://www.theatlantic.com/family/archive/2018/06/this-is-the-age-of-grandparents/561527/

Holt-Lunstad, J. (2021, January 12). A pandemic of social isolation? *World Psychiatry*, *20*(1), 55–56. 10.1002/wps.20839

Holt-Lunstad, J., Smith, T. B., Baker, M., Harris, T., & Stephenson, D. (2015, March). Loneliness and social isolation as risk factors for mortality: A meta-analytic review. *Perspectives on Psychological Science*, *10*(2), 227–237. 10.1177/1745691614568352

Huxley, A. (2017). *Brave new world*. Harper. (Original work published 1932).

International Longevity Centre Global Alliance. (2023). *About us*. https://www.ilc-alliance.org/about/

John, T. (2018, April 25). How the world's first loneliness minister will tackle 'the sad reality of modern life.*Time*. https://time.com/5248016/tracey-crouch-uk-loneliness-minister/

Joint Center for Housing Studies of Harvard University. (2019). Housing America's older adults 2019. Harvard University. https://www.jchs.harvard.edu/sites/default/files/reports/files/Harvard_JCHS_Housing_Americas_Older_Adults_2019.pdf

Kautzman-East, M., & Joseph, M. A. (2020, October 31). *Mental health in the United States: A reference handbook*. ABC-CLIO, LLC.

Morrison, M., & Roese, N. J. (2011, March 14). Regrets of the typical American: Findings from a nationally representative sample. *Social Psychological and Personality Science, 2*(6), 576–583. 10.1177/1948550611401756

National Academies of Sciences, Engineering, and Medicine. (2020). *Social isolation and loneliness in older adults*. The National Academies Press.

National Institute on Aging. (2019, April 23). *Social isolation, loneliness in older people pose health risks*. U.S. Department of Health & Human Services. https://www.nia.nih.gov/news/social-isolation-loneliness-older-people-pose-health-risks

Segal, D. L., Qualls, S. H., & Smyer, M. A. (2018), *Aging and mental health* (3rd ed.). Wiley-Blackwell.

Senior Lifestyle. (2023a). *Top 7 benefits of retirement communities*. https://www.seniorlifestyle.com/resources/blog/top-7-reasons-to-live-retirement-in-a-retirement-community/

Senior Lifestyle. (2023b). *Infographic: Are retirement communities safer than at home care?* https://www.seniorlifestyle.com/resources/blog/infographic-are-retirement-communities-safer-than-at-home-care/

Stanley, A. (2020). *Better decisions, fewer regrets: 5 Questions to help you determine your next move*. Zondervan.

Strom, P. S., & Strom, R. D. (2021). *Adolescents in the Internet age: A team learning and teaching perspective* (3rd ed.). Information Age.

Strom, R. D., & Strom, P. S. (2016). Grandparent education for assisted living facilities. *Educational Gerontology, 43*(1), 11–20. 10.1080/03601277.2016.1231518

Strom, R. D., & Strom, P. S. (2017). Grandparent learning and cultural differences. *Educational Gerontology, 43*(8), 417–427. 10.1080/03601277.2017.1314642

Strom, R. D., & Strom, P. S. (2020). Productive aging: Peer influence and retirement. *Educational Gerontology, 46*(11), 678–687. 10.1080/03601277.2020.1807085

Strom, R. D., & Strom, P. S. (2021). Learning throughout life about the needs of all generations: Recognizing and counteracting generational isolation. In M. London (Ed.), *The Oxford handbook of lifelong learning* (2nd ed.) (pp. 183–206). Oxford University Press. 10.1093/oxfordhb/9780197506707.013.9

Tokyo, J. R. (2021, April 23). Japan: 'Minister of loneliness' tackles mental health crisis. *DW*. https://www.dw.com/en/japan-minister-of-loneliness-tackles-mental-health-crisis/a-57311880

Vespa, J., Armstrong, D. M., & Medina, L. (2020, February). *Demographic turning points for the United States: Population projections for 2020 to 2060*. U.S. Census Bureau, Report Number P25-1144. https://www.census.gov/library/publications/2020/demo/p25-1144.html

Whittier, J. G. (1912). Maud Muller. In T. R. Lounsbury (Ed.), *Yale book of American verse*. Yale University Press. https://www.bartleby.com/102/76.html (Original work published 1854).

10 Family Expectations of Grandparents

Goals for Grandparents

Potential of Grandparents

Some people have been identified as the "World's Greatest Grandmother" or "World's Greatest Grandfather." The recognition is observed on t-shirts, hats, coffee cups, greeting cards, and car bumper stickers. Grandparents are grateful for this display of affection from younger relatives and appreciate the meaning these symbols are intended to represent. However, what grandparents say they want most is to be a source of support their family can always rely on.

Most grandparents have the potential to become a valued resource for younger relatives. However, whether individuals are viewed in this way depends on meeting specific conditions. Successful grandparents have goals in common that their peers can attain if they choose to pursue them. Certain of these desirable qualities might describe someone's current behavior. There may be other qualities that grandparents can acquire by deciding to make changes (Thaler & Sunstein, 2021; Westrick-Payne, 2023).

Expectations for grandparents vary by culture and generation. The results of international studies of three generations (grandparents, parents, and grandchildren) have determined that there are greater differences between the perceptions of generations than among cultures (R. D. Strom & Strom, 1983/2006; R. D. Strom & Strom, 2017; R. D. Strom et al., 1999). The following ten goals are recommended for consideration (R. D. Strom & Strom, 1997, 2021).

1 Spend Time Getting to Know Each Grandchild

Time spent with a grandchild is generally undervalued as a source of influence on child development. Studies by R. D. Strom and Strom (2018, 2021) have found that time together has more significant influence than all other measured factors in three-generational investigations with similar results obtained across ethnic groups and cultures. The *Grandparent Strengths and Needs Inventory* (Collinsworth et al., 1991; Strom & Strom, 2009) presents 60 items divided into six subscales of ten items each representing the following topics.

1 Satisfaction – experiences of being a grandparent that are pleasing,
2 Success – ways that grandparents successfully perform their role,
3 Teaching – kinds of lessons grandparents are expected to provide,
4 Difficulty – problems encountered with grandparent obligations,

DOI: 10.4324/9781003401261-14

5 Frustration – grandchild behaviors that upset the grandparents, and
6 Information needs – essential knowledge about each grandchild.

Results from an experimental and control intervention that involved 400 grandparents, their children, and grandchildren underscores the importance of time spent with grandchildren. The demographic variable that has predicted grandparent success most consistently is time spent together. Those spending more time interacting or doing things with grandchildren (less than or greater than 5 hours a month) were identified as most successful in the observation of grandchildren, parents, and grandparents. Greater time in contact matters more than has been recognized by researchers who usually focus on independent variables that cannot be modified such as level of education or income. Grandparents cannot change their level of formal education or amount of income but can choose to benefit from the advantage that comes from spending more time with grandchildren they love.

Sometimes older adults describe a grandchild by declaring, "She (or he) is one of a kind." This suggests someone is unique by possessing attributes that distinguish her from other people. Every child ought to be seen this way. In contrast, individuality of grandchildren is denied when grandparents contend, "I want to be fair and not play favorites. I treat all of my grandchildren the same." Instead, if the goal is to show equality toward younger relatives, it is sensible to identify, accept, and encourage the differences that are bound to exist in grandchild talents and interests. When each grandchild is recognized as an individual, there is greater motivation to remain in touch with each of them.

One of the joys grandparents can experience is building a close and durable relationship with each grandchild. Achieving this goal becomes more difficult with an increase in the number of grandchildren. There is no merit in counting grandchildren as though they were status symbols. One grandmother might tell her friends she has four grandchildren. The friend could respond by stating she has eight grandchildren. What matters most is to be well informed about each grandchild so that it is possible to support distinctiveness, individual goals, and comment about progress that differs from the scope of feedback students get on their school report card.

2 Reinforce Parenting Goals For Their Children

Margaret was invited by her friend to attend a grandparent education class at the senior center. In response Margaret said, "Why should I take a class about being a grandparent when it comes naturally to me. I brought up three children. Each of them is successful so I must have known something." Margaret is right. Raising three children who become responsible adults is an important accomplishment. However, being a successful parent does not ensure that the same person will also be a successful grandparent. Relatives should help grandparents define what the family expects of them. The goals that parents have for raising their children should become a basic guide for grandparents. When grandparents are familiar with parent goals, they are more able to reinforce the child lessons parents are trying to teach. This knowledge is not revealed to older adults by intuition and it does not come naturally.

On the contrary, what seems to come naturally for many grandparents is enthusiasm for a relationship with grandchildren that focuses on entertainment instead of concern about being a partner with parents for providing care and guidance. Doing what comes naturally might mean not giving enough attention to being a resource for the family. Grandparents who suppose their purpose is to fulfill grandchild wishes unintentionally support selfishness, narcissism, and self-absorption, attributes that detract from healthy progression of child and adolescent development. Encouraging grandchildren to discover and respond to needs of relatives is an important lesson to favorably influence personality development. Grandparents can support parent lessons if they are familiar with their intentions. Some grandparents announce, "I don't want to interfere in the lives of my adult children; they should raise their daughters and sons the way I did, without outside interference." However, grandparents are bound to interfere when they misunderstand or choose to ignore goals of their grandchild's parents. The grandparent role should be a partnership with parents, helping them achieve their goals for bringing up children. This agreement might require some negotiation.

Many grandparents underestimate their possibilities to influence grandchild socialization. Participants in grandparent classes are asked about whether their role is easier or more difficult than was anticipated. The common response is that being a grandparent is easier and it is less demanding because parents have all the responsibility. On the other hand, mothers and fathers rarely report that being a parent is an easy role. In many families, the responsibility to contribute to younger relatives' well-being is disproportionate with grandparents assuming less than their appropriate share of responsibility. There are exceptions where the grandparents have too heavy a load, especially when they become the main source of guidance to raise grandchildren by themselves. About three million grandparents are the primary caregivers and teachers of their grandchildren (Westrick-Payne, 2023). However, there is a substantial difference between being the main caregiver for grandchildren and the much more prevalent situation of older adults being insufficiently involved in helping to guide younger relatives. Sharing some responsibilities to help raise grandchildren is usually an appropriate expectation (R. D. Strom & Strom, 1997).

3 Family Discussion About Grandparent Rights and Responsibilities

Grandparents commonly express disappointment because their status in the family has eroded, become unclear, and appears to be declining in importance. They want to think well of themselves but this is a difficult task when self-esteem depends upon responsibilities that are poorly defined. Establishing a role requires setting goals, pursuing a course of direction, and periodically trying to assess the extent to which progress is being made. Unless grandparents strive to carry out specific responsibilities, they cannot reasonably claim success in achieving them. This is the dilemma of grandparents – they want to succeed but commonly lack a set of rights and responsibilities to apply as criteria for self-evaluation. Consider the following *Rights and Responsibilities for Grandparents* (R. D. Strom & Strom, 1991, pp. 24–25).

RIGHTS OF GRANDPARENTS*
As a grandparent, I would like the right to …

1 Hear from my grandchildren on a regular basis.
2 Spend some time alone with my grandchildren.
3 Pursue my own personal interests and hobbies.

(Continued)

4 Say "No" when requests are made for babysitting.
5 Participate in special events of grandchildren.
6 Give advice to my sons/daughters.
7 Give advice to my grandchildren.
8 Be informed of grandchild's problems and successes.
9 Know the school progress of my grandchildren.
10 Maintain rules of my home during family visits.
11 See grandchildren if there is a divorce.
12 Express my religious and moral points of view.
13 Refuse to give financial help to family members.
14 Share financial resources with my grandchildren.
15 Live my life without having to raise children again.
16 Choose a lifestyle of my own preference.
17 Expect reasonable assistance from my family.
18 Know the parenting goals of my sons/daughters.

RESPONSIBILITIES OF GRANDPARENTS
As a grandparent, I would like the responsibility to ...

1 Acquaint grandchildren with their parents' childhood.
2 Share family history and traditions.
3 Give advice to sons/daughters.
4 Give advice to grandchildren.
5 Provide an example of religious faith.
6 Cooperate with my grandchildren's other grandparents.
7 Keep learning for personal development.
8 Find out my grandchildren's views and feelings.
9 Care for grandchildren if their parents cannot do so.
10 Use leisure time in constructive ways.
11 Set rules for my family when they visit.
12 Know current principles of raising children.
13 Share financial resources with grandchildren.
14 Communicate regularly with my grandchildren.
15 Be an example of personal stability.
16 Support better schooling for children.
17 Be honest about my feelings and needs.
18 Reinforce the parenting goals of my sons/daughters.

In addition, the **GENERATIONAL PERSPECTIVES ACTIVITIES** section of this chapter presents this list of 18 Rights and 18 Responsibilities for three generations (grandparents, parents, and grandchildren) to share their observations of grandparents. The results of this family discussion can help grandparents make decisions about adjustments to their evolving role.

4 Express Feelings, Opinions, and Concerns

Generally, we ask members of grandparent classes to estimate the closeness of their relationship with grandchildren. Typically, they portray the bond as being much closer than is described when we ask the same question of their grandchildren. One explanation for this difference in perception is that children are usually more willing to express their opinions and feelings. In contrast, many older adults find it difficult to talk about emotions so they are unwilling to make their feelings known. When grandparents do not share their opinions, they forfeit the give and take in conversations that could help them be better understood, look at things in new ways, and change their minds about particular ideas, events, and situations (Floyd, 2019; Levine, 2020).

Ralph wants to adopt a new perspective because he recognizes some customs are changing for the better. He observed, "I cannot remember my grandfather ever saying to me 'I love you, Ralph.' Instead, my grandfather was stern, serious, and avoided showing any affection. In contrast, my 14-year-old grandson Darin often says when we are together on the iPhone or texting, 'I love you, Grandpa.' I am grateful to Darin for teaching me this valuable lesson and have told him so."

Relationships also suffer when grandparents build a reputation for intolerance about how other people feel or interpret situations. Eleanor learned this important lesson the hard way. After spending a week with her son's family, she woke up early and noticed that 4-year-old Joyce was playing in the backyard sandbox. As they talked Joyce said, "Grandma, I have to be good only two more days." Eleanor asked, "Why is that?" Joyce replied, "Because that's when you will go home." Some families do not behave in a normal way when the grandparents come for a visit. Instead, a concerted effort is made to put on a performance because there is an assumption that grandparents are unable to accept differences in the way families behave now as compared to how things were years ago. Parents explain that a temporary suspension of family daily routine is easier than for the grandparents to accommodate aspects of a lifestyle that differs from their own. The results of this charade are that grandparents are misled, lessons they should learn do not happen, and older relatives are seen as incapable of adjusting to shifts taking place in the modern family.

5 Consider Grandchildren Sources to Learn From

Social change presents opportunities to develop closer relationships between generations. Grandparents often admit that getting to know grandchildren is difficult for them. This lack of knowledge can be costly because youth seek advice from people they believe understand their struggles, goals, and concerns. It is a contradiction to recognize grandparents as the most mature members in the family and then nullify their potential influence by failing to keep them informed about the satisfactions and disappointments of their grandchildren. There is a related obstacle. Mary describes a familiar experience.

I do not like it when my daughters become the reporters about the experiences of my school-aged grandchildren. They tell me all of the good things happening, accomplishments that occur in school, victories on sports teams, and other aspects of life where my grandchildren are successful. I recognize this is only a partial picture and not the whole story. There are never news reports of disappointing situations even though I realize grandchildren must have such experiences. Fears and failures are not mentioned because parents suppose I should experience only pride and avoid worry. Being fully informed is important so I can encourage grandchildren when they face hard times. That is when I am needed most but am unable to respond if uninformed. I cannot be a listener or a source of comfort when the news is always "Everything is just fine." My grandchildren must wonder why I never console them when emotional support and assurance is needed from people who love them.

Partial or biased parental reporting prevents grandparents from awareness they need and denies them an opportunity to support resilience to offset predictable setbacks experienced by everyone. Reports from parents that leave out the struggles of children cause some grandparents to suppose that growing up is relatively easy these days, without worry or stress. This situation reflects the way expectations of grandparents are poorly defined in many families. Grandparents should challenge why their daughters and sons are unwilling to take them into their confidence. Even friends share more with each other than just reports regarding the good times. Grandparents should inform the whole family they want to hear directly from grandchildren because this is the only way for them to foster a supportive relationship. Grandchildren should speak for themselves without having parents act as the family messengers or interpreters because children are too busy to maintain communication with older relatives (Katz et al., 2021; Perry, 2020).

Parents should tell daughters and sons that grandparents want to be helpful but are unable to offer emotional support or advice when they lack information that is needed. Grandchildren willing to share their experiences can acquaint older relatives with the difficulties of growing up and also stimulate involvement with problem solving. Grandchildren will decide for themselves the extent to which they share feelings but willingness commonly increases when grandparents demonstrate a similar readiness to share the experiences they find satisfying and struggles they have to overcome. That is what relationships are all about, sharing personal experiences. Every chapter in this book has a section about conversations with grandchildren to apply in understanding them as individuals.

6 Identify Grandchild Responsibilities to Grandparents

What responsibilities do you expect from your grandchildren? These are some of the responses that were provided by members of a grandparent class.

Alice, who had assigned herself a lengthy number of tasks on the list of grandparent responsibilities pointed out, "I don't feel my grandchildren should have any obligations toward me." Then Alice was asked by Amy, "How can your grandchildren become responsible if you deny them a sense of obligation toward their older relatives? When adults expect grandchildren to show concern for loved ones, they are more likely to grow up with caring attitudes toward others." Linda expressed her opinion, "As I think about the obligations of grandchildren, I would like to receive compassion whenever I am sick or don't feel well." A lady next to Linda wondered out loud "How do grandchildren who live far away know when you do not feel well?" Linda admitted, "They probably don't know because I would never tell them, supposing that it might cause worry."

Just as grandparents want to know when grandchildren are discouraged and they need emotional support, younger relatives should be made aware when grandparents are distressed and need cheering up. Mutual self-disclosure and being able to count upon one another are the basis for long-term intimate relationships.

7 Convey Optimism As A Quality For Good Health

The optimism of children reminds us we should exemplify this same basic attitude.

Betty stopped by the apartment of her recently divorced son who had been awarded custody of Justin, his 7-year-old son. Betty arrived early to pick up Justin, knowing that it might require some effort to get him ready for church the next morning. I felt confident that whatever clothes Justin might need would be in the large sack of dirty laundry that I would bring home to wash. Then the discovery -- there was no underwear in the pile that I was going to wash, not even one pair."

"There are no undershorts in the laundry sack Justin," Betty said as she headed to the bathroom. "I'll wash the ones you have on while you take a shower and get ready for bed." "But I don't have any undershorts on, Grandma," Justin explained. "There haven't been undershorts in my drawer all week so I just didn't wear any." "You mean you went to school all week without wearing underwear?" Betty asked while scrambling to think of nearby stores that might still be open on Saturday night. "Don't worry, Grandma," Justin said. "My pants are thick, and tomorrow no one is going to know I don't have underwear on except you and me." So, we went to church without anyone knowing but us. The willingness of Betty to share Justin's sense of possibility, to make the best of an undesirable situation, was an effective way to handle it. Later she took steps to make certain that more underwear would be available, and this was done without undermining Justin's respect for his Dad.

Attitudes qualify the people children choose as sources of emotional support. Whether grandparents are optimistic or pessimistic, these attitudes are a memorable aspect of their legacy. More is involved than just a difference in point of view. Think about optimism and pessimism as explanatory styles that people rely on as they try to interpret troublesome situations. Studies have determined that optimists perform better in school and on the job because they cheerfully persist when encountering setbacks whereas pessimists with equal abilities choose to give up. Research has also found that, from midlife (age 40) onwards, pessimists generally have weaker immune systems, higher incidence of infectious diseases, greater health related issues, are more likely to suffer depression, and less able to generate resilience needed to recover from setbacks. People usually report that being around pessimists is uncomfortable. All grandparents should affirm optimism is their basic attitude toward life, family relationships, and reaction to problems they face in daily affairs. Mental health depends on it and chances to favorably influence others as well (Kellerman & Seligman, 2023; Strom, 1989).

Consider a longitudinal study by Hernandez et al. (2015). The subjects included 5,100 men and women, ages 45 to 84, from six regions of the United States; demographics were 38% White, 28% Black, 22% Latino, and 12% Asian. Cardiovascular health of subjects was checked at 18-month intervals over a time span of 11 years. Each health assessment consisted of seven conditions including blood pressure, body mass index, fasting plasma glucose, cholesterol, dietary intake, physical activity, and tobacco use. These are the same metrics that the American Heart Association applies to define heart health. Participants completed surveys to evaluate their mental health, optimism, and physical health based on self-reported medical diagnoses of liver and kidney disease and arthritis. This was the first large-scale investigation ever to examine the association between optimism and cardiovascular health involving a multi-ethnic population. Results showed individuals with the highest levels of optimism, regardless of race, gender, or income, were twice as likely to be in ideal cardiovascular health compared with pessimistic peers and 55% more likely to have a total health score in the intermediate or ideal ranges respectively.

The relationship between mental attitude and mortality was often a subject of conjecture until it was examined by a Leisure World Cohort Study that began in 1981. At that time, nearly 14,000 of the volunteer participants were average age 74. Each participant completed a survey containing seven positively stated items from the Zung Self-Rating Depression Scale (Zung, 1965). Age-adjusted for lifestyle and conditions of disease, the hazard rates for death were calculated for the women ($N = 8,682$) and men (N = 4,992). Thirty-five years later, when the study ended in 2016, 98% of subjects had died at an average age of 88. Findings showed that positive mental attitude for both men and women was statistically significantly related to having a lower 35-year mortality rate. Persons with negative attitudes had an increased risk of death, even after many years of follow-up. One implication is that education to improve outlook on family relationships may increase longevity and improve the quality of life (Paganini-Hill et al., 2018).

If the grandparent role, particularly in middle class White families, continues to decline in importance, grandchildren will lose access to a valuable resource and their grandparents will become more vulnerable to feelings of pessimism and depression because of the loss in their sense of purpose and potential influence. An important observation is that, when children are continually exposed to pessimism, the creative capacity to perceive possibilities in situations, including their own happiness, can be lost (Amigoni & McMullan, 2019). Grandparent optimists are an example for adopting a favorable outlook about the future (American Association of Retired Persons, 2023; Aronson, 2019).

8 Demonstrate Values As Evidence Of Maturity

Religious beliefs are a source of values for many grandparents and the focus of lessons they would like to teach grandchildren. Communicating religious beliefs is not like providing instruction in a classroom where it is possible to quickly give a test to evaluate comprehension. Evidence that beliefs have been learned may require years to confirm and sometimes happen after the grandparent teacher has passed away. Teaching values depends on the consistency of how grandparent enact their faith principles. When statements of belief are reflected by acts of kindness, compassion, patience, and forgiveness, the credibility of grandparent examples will be remembered for a long time.

The term *generativity* is defined as a reduction in preoccupation with self in favor of a balance that includes caring more about the well-being of others, providing help when it is needed. Julia showed this commitment. After her daughter, son-in-law, and grandchildren (ages 5 and 7) moved from Dallas, Texas to Auburn, Alabama, they invited Julia to leave Dallas and join them. Now she has two grandchildren to pick up after school and supervise until the parents come home from work. Her family is pleased and grateful. Julia is glad too knowing she contributes to her family.

The cost of group care for young children is greater than most age groups know and can present an enormous financial challenge. There are 11 million children under age 5 who attend day care or preschool. According to ChildCare Aware of America (2022), the largest trainer of daycare and preschool personnel in the country, group care in many states is actually more expensive than college tuition; 10% of median income for a married couple family; and 35% of median income for a single parent. The United States government considers 7% of parent income a suitable cap for defining affordable child care. None of the 50 states are below this threshold.

When grandparents are between ages 55 and 80, they often experience self-conflict about how to spend time and energy. They compare the amount devoted to self-interests with efforts provided to meet the needs of relatives. No single formula can be recommended for making choices about how much help individuals should provide for their loved ones. However, grandparents who do not invest in the well-being of younger relatives while the elders are still energetic and have much to offer should recognize that a corresponding low level of support may be given to them when their independence is in decline. If grandparents are willing to share responsibilities while they are still healthy and independent, adjusting to their frailty later on can be easier for everyone. Families should merge two questions for reflection: (1) What can parents and grandchildren expect of grandparents? and (2) What can grandparents expect of younger relatives?

9 Encourage Gender Equity Among Relatives

Everyone appreciates microwave ovens, dishwashers, and other labor-saving devices. However, more grandmothers and grandfathers, mothers and fathers, should share domestic chores. This transition appears to be particularly difficult for older men who seem content to have housework done by women only. In these families, wives take care of virtually all the domestic tasks without help from their husbands. The reasons grandfathers should become involved is because it helps wives and gives younger relatives a chance to observe them as being a constructive marriage partner. In contrast, if grandfathers maintain old fashioned expectations about the division of labor, their grandchildren – often without comment – usually dismiss them as credible sources of advice on gender relationships (Biggs & Lowenstein, 2011).

Children are being oriented to a more equitable model based on interdependence and cooperation. The lesson that media, schools, classmates, and parents try to teach is that gender equality is necessary. For this reason, grandchildren do not like to observe grandmother alone do all the cooking, shopping, washing, ironing, vacuuming, and other household chores without help from grandfathers who define their duties as only lawn chores outside the house. Children interpret this situation as gender inequity that leads them to devalue advice from grandfathers (Samuel, 2017).

More is involved than husbands being resistant to change. Attitudes of spouses are also implicated. When husbands first try some household tasks, the initial performance does not approach the standard held by wives. Instead of expressing the judgment "you're hopeless in the kitchen" or "it's easier to do the job myself", wives should provide responses that are more motivating. By showing several times how to perform a task, providing constructive feedback, encouraging another try after making a mistake, and offering favorable comments when there is a positive outcome, grandmothers can help grandfathers share the load and become an example of mutual support (Thaler & Sunstein, 2021).

10 Continue Learning For Self-Improvement

Women and men in grandparent classes are asked to describe what caused them to become a participant. Esther explained her motivation:

When my daughter and 9-year-old granddaughter heard I was planning to enroll in the grandparent education class, they told me "Grandma, you don't need that course. We love you just the way you are." These comments were meant to be a compliment so I replied, "I'm glad that you feel I am successful but realize that learning continues to be important at my age. I have to try to understand changes in society and what these shifts mean for me so that I can adjust with the rest of the family. Education is the key to adjustment. So, encourage me to grow; I will appreciate it more than being told I do not need to learn."

Esther took the initiative to establish reasonable expectations for her development. She resembles others who have been told by friends or relatives that "Your behavior is acceptable to us so you don't have to take a grandparent course." Despite the good intentions motivating such remarks, they do not recognize that improving your understanding will increase your success. In effect, the potential for self-improvement is underestimated. One challenge for the older generation is to establish a higher standard of learning for their peers.

When younger relatives encourage grandparents to pursue further education, older adults should interpret the recommendation as a vote of confidence in their capacity to keep learning. Grandparents can understand that loved ones want them to provide an example that continued learning is essential for healthy adjustment. Parents and children should tell grandparents they expect them to demonstrate a commitment to personal development, devote time to the family, provide guidance to younger relatives, and actively demonstrate concern for their community. When grandparents are expected to contribute talent and energy, they experience a sense of purpose and sustain influence in the family and society (R. D. Strom & Strom, 2021).

Conclusion

Retirement can bring an unexpected loss of purpose, lack of direction, and need to obtain guidance. The possibility to become a well-informed advisor increases with understanding about current challenges and joys of raising children. Attending grandparent classes focused on family development, joining grandparent group discussions, and volunteering to help elementary school students can improve awareness about the current processes involved with growing up. These sources provide general knowledge.

In addition, each grandparent should consult with the parents of their own grandchildren in order to become aware of lessons they want them to learn. Staying in continuous contact with grandchildren is necessary because these conversations can enable the discovery of changing goals, worries, and satisfactions of individual grandchildren. The grandparent and grandchild bond strengthens through reciprocal learning.

Key Concepts

1 Setting goals is essential for success. Defining your role in cooperation with relatives clarifies expectations, provides a sense of direction, and determines priorities. Grandparents can gauge personal growth better when self-evaluation focuses on how specific goals set earlier are fulfilled. Younger relatives should be asked for their feedback about success and learning needs.

2 The grandparent role should be based on reinforcing the childrearing goals of parents. Developing a partnership with parents is more possible when their plans for child guidance are known, accepted, and encouraged by grandparents.

3 Couples should adjust to societal change. People who can adapt are seen as potential sources of advice. More grandfathers need to think about how shifts in gender role expectations implicate their behavior. Sharing household tasks is a way grandfathers can reduce the workload of grandmothers, grow as individuals, and qualify as examples of adjustment for younger relatives.

4 Getting to know each grandchild as an individual is essential to provide support and mature guidance. Treating all grandchildren as if they were the same denies individuality. The way to demonstrate equality is to identify, accept, and encourage the differences in talent, interests, and motivation of grandchildren.

5 Communicate directly with grandchildren. Personal relationships are closer when they do not depend on third-party involvement. In the presence of the entire family, clarify that you want to hear from grandchildren directly instead of being given second-hand reports by parents.

6 Accept your share of responsibility. Grandparents have less responsibility than parents for children. Recognizing the difference does not mean grandparents should underestimate their obligations. If grandparents define their family role as easy, this is often because they have insufficient responsibility.

7 Sharing some responsibility for the education of grandchildren is a wonderful opportunity for grandparents. Older relatives can choose to help with childcare, emotional and social support, and perhaps provide financial assistance that may be needed by adult children and grandchildren.

8 Grandchildren should feel responsible to keep grandparents continually informed about what is going on in their lives, including both pleasant and disappointing experiences. If grandchildren do not stay in touch, grandparents cannot know when support is needed and are less likely to be chosen as a source of advice, encouragement, and comfort.

9 Maintain an optimistic attitude. The way grandparents view people and interpret events is an important aspect of their influence and future legacy. Focusing on the possibilities you see in people, situations, and events enables you to be an example of how everyone should manage problems as they arise.

10 Broaden your goals for self-improvement. Physical exercise, travel, entertainment, and hobbies are worthwhile. Time should also be devoted to education about your family role. By balancing what you like to learn with what you need to know, you will become a more favorable resource for members of your family and the community.

Generational Perspectives Activities

10.1 Family Discussion About Grandparent Rights and Responsibilities
10.2 Team Discussion
10.3 Agenda for Interviews with Grandparents
10.4 Interview a Grandparent and a Grandchild
10.5 A Scenario: Reasoning and Problem Solving
10.6 Team Chapter Review
10.7 Criteria for Self-Evaluation of Grandparents

10.1 Family Discussion About Grandparent Rights and Responsibilities

The purpose for considering **Grandparent Rights And Responsibilities** is for relatives to make known what goals can be important and helpful to the family. After reflection, college students *(you)* circle the GC (for Grandchild) column beside each of the rights and responsibilities you prefer. Then show the circled list to your parents. They can make their opinions known by circling the P (for Parent) column, and GP (for Grandparent) column beside the items they expect of Grandparents. After the three generations circle their feelings, spend time discussing the topics together. There will likely be some differences between the results for grandmothers compared to grandfathers. Enjoy talking with your family about the outcomes.

RIGHTS OF GRANDPARENTS*	**Family Member**		
As a grandparent, I would like the right to …			
1 Hear from my grandchildren on a regular basis.	GP	P	GC
2 Spend some time alone with my grandchildren.	GP	P	GC
3 Pursue my own personal interests and hobbies.	GP	P	GC
4 Say "No" when requests are made for babysitting.	GP	P	GC
5 Participate in special events of grandchildren.	GP	P	GC
6 Give advice to my sons/daughters.	GP	P	GC
7 Give advice to my grandchildren.	GP	P	GC
8 Be informed of grandchild's problems and successes.	GP	P	GC
9 Know the school progress of my grandchildren.	GP	P	GC
10 Maintain rules of my home during family visits.	GP	P	GC
11 See grandchildren if there is a divorce.	GP	P	GC
12 Express my religious and moral points of view.	GP	P	GC
13 Refuse to give financial help to family members.	GP	P	GC
14 Share financial resources with my grandchildren.	GP	P	GC
15 Live my life without having to raise children again.	GP	P	GC
16 Choose a lifestyle of my own preference.	GP	P	GC
17 Expect reasonable assistance from my family.	GP	P	GC
18 Know the parenting goals of my sons/daughters.	GP	P	GC

RESPONSIBILITIES OF GRANDPARENTS*	**Family Member**		
As a grandparent, I would like the responsibility to …			
1 Acquaint grandchildren with their parents' childhood.	GP	P	GC
2 Share family history and traditions.	GP	P	GC
3 Give advice to sons/daughters.	GP	P	GC
4 Give advice to grandchildren.	GP	P	GC
5 Provide an example of religious faith.	GP	P	GC
6 Cooperate with my grandchildren's other grandparents.	GP	P	GC
7 Keep learning for personal development.	GP	P	GC
8 Find out my grandchildren's views and feelings.	GP	P	GC
9 Care for grandchildren if their parents cannot do so.	GP	P	GC
10 Use leisure time in constructive ways.	GP	P	GC
11 Set rules for my family when they visit.	GP	P	GC
12 Know current principles of raising children.	GP	P	GC
13 Share financial resources with grandchildren.	GP	P	GC
14 Communicate regularly with my grandchildren.	GP	P	GC
15 Be an example of personal stability.	GP	P	GC
16 Support better schooling for children.	GP	P	GC
17 Be honest about my feelings and needs.	GP	P	GC
18 Reinforce the parenting goals of my sons/daughters.	GP	P	GC

From: *Becoming a Better Grandparent* by R. D. Strom & S. K. Strom (pp. 23–25). Sage. Copyright © 1991 by R. D. Strom & S. K. Strom.

10.2 Team Discussion

1 What are the characteristics you admire most about your grandmother or grandfather?

2 What are some rights and responsibilities you feel your grandparents have been denied?

3 How do family members behave differently when the grandparents come for a visit?

4 How willing are your grandparents to accept differences in goals of their grand-children?

5 What things have you learned about faith by observing behavior of your grand-parents?

6 What lessons about gender equality have you observed by the example of grand-parents?

7 How have your grandparents supported the childrearing goals set by your parents?

8 What are some of the responsibilities that you feel grandparents have toward you??

9 Talk about memories of optimism you have observed in behavior of your grand-parents.

10 How have your grandparents made time for you over the years in their schedule?

10.3 Agenda for Interviews with Grandparents

1 How do you suppose that being a parent now differs from your own experience?

2 What do you admire about the ways your children perform in the parent role?

3 What methods do parents of your grandchildren rely on that disappoint you?

4 What aspects of the relationship with your adult children are most satisfying?

5 What should children be taught about grandparent rights and responsibilities?

6 How do you let daughters and sons know the way you feel about their parenting?

7 In what ways are parents now less successful and more successful than in the past?

8 What have your grandchildren been taught about their responsibilities to you?

9 How is being a grandparent easier or more difficult than you had anticipated?

10 How do you suppose family expectations of grandparents are going to change?

10.4 Interview a Grandparent and a Grandchild

1 What are some dreams that you've had for quite a while?

2 What are some dreams that you changed or had to give up?

3 What dreams do you have for other people in your family?

4 Who listens to you when you try to describe your dreams?

5 Which of your dreams will probably not be fully achieved?

6 How do your dreams compare to dreams others have for you?

7 Which of your dreams have already started to come true?

8 What are some goals that you want to achieve at this age?

9 What goals are more important to you now than in the past?

10 What goals would you like to accomplish in your lifetime?

11 What do you know about the dreams of your older relatives?

10.5 A Scenario: Reasoning and Problem Solving

Problem solving scenarios present a chance to consider dilemmas and think of solutions. Your task is to view pros and cons of the stated choices, identify relevant information that might be missing, and provide your reasoning for responses that you consider to be best.

Elizabeth feels increasingly isolated because so many changes are taking place. Her friend Jean acknowledges that adjustment to the unfamiliar is hard at all ages but suggests

a patience can be a helpful asset for learning to do things in new ways.
b everyone needs lessons in cultural evolution and cultural preservation.
c conversations with younger people can lead to a broader perspective.
d helping each generation to meet the needs of one another is essential.
e other _____

10.6 Team Chapter Review

Efforts to assess participant learning, provide feedback, and improve quality of instruction is enhanced by a group review of each chapter.

1 What ideas in the lesson changed the way I think about this topic?
2 What insights from the lesson will I try to apply in my relationships?
3 What is the most important point for me presented in this lesson?
4 What are some aspects of this lesson I would like to better understand?
5 Which aspects of this lesson do I wish that I had known about earlier?

10.7 Criteria for Self-Evaluation of Grandparents

Directions: For each question, place a check beside the statements that describe your feelings. You may give several answers for some items. If your feelings are not on the list of choices, write them on the line marked 'Other.'

1 In order to spend more time with my grandchildren

  a I should learn to text, receive and send photos, use Skype, Face Time, and email.
  b I need to give them higher priority in the way that I manage my time schedule.
  c they should stay in contact with me regardless of how busy their daily life is.
  d we live far apart so being with each is usually limited to summer vacation time.
  e Other _____

2 Some of the ways I should improve my family influence are

  a get to know each of my grandchildren as individuals.
  b share my feelings and ideas more often with relatives.
  c offer advice if I see it needed rather than wait to be asked.
  d setting an example of continued learning through life.
  e Other _____

3 How can I get feedback about my success as a grandparent?

  a My grandchildren tell me they approve of my behavior.
  b My daughters/sons let me know they believe I do well.
  c My friends inform me they think that I am doing well.
  d I have no feedback about my success as a grandparent.
  e Other _____

4 How do I feel about the amount of my responsibility as a grandparent?

  a I have more responsibility than seems reasonable.
  b I have about the right amount of responsibility.

c I have less responsibility than seems reasonable.
d I don't want any responsibility for grandchildren.
e Other _____

5 Getting to know my grandchildren as individuals

a seems impossible since I have so many of them.
b is difficult because we live a long distance apart.
c is easy because I get to interact with them often.
d is easy because they try to keep me informed.
e Other _____

6 The expectations relatives have for my role is

a well defined and reasonable.
b unclear and never expressed.
c not a topic for conversation.
d too much child care time.
e Other _____

7 How do I treat my grandchildren differently than grandparents treated me?

a I am less likely to offer correction and discipline.
b I am more inclined to spoil my grandchildren.
c I spend less time with my own grandchildren.
d I listen more to what my grandchildren say.
e Other _____

8 In comparing my influence with my own grandparents

a I am a more influential grandparent.
b I am a less influential grandparent.
c We have about the same influence.
d They died before I could know them.
e Other _____

9 The ways I find out what is going on with grandchildren are

a from reports provided by their parents.
b direct contact with the grandchildren.
c observation of grandchild activities.
d when it is my birthday or a holiday.
e Other _____

10 My children make sure that the grandchildren

a keep in touch with me regularly.
b are reminded of responsibilities to me.
c recognize when it is my birthday.
d talk about me in family discussions.
e Other _____

References

American Association of Retired Persons. (2023). *Vital voices: Issues that impact U.S. adults age 45 and older, October 2022*. AARP Research. https://www.aarp.org/content/dam/aarp/research/surveys_statistics/life-leisure/2023/vital-voices-2022-national-chartbook.doi.10.26419-2Fres.00524.100.pdf

Amigoni, D., & McMullan, G. (Eds.). (2019). *Creativity in later life: Beyond late style*. Routledge.

Aronson, L. (2019). *Elderhood: Redefining aging, transforming medicine, reimagining life*. Bloomsbury.

Biggs, S., & Lowenstein, A. (2011). *Generational intelligence: A critical approach to age relations*. Routledge.

ChildCare Aware of America. (2022). *Demanding change: Repairing our child care systems*. https://info.childcareaware.org/hubfs/2022-03-FallReport-FINAL%20(1).pdf?utm_campaign=Budget%20Reconciliation%20Fall%202021&utm_source=website&utm_content=22_demanding-change_pdf_update332022

Collinsworth, P., Strom, R. D., Strom, S. K., & Young, D. (1991). The Grandparent Strengths and Needs Inventory: Development and factorial validation. *Educational and Psychological Measurement, 51*(3), 785–792. 10.1177/0013164491513030

Floyd, K. (2019). *Affectionate communication in close relationships*. Cambridge University Press.

Hernandez, R., Kershaw, K. N., Siddique, J., Boehm, J. K., Kubzansky, L. D., Diez-Roux, A., Ning, H., & Lloyd-Jones, D. M. (2015, January). Optimism and cardiovascular health: Multi-Ethnic Study of Atherosclerosis (MESA). *Health Behavior and Policy Review, 2*(1), 62–73. 10.14485/HBPR.2.1.6

Katz, R., Ogilvie, S., Shaw, J., & Woodhead, L. (2021). *Gen Z, explained: The art of living in a digital age*. University of Chicago Press.

Kellerman, G., & Seligman, M. (2023). *Tomorrowmind: Thriving at work with resilience, creativity, and connection -- now and in an uncertain future*. Atria Books.

Levine, M. (2020). *Ready or not: Preparing our kids to thrive in an uncertain and rapidly changing world*. Harper.

Paganini-Hill, A., Kawas, C. H., & Corrada, M. M. (2018). Positive mental attitude associated with lower 35-year mortality: The Leisure World Cohort Study. *Journal of Aging Research*. 10.1155/2018/2126368

Perry, P. (2020). *The book you wish your parents had read (and your children will be glad that you did)*. Penguin Life.

Samuel, L. R. (2017). *Aging in America: A cultural history*. University of Pennsylvania Press.

Strom, R. D. (1989). *Grandparent development: Final report*. American Association of Retired Persons, Andrus Foundation, and Arizona State University.

Strom, R. D., & Strom, S. (1991). *Becoming a better grandparent: A guidebook for strengthening the family* (pp. 23–25). Sage.

Strom, R. D., & Strom, S. (1997). Building a theory of grandparent development. *International Journal of Aging and Human Development, 45*(4), 255–286.

Strom, R. D., & Strom, S. (2009). *Grandparent strengths and needs inventory*. Scholastic Testing Service.

Strom, R. D., Strom, S., Wang, C., Shen, Y., Griswold, D., Chan, H., & Yang, C. (1999). Grandparents in the United States and Republic of China: A comparison of generations and cultures. *International Journal of Aging and Human Development, 49*(4), 279–317. 10.2190/DQFF-LVRU-U6W9-8Q6L

Strom, R. D., & Strom, S. (2006, July 10). Redefining the grandparent role. *Cambridge Journal of Education, 13*(1), 25–28. 10.1080/0305764830130107 (Original work published 1983).

Strom, R. D., & Strom, P. S. (2017). Grandparent learning and cultural differences. *Educational Gerontology, 43*(8), 417–427. 10.1080/03601277.2017.1314642

Strom, R. D., & Strom, P. S. (2018). Education for grandparents in longevity societies. *Journal of Adult and Continuing Education, 24*(2), 208–228. https://doi.org/10.1177/1477971418810652

Strom, R. D., & Strom, P. S. (2021). Learning throughout life about the needs of all generations: Recognizing and counteracting generational isolation. In M. London (Ed.), *The Oxford handbook of lifelong learning* (pp. 183–206) (2nd ed.). Oxford University Press.

Thaler, R., & Sunstein, C. (2021). *Nudge: The final edition.* Penguin.

Westrick-Payne, K. K. (2023). *Grandparents' characteristics by age.* Family Profile No. 02, 2023. National Center for Family & Marriage Research, Bowling Green State University. 10.25035/ncfmr/fp-23-02

Zung, W. W. K. (1965, January). A self-rating depression scale. *Archives of General Psychiatry, 12*(1), 63–70. 10.1001/archpsyc.1965.01720310065008

11   Intergenerational Communication

Challenge Age-Segregated Communication

Sources of Advice

George Orwell's (1949/2014) science fiction novel *1984* was meant to be a warning that communication between the generations should never be taken for granted. The main character, Winston Smith, had become discouraged because it seemed as though all aspects of privacy were being eliminated. Everything people did, even in their own homes, was monitored by telescreens operated by the government. Winston also worried about an additional loss of freedom presented by a new language that the state had invented as a way to control public thought. *Newspeak* was the name given to the politically correct vocabulary designed to reverse the meanings of words that were commonly used during the past. As a result, young people were unable to understand or appreciate values previous generations had relied on to set their goals and guide behavior. The only ways to access these former values was to search past literature or to speak with the few remaining old people.

There was a time when the identity of youth was shaped mainly by nationality, gender, race, religion, and socioeconomic status. Since then, technology has enabled young people to increase the amount of experiences they share with peers no matter where they live or their socioeconomic status. Peers are considered the dominant influence on socialization during adolescence at the same time influence of their parents and other grownups continues to decline. Because generation is such a powerful factor in defining identity, teenagers depend more on their peers for conversation, advice, and modeling. Adults should be aware of how this transition is impacting family relationships (Yung et al., 2021).

There are issues implicating social and emotional development where advice from more mature people is needed to process doubts, manage anxieties, set goals, determine priorities, and make decisions. The social self is too narrow when defined exclusively by peers. Teenagers might suppose that the only people who are able to understand them are others of their age group who have similar experiences. This premise should be challenged by older relatives and friends as they try to convince youth that peers should never be the single source of guidance about how to behave or actions to be taken (Brooks & Lasser, 2018; Davis, 2023; Freedman, 2020).

Many parents shield daughters and sons from responsibilities because they believe youth are not ready to make important decisions by themselves. This denial of experiences needed to grow up causes adolescents to feel disconnected from adults, trapping them in a social context governed by peers and media that shape aspirations, thinking, and direction. Being excessively dependent on peers does not define the whole youth subpopulation. However, it is evident that age-segregated interaction cannot

DOI: 10.4324/9781003401261-15

prepare students for the expectations of employers to collaborate with a wide age range of co-workers (Freedman & Stamp, 2021).

Consider a parent story. The event was a high school graduation party for their son who had invited friends to the house for conversation and cake. As students began to arrive, the parents went to their study where they would be out of the way. Twenty minutes later a girl opened the door, made known her observation that the extensive library was awesome, and asked for advice about career prospects in the field of psychology. The parents listened carefully to her reasons about why psychology appealed to her and were ready to answer questions. However, before they could state their views, a teenager showed up at the door and said, "Carrie, I've been looking all over the place for you. Why are you being anti-social?" Apparently, the young man did not think that Carrie's conversation with people older than herself qualified as a social activity.

Reliance on Social Networks

Pew Research Center surveys have shown that youth are increasing communication with friends while decreasing conversations with older relatives (Vogels et al., 2022). One father talked about taking his 14-year-old daughter and her boyfriend to a movie. As he drove them home, the father could hear the young couple in the back seat giggling and could tell from the rear-view mirror that they were texting each other. His observation was, "Suddenly, I felt really old and effectively screened out of a chance for an intergenerational conversation."

The excessive time that adolescents spend on social networks, texting, and smart phones reflects a growing reliance of adolescents on peers for guidance. They share photos, hopes, and concerns on Snapchat, Instagram, Twitter, and Meta. Texting friends is easier because the focus is on shared experiences and equality of status, two conditions that do not occur during conversations with adults (Katz et al., 2021).

The world is undergoing a shift in how families incorporate mobile technology into their lives. Some individuals adjust in a healthy manner while others adopt dysfunctional patterns. On average, adolescents spend six hours or more each day phoning, texting, communicating with age mates on social networks and e-media (Vogels et al., 2022).

In a study of 1,000 parents and their teenagers, the number of parents who acknowledged they spent too much of their time on mobile devices was 52% (Robb, 2019). More adolescents wish their parents would recognize what is happening and reduce the amount of time they spend on communication devices. The proportion of teens who believe their parents spend too much time on devices was 39%. Teenagers observed that their mothers and fathers provided them with a poor example, citing inattention of parents as a problem because they are preoccupied with cell phones during times families are together (Hari, 2022; Mark, 2023). In a related inquiry, Cole et al. (2021) asked a national sample of parents, children, and adolescents these questions: Do you ever feel like you are being ignored because a relative spends too much time talking on mobile devices, texting, or browsing? A majority of respondents (58%) reported that they had often experienced this situation.

Media Impact on Adolescents

In the opinion of U.S. Surgeon General Vivek Murthy, 13-year-olds are too young to join social media platforms (Ravipati, 2023). Instagram, Snapchat, and Twitter all allow users ages 13 or older on their platforms. Scientists have warned of a connection between heavy social media use and mental health issues in children, saying that the negatives outweigh the positives. Murthy agreed, "Age 13 is an important time for children to be thoughtful about what's going into how they think about their own self-worth. Their relationships and the skewed and often distorted environment of social media often does a disservice to many of those children. If we tell a child, 'Use the force of your willpower to control how much time you're spending,' you're pitting a child against the world's greatest product designers."

James Steyer, Professor at Stanford University and Director of Common Sense Media, a non-profit organization that advises parents across the nation regarding aspects of entertainment technology for youth, issued a statement in response to Dr. Vivek Murthy. Steyer expressed his support for Murthy: "This is exactly the kind of leadership we need from our Federal government when it comes to educating the public on technology's impact and holding large tech companies accountable for the impact of their platforms on the social, emotional and cognitive development of our nation's youth. ... It is time to face the facts: we are facing a youth mental health crisis and we need to address it immediately. We applaud the Surgeon General for his leadership and for bringing much-needed urgency to this critical area of protecting the well-being of kids and teens" (Steyer, 2023).

The explosion of communications technology and online social networking has led some observers to conclude that relationships are blossoming more than ever before. This assumption has been challenged by Sherry Turkle, Professor of Clinical Psychology at the Massachusetts Institute of Technology. Turkle's (2016) book *Reclaiming Conversation: The Power of Talk in a Digital Age* includes an extensive analysis of adolescent text messages. Her observation was that human disconnectedness is occurring at the same time connections are expanding with cell-phones and the Internet.

Anxiety is demonstrated by examples of when teenagers do not get immediate replies to their texts. One girl explained that she always needed her cell phone in case of emergencies. She defined an "emergency" as having feelings but not being able to share them with peers. Turkle's (2016) research about the communication patterns of adolescents led to the following insights:

1 Identity of adolescents is not being sufficiently shaped by self-exploration but instead by how individuals are viewed by members of their online network.
2 Mothers report communication with children is more frequent because of texting but also more trivial and less meaningful.
3 Meta users who focus on status updates devalue the true intimacies of friendships.
4 Video chat like Skype or FaceTime can appear more intimate than is actually the case. What was meant as a mechanism to enrich communication seems to push some people closer to their devices while driving them further away from each other.

Older Adults Screen Time and Social Media

Extent of Participation

Just as adolescents and young adults feel most comfortable when they are communicating with others exposed to similar experiences, the same condition accounts for a bond among older adults who remember the Beatles, Vietnam War, President Nixon, LSD, and Tom Jones. Baby Boomers, born between 1946 and 1964, are a large group of web users.

The social world of older adults is being transformed by the Internet. Women and men report being online helps reduce feelings of isolation, curbs loneliness, and challenges experiences of boredom. Staying in touch with relatives is the main reason older adults give for engaging in social networks. In contrast, young and middle-aged adults report that staying in contact with friends is the most important reason for them to participate in networking.

During the past decade, websites have emerged that cater to the social needs of older adults. For example, some retirees prefer https://www.321chat.com/senior/ because they enjoy webcam chats, like to meet new people, or want to explore prospects for romance. Others want to log on to www.thirdage.com that focuses on health issues for adults who are age 45 and older, a group that is more empowered than previous generations and more often implicated as caregivers for aging parents. This website contains articles on health and fitness, blogs, travel photos, and descriptions of consumer benefits.

Facebook is the most used online social network worldwide (Dixon, 2023). About twenty years ago, Mark Zuckerberg launched Facebook from his dormitory room at Harvard University. Ortutay (2023) stated, "Today, 3 billion people check it each month. That's more than a third of the world's population. And 2 billion log in every day. Yet it still finds itself in a battle for relevancy, and its future, after two decades of existence." Facebook has the challenge of trying to ensure relevancy across an ever-broadening age range of users than when the initial audience was largely limited to young adults. Dealing with the problem of age relevance is illustrated by many Millennials who regard Meta (formerly Facebook) as old fashioned with parents still posting pictures of their children and expressing political views. Therefore, many Millennials have moved on to Instagram (owned by Meta) signing in several times a day.

Older adults (75 years and older) enjoy watching TV. The average daily time they spent watching TV per capita in the United States for the years 2009 to 2021 showed this group watched TV more than any other group; in 2021, their average daily time watching TV was 4.8 hours (Stoll, 2023).

Generational Benefits of Reciprocal Learning

People in the same generation share a unique location in time and resulting exposure to similar world events, pop culture trends, and norms that were established when they grew up. As social change quickens it is imperative to become aware of how younger cohorts see situations, respect principles that guide their behavior, know their vision of the future, and view them as essential sources to learn from regarding their experiences and interpretation of events. These conditions define *reciprocal learning*, mutual growth based on consideration of feelings, ideas, values, and perspectives of a different generation (P. S. Strom & Strom, 2021).

Little is known about the executive function of the brain that people rely on for reflection about the perspectives held by others. However, this mental process has been identified as an important factor in communicating with individuals whose experiences differ from our own. A comparative study involved 121 healthy participants from ages 17 to 84. They performed tasks testing their ability to sustain attention and switch back and forth from the view of one party to the other. Results determined that the ability to engage in perspective-taking diminishes with age (Long et al., 2018).

Perceptions about Parents and Grandparents

Adults often inflate their willingness to learn from younger relatives. This conclusion was based on outcomes from numerous studies using the *Parent Success Indicator* (R. D. Strom et al., 2000, 2008). This instrument evaluates parent performance based on views of two generations, parents and their 10-to-14-year-old adolescents. One item appearing on the adult version states, "I am good at learning from my child." The optional responses include always, often, seldom, and never. The same item within the adolescent version is "My parent is good at learning from me." Significant differences have been found between generational responses of culturally diverse (Black, White, and Hispanic) mothers and adolescents for studies conducted in the United States. Adolescents assigned unfavorable ratings to their mothers for being willing to learn from them. Meanwhile, most mothers assigned themselves high ratings for willingness to learn from their children.

Similar results were found for grandparents who typically declared they are eager to learn from their younger relatives. Again, the contrary report expressed by youth is that older relatives are unwilling to learn from them. The three-generational instrument, the *Grandparent Strengths and Needs Inventory,* has been applied to examine the role performance of thousands of grandparents as perceived by culturally-diverse parents, grandchildren, and grandparents in the United States and overseas (Buki et al., 2003; R. D. Strom & Strom, 2013, 2017, 2018; R. D. Strom et al., 1995, 1997, 2000). Significant differences separate generational perceptions about grandparents' willingness to learn from younger generations. Unless and until this situation modifies, hopes for better communication are unlikely to be met.

Reinforce Importance of Staying Focused

Being Available to Listen

Technology can fragment family relationships when grownups are preoccupied by mobile devices. Catherine Steiner-Adair, Professor of Psychiatry at Harvard University, interviewed thousands of adolescents as a base for her book, *The Big Disconnect: Protecting Childhood and Family Relationships in the Digital Age* (Steiner-Adair & Barker, 2013). She concluded that many parents are unavailable to their children, seem disconnected, and narcissistic as shown by the common practice of constantly gazing into mobile devices, looking for the next text, tweet, or email. One message this egocentric behavior communicates to children is that "Anybody who is somewhere else matters more than you do." Some youth reported they are tired of being the call waiting in their parents' lives. Boundaries that protect work and family life have become blurred, and at great cost to development of intimate relationships (Mark, 2023).

Parents typically remind children to pay attention because they realize that this behavior influences comprehension and learning. But, paying attention is not modeled by many parents. Consider an example from a father's observation regarding his 3-year-old daughter.

> Whenever she is trying to get my attention, wants me to look at something she has created, or asks a question, she knows that if I am focusing on something else my inclination is to make meaningless statements like 'Uh huh,' 'Oh, yeah,' or 'That's neat' without turning my head to see her. In these moments, her tone will become more insistent as she says, 'Daddy, look at me with your eyes.' This may sound so basic, but

it is her method to get my undivided attention in the only way that she knows to confirm it—when I am looking directly at her.

Daniel Siegel, a Psychiatrist at the University of California, reminds adults that children need to have their feelings acknowledged because it contributes to emotional attachment. Paying attention to children is a fundamental ingredient for good parenting whereas distraction interferes with emotional attachment and prevents normal development (Jackson, 2018; Siegel & Hartzell, 2014).

Expectations for Adult Learning

In a longevity society education must go beyond just preparing for employment and workforce competencies to include learning needs during retirement. A common obstacle is that many older adults define retirement as the time when they should get to do only the things that please them. Other older adults suppose they deserve a carefree life as recognition for their years of employment. A more mature outlook recognizes that people stop working when they retire but should continue learning to remain a favorable influence on others.

Retirees are the only subpopulation whose learning needs remain undefined by society. Therefore, the content of adult education classes they enroll in is self-determined instead of based on what the rest of society believes they should learn. This unreasonable practice reflects a lack of consensus goals needed to guide development during later life, cannot support attitudes and skills for adjustment, and prevents the acquisition of knowledge to honor family priorities and attain maturity. Population forecasts show that by 2034 for the first time in history, older adults will be a larger group than the population under age 18 (Freedman & Stamp, 2021; Vespa et al., 2020). Perhaps we should ask ourselves: How will a society characterized by this future thrive? If more emphasis is placed on the pursuit of maturity than on aspirations for anti-aging, grandparent education will receive greater attention so a sensible transformation of their role in the family will become more common.

Community agencies and organizations that provide classes for retirees seldom evaluate the outcomes of their instruction on the premise that the assessment procedures we insist on for younger students would cause anxiety and stress for elders, and perhaps cause them to become dropouts. A more promising view is that, unless evaluation is applied to determine what older adults learn, there is no way to accurately judge effectiveness of programs for them or detect changes needed to make their curriculum more relevant. Public estimates of older adult capacity to learn requires evidence that would support their inclusion in national planning to favorably impact mental and social health for all age groups (R. D. Strom & Strom, 2018).

Common Learning Needs of Generations

Education is important at all ages so people can be aware about the present and future concerns of other age groups and give support to them (R. D. Strom & Strom, 2012, 2018). Some grandparents report that it is difficult to keep a conversation going with their grandchildren because "we seem to have nothing in common." A more reasonable outlook calls for the realization that every generation has some learning needs that can only be met through mutual support. This list of learning needs defines all ages.

 1 Coping with stressful experiences
 2 Reasonable time management plans
 3 Use of technology tools to learn
 4 Intergenerational communication
 5 Setting goals and amending them
 6 Knowing how to resolve conflict
 7 Financial management and saving
 8 Avoid mobile device distractions
 9 Detection and admission of failure
10 Use fair peer and self-evaluation
11 Delay immediate gratification
12 Become a self-directed learner
13 Adopt a lifestyle that is unhurried
14 Protect the natural environment
15 Spiritual and ethical development

Living in the Past, Present, and Future

A Balanced Perspective

Besides communicating more often with older and younger generations, adults should make wise decisions about their perspective of time. The way to avoid living too much in the past, present, or future is to adopt a balanced orientation in viewing time. There are aspects of living where it might seem reasonable to identify primarily with the past as a means to enable cultural preservation. Many people feel this way about their religious faith that is rooted in distant history and serves as a source of current hope for the future. Individuals often decide the spiritual realm is one context where they want to remain fixed on the past and do not care if others consider them old-fashioned. In other sectors of life, however, it may be necessary to leave historical aspects behind to confront current challenges. Practices related to medicine, business, and manufacturing are discontinued when research and innovation reveal more effective ways to accomplish things. This shift is identified as progress or cultural evolution. Similarly, family members should think about whether their interaction with relatives reflects a past orientation and remains sensible for the transformation of roles that is needed to support a modern productive relationship (Gleick, 2017; Kellerman & Seligman, 2023).

One change that characterizes modern nations is planning to ensure equality of access to health care, education, and preservation of the environment. Everyone should look ahead as the basis for personal goals and engage in planning as long as sufficient attention is paid to current needs. For people who become preoccupied with the future, spontaneity does not exist because they embrace the assumption that every activity has to be planned. Individuals who are strictly future-oriented are constantly looking forward to when they graduate, when they get a fulltime job, when they get engaged and married, when they become parents, when they are promoted at work, and set aside enough money for travel. It seems they avoid living in the present. Instead, they wait, they save, they are going to do so many things and have such good times someday – and life goes by (Burkeman, 2021).

Stuck in One Timeframe

Every generation should be on guard against becoming stuck in a single time orientation. Since the past is where most achievements of older adults lie, they are inclined to adopt nostalgia as they look back in time more than may is good for their mental health. By inviting older people to become volunteers. in public elementary schools, they can be motivated to shift from a past orientation to a more comprehensive outlook that also includes the present. This shift is needed because adults who become stuck in the past have difficulty accepting non-traditional goals of society such as equality, gender sharing of domestic chores, respect for the opinions of children, and common involvement with technology. Resisting these attitudes by maintaining a strictly past orientation promotes social isolation. However, this is not a lost cause. Studies of attitude shifts show older adults are more capable of changing their minds than commonly supposed (Kellerman & Seligman, 2023).

Parents of teenagers can also get stuck in the past, especially when they attempt to govern conduct of their children by resorting to outdated forms of discipline. Instead of expecting their children to always obey them, they should teach children to exercise critical thinking, make some decisions on their own, and rely on reasonable criteria to apply for self-evaluation. Other parents reveal they are stuck in the past when they look back at the early stages of their child's life as the best of times. The fact is every age of children can provide opportunities for parents to discover the joys of supporting younger relatives in their process of growing up.

Some adolescents and young adults become stuck in the past by supposing their identity should be based on events that took place before they were born, circumstances they could not have participated in. Ethnicity is a coincidence of birth that results in some people being Irish, German, Hispanic, or Black. Heritage is not a matter of choice nor is one ancestry better than any other. In a global context, pride should emerge mainly from actions taken in the present, not the past, and reflect personal motivation, behavior, and achievements rather than things that were accomplished by ancestors.

Some parents demonstrate they are stuck in the present when they are preoccupied with their jobs and fail to invest enough time in their marriage and guidance of children. Other parents show excessive concern about the present when they spend too much income on entertainment, while failing to set aside money needed for college tuition of children and their own retirement. Adolescents and young adults can also get stuck in the present when they devote excessive time to peer communication, reflecting a serious imbalance in how time should be used to maximize personal potential. While technology has enabled rapid communication, concern is growing about the decline of interaction among generations within families (Freedman & Stamp, 2021; Turkle, 2016).

Adolescents get stuck in the present when they lack long-term goals and sense of vision that is needed to motivate dedication, selective attention, and a focus on productive behavior (Duckworth, 2018; Mark, 2023). Some teenagers are not expected to adopt long-range plans to guide their preparation for a career. Instead of encouraging young people to establish some of their own goals, parents may expect that they will follow the plans made for them by relatives, teachers, or other adults. All of us should recognize an overscheduled life usually results in stress, lack of goals, underachievement, and ill-mental health (P. S. Strom & Strom, 2021).

Another reason adolescents can get stuck in the present is that parents have not taught them to wait and plan for the things they desire. They suppose their wishes should be met immediately and therefore do not develop patience needed to succeed with their tasks and relationships that require continuous attention. For the near and foreseeable future, people of all ages will need to choose a personal path defined by a healthy balance of paying sufficient attention to the past, present, and future. This perspective can contribute to reciprocal learning and mental health of all generations.

Expansion of Criteria for Identity

People around the world are considering whether customary ways of defining personal identity should expand. The growth of technology, equality of aspirations, and mutual quest for interdependence is having an impact on individual self-impression. Identity cannot continue to be as closely related to social status, income, religion, ethnicity, or military power as it was in the past. Many individuals with low income believe their lives are as important as the lives of affluent people. This non-traditional outlook about status means personal growth requires going beyond the previous criteria of cultural identity and demonstrate concern about residents of other nations. In the past, a sense of belonging was generally limited to nationality or culture. Today, in many countries, refugees seen as outsiders and less important in the past are being welcomed. Such changes present immigration difficulties but also provide evidence of cultural progress (Twenge, 2023).

Cultures can still thrive in the future if there is a healthy balance of group identity, greater objectivity, and collective self-criticism. The inclination to refer to cultural differences without taking generational differences into account ignores the basis for internal criticism that is needed to balance important aspects of cultural preservation and cultural evolution.

Conclusion

Families, communities, and nations should encourage shifts in lifestyles that promote progress while ensuring that the values considered essential across time do not get left behind. Cultural preservation and cultural evolution are necessary and can be reconciled when there is sufficient intergenerational communication. Grandparents should realize communication with younger relatives is a way to improve their adjustment. When grandparents are better informed about the lives of younger relatives, this orientation can benefit everyone.

Discovering opportunities for adults and younger people to trade places as mentors will become a challenge from now on. Unless reasonable changes are made young people could restrict intergenerational communication even more to members of their cohort, having been denied adult listeners and respectful status. Successful relationships are reflected by shared dominance instead of unilateral control based on age, gender, or rank. People who value and rely on the strengths of one another reflect the universal need for interdependence.

Technology tools present an opportunity for adolescents to take leadership in improving communication across generations. A major challenge for youth is to improve time management, particularly to minimize age-segregated communication in favor of building a broader outreach that includes older relatives and people of other age groups. An innovative mission for schools should be to increase the amount of time students are expected to spend learning from older relatives and residents in their community. What students learn outside school is essential to equip them for a productive future. Making a shift from the current preoccupation with me, myself, and my peer group to giving greater attention to well-being of others supports further development of maturity. In addition, parents should teach children that responsibility for wise management of time includes sustaining regular contact with older loved ones so that both parties are better informed and offer mutual emotional support and guidance.

Age-segregated communication is easier because conversations include more agreement and less uncertainty. However, this practice has a negative effect of preventing thinking about issues that are considered important by other generations. Older adults should risk disclosing thoughts and feelings in order to make themselves better known and identify personal needs. Spending time together can result in reciprocal learning that can help both generations to build closer relationships and improve mental health.

Key Concepts

1 Conversations between younger and older relatives can increase by reliance on agenda questions that motivate self-disclosure of both parties and enable them to get to know each other better. Some school homework should acknowledge older adults as resources by making students generational reporters allowing them to enhance their perspective on events, ideas, and situations beyond what is acquired when restricted to age-segregated conversations or Internet searching.

2 The caring capacity of adolescents can be motivated by challenging them to assume leadership for improving the communication they have with older adults. Community service and school tasks involving communication with older adults helps students mature by making them aware of their responsibilities toward people outside the family.

3 Every generation should be aware of how other age groups interpret events, appreciate the values that guide behavior, acknowledge their vision about the future, and periodically trade places as sources of learning. Such conditions are met by recognizing that all age groups should be encouraged to participate in reciprocal learning with other generations.

4 During adolescence peers becomes the dominant source of influence for socialization. Because generation is such a powerful factor in shaping identity, youth rely more upon one another for interaction, advice, and direction than was the situation during previous generations.

5 Some important aspects of growing up require guidance from people more mature than the adolescent peer group. Help from adults is needed to process and interpret ideas, doubts, and concerns. The social self is too narrow when defined only by the ideas and feelings of peers.

6 When families are together, some parents are unavailable to children, disconnected as shown by constantly checking cell phones, waiting for a next text, email or Tweet. One message this behavior can convey to children is that the people who are not here matter more than you.

7 The concept of reverse mentoring requires turning around the usual relationship where an older person provides guidance for a younger person. In effect, it means parties trade places by shifting roles as a teacher and learner along with taking turns in sharing dominance.

8 Society should promote continuous education so everyone can remain aware about the present and future concerns of other age cohorts. Accordingly, the mission of schooling should go beyond readiness for a career and workforce competence to also

prepare no longer employed older adults for productive aging and a retirement that benefits their family and community.

9 One way to reduce risks associated with authority inversion is provide adolescents with an orientation to the attitudes and methods that are known to characterize good teaching. Possession of a skill does not ensure someone can help others they teach to acquire particular competence. There is a great need for more adolescents who demonstrate good teaching techniques.

10 Grandparents should assign priority to spending time with grandchildren. Cross-cultural studies have demonstrated that grandparents who spend more time interacting with grandchildren and doing things together are seen by three generations as more successful.

Generational Perspectives Activities

11.1 Team Discussion
11.2 Agenda for Interviews with Parents and Grandparents
11.3 Interview Children about Friendships
11.4 Generational Comparisons
11.5 A Scenario: Reasoning and Problem Solving
11.6 Team Chapter Review
11.7 Criteria for Self-Evaluation of Team Members

11.1 Team Discussion

1 What traditions should we honor and make an effort to preserve?
2 What traditions do we no longer benefit from and should leave behind?
3 What new traditions should we create and pass on as our unique legacy?
4 What aspects of your ethnic heritage should be kept? changed? left behind?
5 What advantages do children have that were not part of your growing up?
6 What growing up advantages did you have that are no longer available?
7 In what ways do older adults seem to be stuck in the past, present or future?
8 In what ways do you personally seem stuck in the past, present or future?
9 How do schools seem stuck in the past, present or future?
10 In what ways do your parents seem stuck in the past, present or future?

11.2 Agenda for Interviews with Parents and Grandparents

1 What are some aspects of growing up now that you would like to better understand?
2 What advantages and disadvantages appear to be associated with age-segregation?
3 What social benefits have you gained from online communication with your friends?
4 How is online communication with teenagers different from face-to-face talk?
5 What aspects of communication could you improve in relating to teenagers?
6 How does school homework of adolescents involve you as a source for learning?
7 How do you feel about having equal representation of adult age groups in Congress?
8 How do you suppose teenagers perceive their role as teachers of older relatives?
9 What are some lessons that you would like to be taught by your teenagers?

11.3 Interview Adolescents about Friendships

1 How frequently do you and friends send online messages to each other?
2 What is it about your friends that makes you like them more than others?
3 What are the biggest problems you have experienced with your friends?
4 What are the important conditions needed to build a lasting friendship?
5 What things do you talk to friends about but do not share with adults?
6 How do you solve a problem when friends disagree about something?
7 How willing are parents to consider you a source for their learning?
8 Why does your age group communicate more with friends than relatives?
9 In what ways will communication between age groups change in the future?
10 How willing are grandparents to consider you a source for their learning?

11.4 Generational Comparisons

Grandparents, parents and grandchildren are the only authorities about their own personal history. Cooperative learning teams can choose two or three adolescents and parents willing to answer questions on the cell phone, text, email or face-to-face. Provide them the agenda questions ahead of time so they can respond with relevant answers and schedule a convenient time. Make notes about your own answers you intend to give for each question because reciprocal learning is the goal.

1 Who are some famous people that you have admired and wanted to become like?
2 What have you liked most and disliked about your experiences in the classroom?
3 What things should older people learn so they understand people who are young?
4 What are the most important achievements that you have already accomplished?
5 How will things change in our country as more people become able to live longer?
6 What are some goals and dreams you continue to have and hope can be achieved?
7 What do you admire the most about your parents, grandparents, or grandchildren?
8 What can people of your age do to improve life for older people or younger people?
9 What are some favorite activities that you enjoy and look forward to doing?
10 What should the community and nation expect of people when they are retired?

11.5 A Scenario: Reasoning and Problem Solving

Problem solving scenarios present an opportunity to consider dilemmas, devise solutions, and engage in perspective taking by considering the views of others. Your task is to look at the pros and cons of stated choices, create more options, identify relevant information that may be missing, and defend reasoning for the advice that you consider best.

Kim is eating out with her daughter, son-in-law, and their two teenage sons. As soon as everyone tells the waitress their order, the boys and father begin gazing at their mobile devices and are speechless. Kim wonders how she should respond to this increasingly familiar situation during family time together.

a Tell everyone you hoped this time together could be spent on catching up.
b Shut up and accept an emerging lifestyle that is focused on distractions.

c Talk with her daughter only while the other relatives occupy themselves.
d Question why screen distractions should take precedence over the family.
e Other _____

11.6 Team Chapter Review

Efforts to assess participant learning, provide feedback, and improve quality of instruction is enhanced by a group review of each chapter.

1 What ideas in the lesson changed the way I think about this topic?
2 What insights from the lesson will I try to apply in my relationships?
3 What is the most important point for me presented in this lesson?
4 What are some aspects of this lesson I would like to better understand?
5 Which aspects of this lesson do I wish that I had known about earlier?

11.7 Criteria for Self-Evaluation of Team Members

Directions: For each question, place a check beside statements that reflect your feelings. You may give several answers on some items. If your feelings are not on the options list, write them on the line marked 'other.'

1 I believe some consequences of age-segregated communication are

  a students begin employment lacking experience in working with adults.
  b students rely more on their peer group for advice than they do on adults.
  c misunderstanding about strengths, goals, and values of other age groups.
  d loss of social and emotional support that is necessary for mental health.
  e Other _____

2 Bringing people of different age groups together for conversations

  a should become a priority of schools for some homework tasks.
  b could feature youth leadership since they are most tech savvy.
  c might involve talk shows with teenage to old age participants.
  d would identify mutual concerns and some issues that are unique.
  e Other _____

3 The greatest obstacle(s) to intergenerational communication are

  a adolescent engagement with social networks.
  b finding something in common to talk about.
  c willingness of older adults to self-disclose.
  d breaking away from old time priority habits.
  e Other _____

4 When children have tried to teach me things

  a I have been able to learn and express my gratitude.
  b They do not give enough time to practice a skill.

c I find they are motivated to help and encourage me.
d I have not requested help and none has been given.
e Other _____

5 The homework assignments of children

a sometimes direct them to ask me questions.
b never identify me as a source of perception.
c ignore only views of experts as important.
d rely only on the Internet and print sources.
e Other _____

6 When we spend family time together, cell phones

a should be turned off by all family members.
b interfere with paying attention to each other.
c distract the parents from talking to children.
d prevent adolescents from talking to parents.
e Other _____

7 When talking with younger relatives

a I have difficulty trying to keep our conversation going.
b I am less willing to share feelings than the children.
c I am always able to think of topics for us to explore.
d I learn more from the child than s/he learns from me.
e Other _____

8 When I communicate with younger relatives

a I rely on texting because s/he prefers this method.
b I use email because I like this method the best.
c I use Skype or FaceTime so we have face-to-face.
d I only like to use the telephone for conversations.
e Other _____

9 The cell phone habits of my younger relatives are

a excessive and take away from more important things.
b carefully monitored by the parents to avoid excess.
c similar to the overreliance shown by their parents.
d reasonable in amount of time spent on this activity.
e Other _____

10 I appreciate selfies sent by members of the family

a but feel they should not be used as substitutes for messages.
b and send pictures to them of things I do and places I visit.
c and share photos they take with my friends and acquaintances.
d but do not believe that a picture is worth a thousand words.
e Other _____

References

Brooks, M., & Lasser, J. (2018). *Tech generation: Raising balanced kids in a hyper-connected world.* Oxford University Press.

Buki, L. P., Ma, T-c., Strom, R. D., & Strom, S. (2003). Chinese immigrant mothers of adolescents: Self-perceptions of acculturation effects on parenting. *Cultural Diversity & Ethnic Minority Psychology*, 9(2), 127–140. 10.1037/1099-9809.9.2.127

Burkeman, O. (2021). *Four thousand weeks: Time management for mortals.* Farrar, Straus and Giroux.

Cole, J. I., Suman, M., Schramm, P., & Zhou, L. (2021). *2021 Digital Future Project: Surveying the digital future, Year Seventeen.* Center for the Digital Future University of Southern California Annenberg. https://www.digitalcenter.org/wp-content/uploads/2021/02/Digital-Future-Project-2021-edition.pdf

Davis, K. (2023). *Technology's child: Digital media's role in the ages and stages of growing up.* MIT Press.

Dixon, S. (2023, August 2). *Share of Facebook users in the United States as of August 2023, by age group.* Statista. https://www.statista.com/statistics/187549/facebook-distribution-of-users-age-group-usa/

Duckworth, A. (2018). *Grit: The power of passion and perseverance.* Scribner.

Freedman, M. (2020). *How to live forever: The enduring power of connecting the generations.* Public Affairs.

Freedman, M., & Stamp, T. (2021, March 15). Overcoming age segregation. *Stanford Social Innovation Review.* 10.48558/49jk-2k30

Gleick, J. (2017). *Time travel: A history.* Vintage.

Hari, J. (2022). *Stolen focus: Why you can't pay attention -- and how to think deeply again.* Crown.

Jackson, M. (2018). *Distracted: Reclaiming our focus in a world of lost attention.* Prometheus Books.

Katz, R., Ogilvie, S., Shaw, J., & Woodhead, L. (2021). *Gen Z, explained: The art of living in a digital age.* University of Chicago Press.

Kellerman, G., & Seligman, M. E. P. (2023). *Tomorrowmind: Thriving at work with resilience, creativity, and connection -- now and in an uncertain future.* Atria.

Long, M. R., Horton, W. S., Rohde, H., & Sorace, A. (2018, January). Individual differences in switching and inhibition predict perspective-taking across the lifespan. *Cognition, 170,* 25–30. 10.1016/j.cognition.2017.09.004

Mark, G. (2023). *Attention span: A groundbreaking way to restore balance, happiness, and productivity.* Hanover Square.

Ortutay, B. (2023, May 8). *Facebook has 3 billion users. Many of them are old.* https://apnews.com/article/facebook-teenagers-tiktok-instagram-young-adults-fc9f6daa605e7c7f6fd5f4eaa90141fa

Orwell, G. (2014). *1984.* Harper Perennial. (Original work published 1949)

Ravipati, S. (2023, January 29). *Surgeon General: 13-year-olds too young to join social media platforms.* AXIOS. https://www.axios.com/2023/01/29/us-surgeon-general-vivek-murthy-youth-social-media

Robb, M. B. (2019). *The new normal: Parents, teens, screens, and sleep in the United States.* Common Sense Media. https://resources.finalsite.net/images/v1560519249/fcis/snttiqmx155f0fvzw8yp/2019-new-normal-parents-teens-screens-and-sleep-united-states.pdf

Siegel, D. J., & Hartzell, M. (2014). *Parenting from the inside out: How a deeper self-understanding can help you raise children who thrive.* Penguin Group.

Steiner-Adair, C., & Barker, T. H. (2013). *The big disconnect: Protecting childhood and family relationships in the digital age.* Harper.

Steyer, J. P. (2023, January 30). *Statement on Surgeon General saying 13 is too young for social media.* Common Sense Media. https://www.commonsensemedia.org/press-releases/statement-on-surgeon-general-saying-13-is-too-young-for-social-media

Stoll, J. (2023, April 20). *Average daily time spent watching TV per capita in the United States from 2009 to 2021, by age group.* Statista. https://www.statista.com/statistics/411775/average-daily-time-watching-tv-us-by-age/

Strom, P. S., & Strom, R. D. (2012). A paradigm for intergenerational learning. In M. London (Ed.), *The Oxford handbook of lifelong learning* (pp. 133–146). Oxford University Press. 10.1093/oxfordhb/9780195390483.013.0049

Strom, P. S., & Strom, R. D. (2021). *Adolescents in the Internet age: A team learning and teaching perspective* (3rd ed.). Information Age.

Strom, R. D., Strom, S., Collinsworth, P., Sato, S., Makino, K., Sasaki, Y., Sasaki, H., & Nishio, N. (1995). Grandparents in Japan: A three generational study. *The International Journal of Aging and Human Development*, *40*(3), 209–226. 10.2190/KYFJ-DGWF-WJB8-FLYR

Strom, R. D., Buki, L. P., & Strom, S. (1997). Intergenerational perceptions of English-speaking and Spanish-speaking Mexican-American grandparents. *International Journal of Aging and Human Development*, *45*(1), 1–21. 10.2190/L0AV-0MU6-BK74-CE1B

Strom, R. D., Strom, S., Strom, P. S., Makino, K., & Morishima, Y. (2000). Perceived parenting success of mothers in Japan. *Journal of Family Studies*, *6*(1), 25–45. 10.5172/jfs.6.1.25

Strom, R. D., Strom, P. S., & Beckert, T. (2008,Fall). Comparing Black, Hispanic and White mothers of adolescents with a national standard of parenting. *Adolescence*, *43*(171), 525–546. PMID:19086668.

Strom, R. D., & Strom, P. S. (2013). Grandparents and reciprocal learning for family harmony. In P. Hughes (Ed.), *Achieving quality education for all: Perspectives from the Asia-Pacific region and beyond* (pp. 139–145). Springer.

Strom, R. D., & Strom, P. S. (2017). Grandparent learning and cultural differences. *Educational Gerontology*, *43*(8), 417–427. 10.1080/03601277.2017.1314642

Strom R. D., & Strom, P. S. (2018). Education for grandparents in longevity societies. *Journal of Adult and Continuing Education*, *24*(2), 208–228. 10.1177/1477971418810652

Turkle, S. (2016). *Reclaiming conversation: The power of talk in a digital age*. Penguin.

Twenge, J. M. (2023). *Generations*. Atria.

Vespa, J., Medina, L., & Armstrong, D. M. (2020). *Demographic turning points for the United States: Population projections for 2020 to 2060*. United States Census Bureau. https://www.census.gov/content/dam/Census/library/publications/2020/demo/p25-1144.pdf

Vogels, E. A., Gelles-Watnick, R., & Massarat, N. (2022, August 10). *Teens, social media and technology 2022*. Pew Research Center. https://www.pewresearch.org/internet/2022/08/10/teens-social-media-and-technology-2022/

Yung, A. R., Cotter, J., & McGorry P. D. (2021). *Youth mental health: Approaches to emerging mental ill-health in young people*. Routledge.

12   Death, Grief and Recovery

Looking at Tomorrow

Think about Widowhood

Husbands and wives can help each other by regularly reviewing their affairs. Both partners along with sons and daughters should know where the estate papers are kept. Spouses should know what to do at the time of death. Making a will and assigning power of attorney is an important responsibility for a couple, hopefully long before either of the partners becomes terminally ill (Hoyt & Goldy-Brown, 2022; Mayo Clinic, 2023).

Both spouses should be informed about family commitments. This knowledge will help when s/he must assume new responsibilities. Sharing takes time but can reduce the burden later for a spouse. Depend on each other but maintain the ability to fend for oneself. For example, this means that women should continue driving instead of always relying on husbands. And husbands who do not know how to cook should commit to learning. Research shows that in the year after losing a spouse, men were 70% more likely to die than similar age men who did not lose a spouse, while women were 27% more likely to die compared to women who did not become widowed (Weiss, 2023). Support the personality development of your spouse and take pride in his or her growth and achievements. Have good times together and let each other know how grateful you are for your partnership. Build memories because they will be the most important gifts that are left to your spouse, children, and grandchildren.

Benefits of Hospice Care

Hospice is a program of care and support for people who are terminally ill (with a life expectancy of six months or less, if the illness runs its normal course) and their families. Here are some important facts about hospice (Centers for Medicare & Medicaid Services, 2022, 2023):

- The focus is on comfort (palliative care), not curing an illness.
- Services typically include physical care, counseling, drugs, equipment, and supplies for the terminal illness and related conditions.
- A specially trained team of professionals and caregivers provide care for the "whole person," including physical, emotional, social, and spiritual needs.
- Care is generally given in the home.
- Family caregivers can get support.
- Hospice isn't only for people with cancer.

DOI: 10.4324/9781003401261-16

Palliative care is the part of hospice care that focuses on helping people who are terminally ill and their families maintain their quality of life. If you're terminally ill, palliative care can address your physical, intellectual, emotional, social, and spiritual needs. Palliative care supports your independence, access to information, and ability to make choices about your health care (National Institute on Aging, 2021). Medicare, Medicaid, most private insurance plans, HMOs, and other care organizations cover hospice care, and pay all or most of the expenses.

Balance in Daily Life

Strive for balance in your experiences as a couple. In this context, Elisabeth Kübler-Ross (1926–2004), author of grief stage theory, provided a valuable lesson. She wrote, "While growing up in Switzerland, I was educated with the basic premise of work, work, work. You are a valuable human being only if you work. Looking back, I realize this guideline was utterly wrong. Half working and half dancing – that seems about the right mixture. I myself have danced and played too little." Her gravesite at the Paradise Memorial Gardens Cemetery in Scottsdale, Arizona, has this message on the headstone: "Loving mother, and grandmother, compassionate friend, teacher and student. Graduated to 'dance in the galaxies' on August 24, 2004. We'll be loving you always" (Kübler-Ross, 1969).

A related viewpoint comes from Michael Josephson, former Professor of Law at the University of Michigan and Assistant District Attorney in Los Angeles. Later, he established the Josephson Institute of Ethics in Los Angeles that monitors youth development nationally and provides instruction in character development. Josephson wrote a poem that urges reflection by adults about the way they spend their time. Josephson's (2003) poem is entitled *What Will Matter**.

Ready or not, some day it will all come to an end.
There will be no more sunrises, no minutes, hours or days.
All the things you collected, whether treasured or forgotten will pass to someone else.
Your wealth, fame and temporal power will shrivel to irrelevance.
It will not matter what you owned or what you were owed.
Your grudges, resentments, frustrations and jealousies will finally disappear.
So too, your hopes, ambitions, plans and to do lists will expire.
The wins and losses that once seemed so important will fade away.
It won't matter where you came from or what side of the tracks you lived on at the end.
It won't matter whether you were beautiful or brilliant.
Even your gender and skin color will be irrelevant.
So what will matter? How will the value of your days be measured?
What will matter is not what you bought but what you built, not what you got but what you gave.
What will matter is not your success but your significance.
What will matter is not what you learned but what you taught.
What will matter is every act of integrity, compassion, courage or sacrifice that enriched, empowered or encouraged others to emulate your example.
What will matter is not your competence but your character.
What will matter is not how many people you knew, but how many will feel a lasting loss when you're gone.
What will matter is not your memories, but the memories of those who loved you.
What will matter is how long you will be remembered, by whom and for what.

Living a life that matters doesn't happen by accident.
It's not a matter of circumstance but of choice.
Choose to live a life that matters.
*From: Josephson, M. (2003). *What will matter*. Josephson Institute of Ethics.
https://josephsoninstitute.org. Copyright © 2003 by Michael Josephson.
Reprinted with permission.

Elements of Adjustment

Most people accept the concept of uniqueness as it applies to the physical world. For example, fingerprints are one of a kind. Still, people often deny the possibility of uniqueness in the realm of emotional experience. However, the fact is widowed women and men vary in the way they manage grief, duration, intensity, and sequence of grieving stages, outlook they bring to a tragedy, and the pace of recovery. Therefore, it is wise to accept first-hand accounts about the way a widowed individual feels rather than believing the person is over-reacting, or not behaving as they should be based on our experience in observing how other people managed grief. There are many factors that impact coping including the previous losses a person has faced, support they receive, closeness of relationship with the deceased, role that the spouse had in their life, circumstances surrounding the death, religious beliefs on what happens after death, age of both parties, and other aspects of experience. All these factors urge consideration of the individual. Consider some practical guidelines that can ease adjustment process for widowhood persons (Cain, 2022).

Take Time to Grieve

Some men and women whose lives correspond with the current rapid pace of living reject the traditional saying that "Time heals all wounds." These people are accustomed to expecting quick solutions for most problems and tend to be impatient with situations that require prolonged effort before progress is evident (Roberts, 2015). There is no doubt that many inventions we rely on to speed up processes such as microwave cooking have led to greater convenience. In contrast, an emphasis on speed can impair mental health if this strategy is applied to emotional recovery (Gleick, 1996, 2017). What happens is that people appear willing to accept someone else's grief providing the individual works through the recovery process in a short time. Sometimes this rush to bring grieving to an end can come from relatives. If they expect a family member should resume a normal life before it is possible, recommend they read this chapter to become aware of the slow recovery process needed to adjust to the crisis of attachment. Most widowed persons require a year and sometimes even more to adjust to their new situation. Even then, special events like birthdays, anniversaries, and holidays retrigger feelings of grief (Carr, 2016).

Most people are poorly informed about the grieving process so they persist in believing that widowed persons should feel obliged to recover in a short time. Co-workers and employers are the most likely to avoid someone in grief because they feel uncertain regarding what to say or how to relate to the person. The insensitive statements they make can be an unintended source of stress and cause feelings of alienation and hurt (Devine & Nepo, 2017; James & Friedman, 2017).

Continue to Share Feelings

Husbands and wives usually count on their spouse as the person who listens to their concerns, cares for them if they are ill, helps make decisions, monitors quality of their thinking, provides corrective feedback on their behavior, shares meals and conversations, sets goals and plans with them, participates in leisure activities together, looks out for their safety, and promotes self-esteem. These basic needs continue after a spouse dies but must be met by someone else (Mabry, 2017). Telling relatives and friends about feelings makes them more aware and can diminish the sorrow of someone who is grieving. The new listeners must be willing to hear negative feelings that are brought on by occasional depression. Recognize that joyful experiences can still be shared, even though the grieving process continues (Cain, 2022; James & Friedman, 2017).

Keep Making Decisions

When healthy widowed persons review their process of recovery, they usually conclude that maintaining a degree of independence was important in helping them to overcome grief. At the time, it would have been easier to allow other relatives to make decisions for them. However, it is better to accept some assistance initially such as when relatives help take care of aspects of funeral arrangements but leave the choice of coffin, nature of burial service, and other details to the widow/widower. A close friend or relative who can look out for the best interests of the family should accompany someone who is grieving. Taking this approach leads to learning important procedures like knowing how many death certificates are needed to settle financial affairs, how to change or end social security payments, and prepare insurance forms. Time on such tasks provides distraction from self-examination, and confirms the person is capable of managing personal affairs. A trusted friend can help with processing medical cost statements incurred during the final period of life. Medicare and insurance bills should be examined but survivors are commonly distracted and find this task an additional source of stress (Carr, 2016).

Making major decisions should be avoided, especially ones that involve lifestyle like moving to another place, selling the house, or getting married again. These judgments are premature during the first year after the death of a spouse and frequently lead to regret. People who make such choices too soon usually do so because they hope that it will reduce feelings of loneliness. However, being lonely is a continuous burden for widowed persons no matter where they may go, and it will persist until they recover (Holt-Lunstad, 2017, 2021).

Newly widowed persons are able to handle everyday choices but should not overestimate their emerging capacity to deal with issues that may involve greater significance. This is a time when there is often insomnia, absentmindedness, problems trying to concentrate, failure of memory, the intrusion of unpleasant thoughts, and a tendency to repeat things over and over again. In combination, such limitations make it too difficult to sort out or evaluate long-term choices. It is better to wait until a sense of perspective returns.

Stages of Grief

Elisabeth Kübler-Ross was a psychiatrist and medical director of the Family Service and Mental Health Center in Chicago. She was also co-founder of Hospice in the United States. After she conducted interviews with 500 patients who were terminally ill, Kübler-Ross (1969) determined that survivors left behind to grieve generally experience similar emotional stages. People differ in the length of time they remain in each stage, the intensity of feelings they experience, sequence in which stages are encountered, and how often certain stages are repeated. The stages do not have a predictable progression. Nevertheless, there is agreement that these stages are an accurate portrayal of the usual grieving process and offer insight for anyone seeking to provide emotional support for survivors. The Kübler-Ross five stages of grief include (a) denial, (b) anger, (c) bargaining, (d) resignation, and (e) acceptance, and are described here.

Denial

Usually the first response of people who are grief-stricken is shock. Their typical reaction is, "No, it can't be true. I do not believe it." The benefit provided by shock is that it temporarily protects people from becoming overwhelmed with sorrow and having to face the truth all at once. Terrible news takes time to be fully accepted. This means denial is a healthy form of escape from reality provided it lasts only a few days. Friends are often misled by the behavior of a widow at the funeral. What they suppose is an example of courage and presence of mind is actually a result of numbness, a buffer effect induced by denial. This natural defense helps individuals get through public obligations before they are allowed to withdraw and proceed with the process of grieving.

Initially, it is common for a widowed person to want to frequently visit the cemetery, be near the body of the loved one. The survivor may stand beside the grave and try to communicate, even though it is a one-way conversation. This evidence of denial is normal and shows that the grieving person remains unwilling to fully concede the separation. Relatives and friends should not discourage gravesite visits unless the practice becomes a compulsion and the widow feels it must be incorporated into the daily routine.

Anger

Sorrow is sometimes accompanied by feelings of anger. The target for anger might be anyone, including the deceased. If the widowed person is accustomed to suppressing anger, s/he can become stuck for a longer time in the denial stage (Filomena, 2017). For example, Jane's husband recently died of lung cancer but she cannot bear to show anger toward him so she rationalizes his two-pack a day cigarette habit was not enough to cause the disease. In contrast, MaryAnn's husband also died of a lung disorder and she is furious with him for ignoring her pleas to stop smoking when he knew the possible consequences. Regardless of whether widows or widowers are religious, they often inform God that He is to blame for the injustice of taking their spouse from them when the world has so many bad people who should have been chosen instead.

Sometimes widowed persons express anger about their own behavior, supposing that, if they had done certain things, the deceased would still be alive. Anger can also implicate friends who have not bothered to visit since the funeral or relatives inclined to treat the bereaved person like a child. At times anger centers on what is seen as an unreasonable effort by the doctors to keep a terminally ill and suffering person alive. Grieving persons need someone to help them monitor their response of anger and tell them when this behavior becomes excessive (Hertz, 2021).

Bargaining

Death is the end of life, a condition that cannot be changed. Nevertheless, some widowed persons convince themselves that the loss they suffer might have been prevented so they punish themselves with comments like: "If only we had gone to the Mayo Clinic for the best diagnostic testing, she would still be alive," "If only he had taken the early retirement option when I wanted him to," "If only he would have stayed on the low cholesterol diet that the doctor recommended." Whether these precautions would have altered events will never be known and no longer matter after the death.

Since God has not responded to angry pleas, it is supposed that He may consider a more kindly request. Therefore, widowed persons, or those with a terminally ill spouse may resort to promises of good behavior, public service, and compensation to the community if the dying person is allowed to live longer. Such attempts to bargain for more time reveal that a grieving person is locked into thinking about the present and still cannot deal with their future. The best thing relatives and friends who listen to a bereaved person pray for the impossible is to provide comfort, demonstrate affection, and pray themselves with a focus on thanksgiving for the life of the deceased and appeals for strength so the survivor can endure the loss (James & Friedman, 2017).

Resignation

When people abandon hope of being reunited with a loved one, they often experience depression. Feelings of depression are shown by lack of interest in the future. During such times, people report feeling useless. This outlook suggests that life no longer has purpose and will never again provide a sense of meaning. Fortunately, it is possible for most people to be occasionally distracted from dwelling on their personal situation by experiencing short intervals of joy. Then a memory, familiar place, or event activates depression once again. Studies have found that, from 15% to 30% of survivors, experience clinically significant depression in the year following death of a spouse. Some of the signs that depression is continuing too long are neglect of personal appearance, poor eating habits, and withdrawal from interaction with others. These symptoms suggest consideration of seeking professional counseling (National Institute on Aging, 2020).

The goal at this stage of grieving is to assume greater control of life, achieve a balance of moods so that satisfaction can become more prevalent in the overall outlook about life. This is difficult because a lot of energy is devoted to feeling sorry for self. A helpful way to offset the poor self-impression that typically comes with depression is to spend time with others who are able to stimulate a positive picture of self-worth. This can happen by involvement with support groups like the American Association of Retired Persons Widow to Widow program and by volunteering at an elementary school. Young children are often the most persuasive source to confirm for a survivor that s/he still has value as a single person. Spending time trying to help children does not end personal sorrow but can renew joyful feelings, boost self-esteem, and provide the orientation bereaved persons need to regain an optimistic perspective about their future.

Acceptance

There comes a time when the widowed person recognizes, "I have survived and can go on living without someone who was very important to me. I am ready to resume my interest in the future, establish new goals and identity for myself, and invest more energy in relationships again." This constructive attitude is possible because emotional balance has gradually replaced a one-sided pessimistic view of life. The person is no longer preoccupied with events of the past nor overcome by uncertainty regarding their future.

They enjoy certain aspects of the present, express feelings to other people, and show greater confidence in making decisions instead of always guessing what their spouse would want them to do (O'Connor, 2023).

Of course, the habit of planning with two people in mind is difficult to break, because it calls for looking at tomorrow from a new and independent perspective. No one becomes the old self again because identity has changed. This means that, for a while, it is best to look ahead only a short distance and set goals that can be achieved within a matter of hours, days, or weeks. Dealing with more than one task remains difficult, so it can help to write lists of chores that must be done and then decide the order of their priority. This simple procedure can ensure that daily obligations are taken care of without experiencing the feeling of being overwhelmed (Devine & Nepo, 2017).

Recovery

Friends and Loneliness

Widowed persons identify loneliness as their most difficult problem (Hertz, 2021; Holt-Lunstad, 2017, 2021; Holt-Lunstad et al., 2015). Eight months after the death of her husband, Pearl wrote this note to her nephew:

> "It is so lonesome without Gordon that some days I wonder whether I can make it. My life seems to have no future. Then I scold myself and remember what good children I have, wonderful friends standing by me, and my church. After that I thank God for all of my blessings." During widowhood, the most important relationship in life is gone, and can never be replaced. However, by developing new friendships, experiences can still be shared. Whether or not your family lives close by, make an effort to meet new people.

Studies have shown that widows adjust better socially than widowers (The National Academies of Sciences, Engineering, & Medicine, 2020). One reason may be that the identity of women, until recently, has centered on their husband, as symbolized by taking his last name to become their own. When a husband dies, his wife's lifestyle radically changes because, until recently, fewer women had continuous employment careers. Problems of making decisions, handling finances, concerns about personal safety, and worry about dependent children seem to outweigh the difficulty widowers have learning to get by in the kitchen and managing a household (Holt-Lunstad, 2021; Weiss, 2023).

Widows frequently complain that friends they have known for years, particularly couples, exclude them from their activities. The explanation widows usually give is that women friends consider them to be a potential threat to their marriage. It is less often recognized that being around a widow reminds a couple of the husband's mortality and the condition his own wife may someday have to face. It is not surprising that widows would like to spend some time with men. However, instead of blaming old friends, try to make new ones. Some new friends might be younger and can do much to enlarge perspective. It takes initiative to enlarge the social circle.

Attend a Support Group

So much of grieving is talking about confused feelings that it is worthwhile to seek out those willing to give their undivided attention. Some of the best listeners are women or men who have been widowed. They have already endured the suffering, confused feelings, and loneliness. People often say, "I just didn't feel I could make it until I heard the stories of other widowed persons." Sharing stories is the essence of a support group. Members can provide evidence that others have traveled a similar difficult path and emerged as independent persons (James & Friedman, 2017).

Support groups also provide assurance that to worry about one's mental state is normal. There is often fear about the unknown workings of the mind. When a person knows what to expect ahead of time, s/he is less likely to be overwhelmed. During grief, even supernatural events seem to be common. From 20% to 50% of widowed persons report seeing, hearing, or sensing the presence of the deceased. They seldom report these experiences because grievers believe other people will consider them mentally ill. Some men and women prolong their grief by staying home to avoid the prospect that others will discover their mental confusion. They want to reduce the risk of being seen as a fool in public. Nevertheless, the risk of making mistakes, learning new things, and sharing feelings with others are worth taking. Withdrawal is not the key to recovery; the gradual acquisition of a new perspective is what matters most (National Institute on Aging, 2020).

Besides family, friends, and other widowed persons, talking to a family counselor who is trained to work with bereaved persons can help. Wives that have forewarning of their husband's death usually adjust better than those who are widowed unexpectedly. The critical advance time appears to be two weeks which gives people a chance to say goodbye, express affection, ask for forgiveness, renounce regrets, reconcile, make promises, say things that should be told, and try to settle issues that were previously unresolved (Mabry, 2017).

Jane's story reminds us that grandchildren can be important sources of comfort. After she was widowed, Jane visited her son and his family in New York. The granddaughters were 9 and 12 years old. "The nine-year-old Tiffany wanted me to sleep with her. After we were in bed and said our prayers, Tiffany put her arms around me and said, 'Now, Grandma, I know that you miss Grandpa Lou. But if you want to talk anytime, I will be here to listen.' I replied, 'Well, it's good to know that. Thank you.' The next morning, I asked my son and his wife if they had told Tiffany to talk to me. They knew nothing about it. I said, 'She's had wonderful training from you as her parents and passed it on to her grandmother.' I still get choked up whenever I tell my friends this beautiful story."

The average age for becoming a widow or widower is 59 (Gurrentz & Mayol-Garcia, 2021). There are 12 million widows and 4 million widowers in the United States. More older men than women remarry after the death of a spouse. Some explain this difference by suggesting that men have more opportunities to remarry. A view less often mentioned is that older women prefer not to remarry because they know how to take care of themselves and have close ties with their children and grandchildren. Some women also prefer to be free of previous constraints, do not want to take care of another man who is ill, and may fear possible objections from their children. Daughters and sons frequently disapprove of remarriage for their mother because they idealize the deceased father, question motives of a boyfriend, and have concerns about their own inheritance (Heston, 2021; Weiss, 2023).

Keep in Touch

Phone a widow a few days after the funeral to ask whether you can come to visit. If s/he prefers to wait a while, then plan to call back later. There is nothing anyone can say that matters as much as "I care about you." Listen to the person's feelings, provide comfort, and make known that you will be available whenever she wants to have a talk. Sometimes there may be little conversation but it helps to sit together, watch a television program, or take a walk. If the widow expresses concern about personal safety and does not have family living nearby, offer to establish a phone check-in system so someone is there if needed. Find out the person's favorite food, and bring it in a disposable container so s/he will not worry about returning it. Help the person get out of the house by taking a walk in the mall, going out for coffee or lunch, visiting church, or running errands. Plan to watch a movie or attend some sporting event together.

Always express optimism; it can often have a therapeutic effect. Talk about the deceased and the good times that are remembered, funny things that happened, and special qualities that were admired about the person. It is wrong to say nothing about the deceased and pretend as though s/he never existed. The departure of someone should not end sharing memories about him or her. Seneca, the Roman philosopher, expressed this insight, "As a story, so is life: not how long it is, but how good it is that matters." Knowing how to spend time with a widowed person may be difficult but realize that being there shows concern about welfare and confirms s/he is important. Being the friend needed can be of great benefit (Kellerman & Seligman, 2023).

Consider Bill, a retired publisher whose wife Alice recently died. His letter to Bob and his wife illustrates the importance of just being with a widowed person and the struggles involved in trying to learn things more wives and husband should try to teach each other. Bill wrote this thank you note:

> I had a great time on Saturday with the two of you. A good lunch conversation at Coco's and a wonderful get-together at my home afterward that brought back memories of past years when Alice and I enjoyed having coffee, rolls, and meaningful conversation at your home. And, thanks too for the oh-so-good date bread you left along with the grapefruit. The date bread topped with cream cheese spread did not last long. At this stage of my life I am latching onto every recipe I can get my hands on and am asking if you would share that recipe with me. I would not ask for something that good, for nothing. So, I am attaching a recipe I found in Alice's recipe box I have liked over the years, and which I have finally mastered after a few trial runs. There is a story that goes with this recipe. I searched for it for some time, and finally finding it I set about to bake 'from scratch' for the first time ever. It was a fiasco, or I should say a succession of fiascos. The first lesson learned was that baking powder and baking soda are not the same thing. The first effort was a delightful taste that halfway filled the baking pan and was quite solid in texture. The second time around it was twice the size of the baking pan, and even though partway through the baking process I took a spatula and shaved the top part off, it still spilled over the edge of the pan. But it was good. By the third trial run, I figured out that Alice did not write "makes two loaves" on this particular recipe. The enclosed recipe is so identified. My love to you both. Bill.

Conclusion

Most people do not want to think about the prospect of their own death. Exceptions are those who suffer from severe pain related to illness, injury, or psychological trauma. Healthy emotional development through life improves adjustment to bereavement and reduces fear and anger. This increased level of being able to accept loss is fortunate because rates of death rise significantly among people who reach the age of retirement.

The mental health of widowed persons can improve when family and friends are informed about evolution of the grieving process. Those who mourn the death of a loved one typically experience predictable grieving and mourning stages that include denial, anger, bargaining, resignation, and acceptance. It is helpful for grieving persons to follow practical guidelines to ease their adjustment. Some important considerations are to: take time to complete the grieving process even though others may try to hurry the length of this ordeal; continue to communicate feelings and rely on new confidants to provide feedback; keep on making decisions to maintain a sense of control and gradually regain independence; take initiative to enlarge the personal circle of friends; seek comfort from others who are widowed and able to confirm the normality of your experience; respond to acquaintances as they struggle with loss of someone dear to them; think about widowhood ahead of time by reviewing family responsibilities and financial planning; and, acknowledge the relationships for which you are grateful.

Key Concepts

1 Couples should review family affairs several times a year, ensure financial records are up-to-date, and information is shared with chosen relatives. Planning includes making a will, assigning power of attorney, and clarifying end-of-life preferences. This acquaints both partners with each other's wishes and makes decisions less difficult for the survivor.

2 Everyone should become familiar with stages of grieving so they can support people coping with loss. No words can eliminate sadness and loneliness felt by survivors but they are grateful for emotional support of friendship and being allowed to recover at their own pace.

3 The loss of a spouse forces a change in personal identity and narrows perspective because processing ideas and feelings must occur without the partner. Initially, life seems to have lost its meaning so no attention is given to looking ahead. This outlook can change with a commitment to resume making plans. The agenda may require trying new activities, meeting new people, and exploring new places. Healthy change can also involve more interaction with familiar and satisfying activities, especially spending additional time with the family.

4 Relatives and friends who are well-intended often express a willingness to act in a widow's behalf to ease burdens. However, retaining independence is necessary since it confirms that a person is still able to manage personal affairs. Major decisions like selling a house or moving should be deferred until normal perspective is restored. Changing an address cannot prevent loneliness.

5 During visits with a survivor mention the good times remembered about the deceased, funny things that were enjoyed together, and admirable qualities about that person. The passing of someone you know and care about should not end conversations recalling pleasant memories about them.

6 Being able to perform the tasks normally done by a partner requires a willingness to participate in reciprocal learning. The resulting knowledge enables a comprehensive view of domestic and financial obligations that can help the survivor. Sharing takes time but prepares the partner and later reduces scale of the burden.

7 Talk about the balance of work and play you and your spouse want to achieve together. Imbalance often results in regret. But you can change ways your time is

spent so greater attention is given to activities that offer opportunity to improve communication, understanding, and mutual satisfaction.

8 Stay in touch with widowed persons who are living alone. You can use Skype, FaceTime, texting, email, and cell phone calls to continue conversations when you are not together in face-to-face situations. Regular contact including visits allows you to reinforce the message that this person is valued, you think about them, and want what is best.

9 Support groups should be recommended for newly widowed individuals. Sharing stories can provide evidence that others have traveled a similar path, worrying about one's mental state of mind is normal, and that others have emerged from this difficult time as independent persons.

10 A wise practice for widows is to avoid major decisions about lifestyle like moving or getting married again. These judgments are premature in the first year after death of a spouse and often lead to regret. Preoccupation with loneliness will continue until recovery and identity is altered.

Generational Perspectives Activities

12.1 Team Discussion
12.2 Agenda for Interviews with Parents
12.3 A Scenario: Reasoning and Problem Solving
12.4 Team Chapter Review
12.5 Criteria for Self-Evaluation of Grandparents

12.1 Team Discussion

1 What situations usually cause feelings of loneliness for you?
2 What ways have you found helpful to cope with loneliness?
3 How does watching television help you deal with loneliness?
4 Who are the dead people you miss more than anyone else?
5 Which of your friends in the past would you like to visit again?
6 In what ways do you try to reduce times of loneliness for others?
7 Who is a person you know that seems to suffer from loneliness?
8 How did you feel when a pet or someone that you loved died?
9 Who do you expect will be the next relative of yours to die?
10 What do you believe happens to people after they have died?

12.2 Agenda for Interviews with Parents

1 What do you suppose will be the most difficult aspects for you of becoming a widower or widow?
2 What should family members do to help a surviving spouse with loss and loneliness?
3 How have you tried to ease the burden of a friend who experienced loss of a spouse?
4 How should friends support someone who is in mourning after s/he becomes a widow?
5 What are your feelings about a relative getting married again after death of a spouse?
6 What do you think about prenuptial agreements for older couples who get married?

7 What can faith-based groups do to facilitate the recovery of widowed persons?
8 What steps have you and your spouse taken together to be prepared for widowhood?
9 What do you know about the benefits of widowed persons attending support groups?
10 What do you know about provision of hospice care and making end-of-life choices?

12.3 A Scenario: Reasoning and Problem Solving

Problem solving scenarios present an opportunity to look at situations that might happen for a family and think about possible solutions. Your task is to look at pros and cons of choices that are stated, think of additional options, identify relevant information that might be missing, find out how teammates view the alternatives, and defend your reasoning about the advice that you consider best.

Alison was widowed six months ago. Her son Michael and his family live a two-hour drive away. They phone Alison once a week on Sunday nights to see how she is doing but seldom come to visit. When friends ask Michael about how his mother is managing her situation, he expresses pride regarding her sense of independence. What would you like to tell Michael?

a Congratulate your Mom for showing she is willing and able to take care of herself.
b Widows should not have to endure more loneliness to prove they are independent.
c You should recognize how the whole family could benefit from having more visits.
d Why can't you and the children stay in touch more often by phone, text, or email?
e You should recommend that your Mom sell her place so she can move in with you.
f Other _____

12.4 Team Chapter Review

Efforts to assess participant learning, provide feedback, and improve quality of instruction is enhanced by a group review of each chapter.

1 What ideas in the lesson changed the way I think about this topic?
2 What insights from the lesson will I try to apply in my relationships?
3 What is the most important point for me presented in this lesson?
4 What are some aspects of this lesson I would like to better understand?
5 Which aspects of this lesson do I wish that I had known about earlier?

12.5 Criteria for Self-Evaluation of Grandparents

Directions: For each question, place a check beside the statements that describe your feelings. You may want to give several answers on some items. If your feelings are not shown here, write them on the line marked 'other.'

1 If my spouse dies before me, I would have to learn

    a how to manage money and deal with financial investments
    b how to cook, clean, wash, and do other housekeeping tasks
    c how to get involved with a variety of new social activities
    d how to maintain the house, grounds, and major appliances
    e Other _____

2 How do you feel about the amount of time your family spends with you?

    a I wish they would spend more time with me but I don't say anything.
    b I am busy with friends so having more time with family doesn't matter.
    c My children and grandchildren are always busy so I try to forget about it.
    d Speaking on the phone and texting is a gift for which I am thankful.
    e Other _____

3 My advice to women and men who are widowed is to

    a become involved with a friendship group at church
    b join a community support group for recovery
    c accept invitations from friends to do things together
    d take your time with recovery and remain prayerful
    e Other _____

4 My feeling about older adult widowed persons who decide to date again

    a seeking companionship is beneficial but avoid another marriage
    b should be discouraged to protect inheritance of the adult children
    c could lead to a satisfying second marriage in a longevity society
    d should be made clear this arrangement is only for social purposes
    e Other _____

5 My daughters and sons have expressed feeling that dating for me

    a is alright if the relationship is recognized as limited to friendship
    b is a breach of the lengthy commitment I had to their other parent
    c is alright and I should be the one to determine my own lifestyle
    d is unacceptable because I am too old for that sort of relationship
    e Other _____

6 What do you suppose would be the greatest challenges for you as a widow?

    a Trying to keep busy to avoid thinking about my loss and new situation
    b Spending too much time looking to the past and feeling sorry for myself
    c Coping with loneliness of being apart from someone who was my life
    d Feeling I have nothing to live for without the partner I loved so much
    e Other _____

7 At my funeral I would prefer that the emphasis will be on

    a reading my favorite bible verses and a declaration of my faith
    b family and friends sharing their memories of our relationship
    c description of my career and achievements at the workplace
    d my gratitude to God for such a wonderful partner and family
    e Other _____

8 As I anticipate the possibility of widowhood, I expect to rely on

    a faith in God and prayer as the main key to help with recovery
    b family and friends to provide the emotional support needed
    c minister as spiritual advisor and prayer by the church family

  d learning from my partner how to perform their family tasks
  e Other _____

9 I know people who have been widowed and my reaction is

  a to visit with them and do things together that we enjoy
  b keep in cell phone contact so safety worries are shared
  c invite them to my place for visiting and meals together
  d express a continual willingness to act as a listener
  e Other _____

10 My experience in trading places that involve doing domestic tasks is

  a I have made little effort to learn some things my spouse manages
  b I have shared with my spouse tasks that s/he needs to understand
  c I have been reluctant to help both of us know tasks of the other
  d I am prepared to take care of all domestic tasks when necessary
  e Other _____

References

Cain, S. (2022). *Bittersweet: How sorrow and longing make us whole*. Crown.

Carr, D. (2016). Grief and bereavement. In M. Meyer & E. Daniele (Eds.), *Gerontology: Changes, challenges, and solutions* (Volume 2, pp. a271–a294). Praeger.

Centers for Medicare and Medicaid Services. (2022). *Hospice*. U. S. Department of Health and Human Services. https://www.cms.gov/Medicare/Medicare-Fee-for-Service-Payment/Hospice

Centers for Medicare and Medicaid Services. (2023). *Medicare Hospice benefits*. U. S. Department of Health and Human Services. https://www.medicare.gov/Pubs/pdf/02154-medicare-hospice-benefits.pdf

Devine, M., & Nepo, M. (2017). *It's ok that you're not ok: Meeting grief and loss in a culture that doesn't understand*. Sound True.

Filomena, J. (2017). *Widowhood: Moving through the pain of widowhood to find meaning and purpose in your life again*. Morgan James.

Gurrentz, B., & Mayol-Garcia, Y. (2021, April 22). *Marriage, divorce, widowhood remain prevalent among older populations*. U.S. Census Bureau: Love and Loss Among Older Adults. https://www.census.gov/library/stories/2021/04/love-and-loss-among-older-adults.html

Gleick, J. (1996). *Faster, the acceleration of just about everything*. Pantheon Books.

Gleick, J. (2017). *Time travel: A history*. Vintage.

Hertz, N. (2021). *The lonely century: How to restore human connection in a world that's pulling apart*. Random House.

Heston, K. (2021). *How to adjust when an adult parent remarries*. wikiHow to do anything … https://www.wikihow.life/Adjust-when-an-Adult-Parent-Remarries

Holt-Lunstad, J. A. (2017, April 27). *Testimony before the United States Senate Aging Committee*, 115th Congress. https://www.aging.senate.gov/imo/media/doc/SCA_Holt_04_27_17.pdf

Holt-Lunstad, J. A. (2021, January 12). A pandemic of social isolation? *World Psychiatry, 20*(1), 55–56. 10.1002/wps.20839

Holt-Lunstad, J. A., Smith, T. B., Baker, M., Harris, T., & Stephenson, D. (2015). Loneliness and social isolation as risk factors for mortality: A meta-analytic review. *Perspectives on Psychological Science, 10*(2), 227–237. 10.1177/1745691614568352

Hoyt, J., & Goldy-Brown, S. (2022). *How to make a will*. Senior Living. https://www.seniorliving.org/finance/estate-planning/how-to-make-a-will/

James, J., & Friedman, R. (2017). *The grief recovery handbook*. William Morrow.

Josephson, M. (2003). *What will matter*. Josephson Institute of Ethics. YouTube. https://www.youtube.com/watch?v=bmcsI1mv8OA

Kellerman, G. R., & Seligman, M. E. P. (2023). *Tomorrowmind: Thriving at work with resilience, creativity, and connection -- now and in an uncertain future*. Atria.

Kübler-Ross, E. (1969). *Death and dying: What the dying have to teach doctors, nurses, clergy and their own families*. MacMillan.

Mabry, R. L. (2017). *The tender scar: Life after the death of a spouse*. Kregel Publications.

Mayo Clinic. (2023). *Living wills and advance directives for medical decisions*. Consumer health. https://www.mayoclinic.org/healthy-lifestyle/consumer-health/in-depth/living-wills/art-20046303

National Academies of Sciences, Engineering, & Medicine. (2020). *Social isolation and loneliness in older adults: Opportunities for the health care system*. The National Academies Press.

National Institute on Aging. (2020). *Mourning the death of a spouse*. National Institutes of Health. https://www.nia.nih.gov/health/mourning-death-spouse

National Institute on Aging. (2021). What are palliative care and hospice care? National Institutes of Health. https://www.nia.nih.gov/health/what-are-palliative-care-and-hospice-care#:~:text=setting%20for%20care.-,What%20is%20palliative%20care%3F,to%20cure%20their%20serious%20illness

O'Connor, M. (2023). *The grieving brain: The surprising science of how we learn from love and loss*. Harper One.

Roberts, P. (2015). *The impulse society*. Bloomsbury Publisher.

Weiss, H. (2023, March 22). Losing a spouse makes men 70% more likely to die within a year. *Time.* https://time.com/6265173/men-dying-after-spouse-dies/

Part IV
Old Age (Ages 80+)

13 Mental, Physical and Social Health

Mental and Physical Health

How Extensive Is the Revolution in Human Longevity?

Archeological records indicate that in ancient time most people had a lifespan of about 20 years, just long enough to ensure survival of the species (Feder, 2019). This shorter lifespan is in sharp contrast to experience in wealthy nations where currently people can, on average expect to live almost 80 years or perhaps longer if born during this millennium. The United States has added 28 years of life expectancy in just the past century (Kawas, 2022).

To explore how longer life could become more common, Buettner (2017) examined conditions where people have the longest lifespan and maintain habits reflecting a healthy lifestyle. People from these so-called *Blue Zones* reach 100 years of age at significantly greater rates than anywhere else in the world. The Blue Zones include (a) Ikaria, Greece, an island off the coast of Turkey, (b) Okinawa, Japan, where women live the longest, (c) Sardinia, Italy, (d) the Nicoya Peninsula of Costa Rica, and (e) Loma Linda, California, with the highest concentration of Seventh Day Adventists in the nation. Buettner (2015) has documented the kinds of foods centenarians eat, company they keep, their daily routines, and outlook on life have been documented. People living in each of the Blue Zones seldom sit down; most of their time is spent moving around. Lessons from centenarians can help others willing to adopt aspects of lifestyle for a chance to extend life by as much as a decade.

What Are the Disability and Risk Factors after Age 90?

Having a long life is a common aspiration but reaching this goal can be accompanied by undesirable conditions, particularly having to manage disabilities. Researchers at the University of California in Irvine have been conducting research for more than two decades with 700 men and women beyond age 90 at six-month intervals to check for changes in incidence of disability and risk factors. Over 40% of participants suffer from dementia and 80% are disabled. Disability is defined by a need for help with daily living activities. Kawas et al. (2021), medical director of the 90 Plus Project, has described some ways to maintain function in old age.

First, half the participants who have died showed no evidence of dementia (deterioration of mental function) at the time of autopsy, even though their brains contained lesions associated with Alzheimer's disease (AD), a degenerative and incurable disease. Most were well-educated and somehow their brains were protected from the ravages of AD.

DOI: 10.4324/9781003401261-18

Economic costs of dementia are greater than heart disease and cancer combined. Alzheimer's rates double every five years after age 70 (Alzheimer's Association, 2023).

A second set of results relates to lifestyle. None of the risk factors for people in their 60s, 70s, and 80s seem to apply after age 90 (Biswas et al., 2023; Kawas et al., 2021). Hypertension, high cholesterol, and statin prescriptions are risk factors for 60-year-olds; however, they appear to protect 90-year-olds from AD instead of increasing their risk for the disease.

Third, physicians often discourage weight gain in younger patients but, in their 70s, 80s, and 90s, weight increase ceases to be a risk and appears to become a protective factor. Perhaps the ability to gain weight is an indicator of robustness. Overweight 70-year-olds live longer than their underweight peers. For unknown reasons the body tries to gain weight in old age. In contrast, being underweight presents a 50% greater risk of mortality. Being thin in old age is undesirable. Extra fat also has a downside because it means blood sugar levels rise six points a decade, making type 2 diabetes a common disease among the elderly (McDonald, 2019).

Another mistaken assumption is that research findings on 60- to 70-year-olds do not apply to people in their 80s and beyond. The reason so little is known about people who are 90 years or older is that they have typically been excluded from studies on the assumption they might not survive until the project would be completed. The reasons why high blood pressure and high cholesterol seem protective against AD for people over 90 are unknown (Kawas, 2022). However, this protection seems to occur only if hypertension originates during the 80s or 90s, not at an earlier age. A good diet is common but no particular foods have been identified as contributing most to health. The 90+ subjects who drink moderate amounts of alcohol as well as coffee live longer. Typically they consume two or three cups of coffee a day; many drink alcohol once or twice a week. Those who exercise also live longer, even walking as little as 15 minutes a day. Thirty minutes is even better and 45 minutes is optimal. Exercise beyond 45 minutes a day does not add to longevity. Exercise reduces body fat, sensitizes body's tissues to insulin, and lowers blood sugar levels. Exercise boosts HDL (good) cholesterol and lower levels of LDL (bad) cholesterol and triglycerides.

A number of international studies are focused on centenarians (100 years or older). Fewer than 1% of Americans live to be 100 years of age. Holstege et al. (2018) at Vrije University in Amsterdam, Netherlands, are studying 340 Dutch centenarians. In this 100-plus study many subjects have performed as if they were 30 years younger in terms of overall cognition, ability to make decisions, execute plans, recreate by drawing a figure they had just looked at, being able to list animals or objects that began with a certain letter, and able to avoid becoming distracted when doing a task or getting lost when they left home. Autopsies of 44 participant have shown that many had substantial neuropathology of the brain common among people with AD yet they remained cognitively healthy up to four years beyond age 100. Some of the commonalities in the group include extensive education, occupations that required continual involvement with complex thinking, consuming a Mediterranean style diet, engaging in leisure activities, socializing with others, and exercising on a regular basis (Beker et al., 2021).

Do People Retain Their Capacity to Learn in Later Life?

Retirement initially became a norm for the United States in the 1970s. Before that time the mental abilities of old people were rarely a focus of study. Individuals who reached old age were usually taken care of by relatives. Those whose families could not provide care were often placed in "old people's homes." As a result, most of the initial studies of mental aging were based on convenience samples of institutionalized elders. Because this population was the main source of knowledge about cognition in old age, the learning potential of older adults was initially underestimated, communicated to society as a norm, and accepted as a limitation of cognitive development (Blazer et al., 2015).

A more favorable impression emerged with longitudinal tracking. A goal of longitudinal research is to record observations of the same persons over a long period of time. Schaie (2013) monitored mental abilities of 500 people from age 25 to 95 for 50 years. Follow-ups were carried out at seven-year intervals to identify changes in mental functioning, assess the timing when detectable age declines occur in cognitive abilities, identify normative extent of loss, and factors that might account for individual differences in age-related changes. Schaie found that, at every re-test, a majority retained competence as they grew older (Schaie & Willis, 2017).

The best known longitudinal study was conducted by British film director Michael Apted (1941–2021). In 1964 he interviewed fourteen 7-year-old English boys and girls from varied socioeconomic backgrounds and reported on them at seven-year intervals when they were ages 14, 21, 28, 35, 42, 49, 56 and 63 (in 2019). The video self-reports, known as the *Up Series*, allow viewers to observe the same children as they grow up and move through adult life (Apted, 2023). Whether the *Up Series* will continue when the subjects reach age 70, in 2026, is uncertain (Coscarelli, 2021).

Even when mental competence begins to decline in some adults, rate of loss can be slowed or even reversed by education. Certain cognitive abilities decline earlier than others and require greater attention for restoration. Accordingly, educational interventions have focused on abilities showing the greatest loss after age 65, particularly reasoning and problem solving (the same skills included in problem solving exercises at the end of each chapter of this book). The mental performance of 200 men and women, from ages 65 to 95, was tracked for 14 years. Half the subjects recorded loss while others remained stable. The conclusion was that mental skills atrophy owing to disuse but mental stimulation can remove some deficits. Schaie and Willis (2017) found that, after just five hours of training, 40% of older adults were able to match or exceed their earlier problem solving skills.

Other studies to determine the enduring benefits of instruction have focused on reasoning and problem solving also underscored significant influence of mental stimulation. Rebok et al. (2014) examined the long-term effects of training specific cognitive abilities. The culturally diverse sample included 2,800 men and women, average age 73. Subjects were divided into three groups with each exposed to a different training focus. One group focused on reasoning and problem solving, another with processing speed, and a third centered on memory. Instruction was provided in ten one-hour sessions. Follow-up assessments were administered at the conclusion of instruction and then annually. When clinical trials ended ten years later, the subjects were 83 years old. Of those who practiced reasoning and problem-solving, 74% showed improvement over baseline scores. Most (62%) in the processing speed group also improved. But memory trained subjects did not improve.

How Does Early Education Impact Thinking in Old Age?

The amount of formal education influences relative risk for AD and other forms of dementia. This has been a consistent finding of independent studies in Australia, China,

Finland, France, Israel, Italy, Sweden, and the United States (Blazer et al., 2015; Calhoun, 2022; Lövdén et al., 2020). The first international study involved 5,500 Chinese in Shanghai, ages 55 to 75. Their overall incidence of AD was 5%; however, other factors being equal, those with no formal schooling had twice the risk of dementia as age peers who had completed elementary or middle school. After comparing effects of education and age, Katzman (1993) speculated that dementia might be delayed 7 to 10 years because of protective effects provided by education.

A Scandinavian longitudinal study by Ngandu et al. (2007) involved 1,400 people for 21 years, from midlife until old age. Participants were categorized in three groups: the lowest level had five or less years of formal education; a medium level had six to eight years of school; and the highest level had nine or more school years. Compared to the low-level group, those with a medium level had 40% less risk of developing dementia and those with a high level had 80% less risk.

The National Institutes of Health reviewed evidence of risk factors for Alzheimer's disease and cognitive decline (Daviglus et al., 2010). Several modifiable factors related to increased risk. One factor, low level of formal education, presented twice the risk for dementia. Data drawn from 146 countries suggested 15% of adults throughout the world have not received any formal education. Another 25% have only had primary education, making a total of 40% classified as low educational attainment. Gutchess (2019) estimated that internationally 6 million cases of AD are attributed to low levels of education.

The Organization for Economic Cooperation and Development (Murtin et al., 2017) examined international inequalities in longevity. Across a multi-national sample, the lifespan forecast for people who were 25-year-olds was eight years longer if they had higher education. For the United States someone with a low education level, defined as elementary and middle school, was expected to live to age 74 while an individual with higher education, defined as some college, was forecast to reach age 82. Some differences in lifespan implicated smoking, obesity, and alcohol. Every nation should provide continuous health education so that all age groups are better equipped to make decisions about choices of lifestyle.

The amount of formal education in childhood and adolescence influences relative risk for AD and other forms of dementia in later life. In this context, a study of 704 older adults (ages 58–98) examined declarative memory, defined as the ability to remember events, facts, and words (Reifegerste et al., 2021). Subjects were shown objects and tested several minutes later to assess their memory of the objects. Results showed that memory deteriorated with age; however, having more education early in life was able to counter losses, especially for women. For men the gains in memory associated with each year of education was two times greater than losses experienced for each year of aging. In women the gains were five times larger. This means an 80-year-old woman with a bachelor's degree would perform as well on declarative memory as a 60-year-old woman with only a high school education. Four extra years of education made up for the memory losses from 20 years of aging. According to the Population Reference Bureau (2023), older adults with more education are less likely to develop dementia; they spend a larger portion of their lives cognitively healthy and fewer years with dementia. In 2019, 5% of older college graduates (ages 70 and older) were living with dementia, compared with 18% of their counterparts with less than 12 years of education.

A systematic review was conducted of studies from 24 countries (Maccora et al., 2020). Results suggested each year of formal education reduced the risk of AD by 8%. Among potentially modifiable risk factors for dementia, low education appears to have the greatest influence on population risk worldwide. United Nations Educational, Scientific and Cultural Organization (UNESCO) reported that of the 787 million global share of children of primary school age, 8% did not attend any school (Roser, 2021). That means over 58 million children did not have a chance to learn to read and write. These children live in South Asia (12.8 million), Middle East and North Africa (2.7 million), Europe and Central Asia (6.2 million), and Sub-Saharan Africa (33.8 million). The two main reasons for this tragedy are warfare in conflict regions and low income.

Can Education for Retired Persons Influence Cognitive Functioning?

The oldest-old (people aged 90 or older) are the most rapidly growing segment of society (Pierce & Kawas, 2017). World-wide the number of oldest-old people is forecast to become 71 million in 2050, a five-fold increase over the current situation. Many studies have found that formal education in childhood and adolescence predict a reduced incidence of cognitive decline during retirement. However, research to determine whether education during retirement impacts cognitive decline remains unexamined. One international study included 84 people without cognitive impairment and 38 individuals with cognitive impairment (mean age 92.4 years). Results found no evidence of an association between past cognitive activity at the ages of 6, 12, 18, and 40 years, and cognitive functioning after age 90. This implies that the protective effects of cognitive activity at early ages may not persist for the oldest-old population (Seblova et al., 2020; Visser & Krosnick, 1998). There is a need to know if provision of relevant education, perhaps offered in different doses between once a week to five times a week, could contribute to sustained protection against negative effects of brain decline.

How Important Is Gender Equality in Education?

A meta-analysis carried out a generation ago compared cognitive abilities of men and women. Researchers estimated women had a 50% higher risk for Alzheimer's and other forms of dementia (Gao et al., 1998). However, studies in this analysis included cohorts born in the 1920s, a time when gender differences in access to school was large. More recently, in 2021, Bloomberg et al. (2021) at University College in London examined 16,000 men and women born between 1930 and 1955 to evaluate the importance of education on memory and verbal fluency, both factors linked to dementia risk. A strength of this investigation is the large sample and more current data base than prior smaller longitudinal studies. Lead researcher Bloomberg explained that findings suggest, among people educated in the first half of the 20th century, gender inequities in access to schooling led to lower education levels among women; this likely negatively impacted cognitive ageing and increased the risk of dementia for women.

However, in the present study there was no evidence of cognitive disadvantage in women after accounting for level of education (Bloomberg et al., 2021). On the contrary, women had better scores on the memory test, and difference was marked at older ages and in women born more recently. Women in the highest education group and latest birth cohort also had better fluency scores than men and slower decline of memory. These findings highlight formal education as a contributing factor for sex differences in cognition, reducing the necessity of considering sex-specific effects in evaluating modifiable factors for cognitive outcomes, and emphasize the importance of equitable access to education for health. Socially constructed gender norms in relation to education are changing. As gender disparities decrease, it will become important to ensure equitable access to education for health, especially in nations where female access to education remains limited.

The National Institute of Aging supported a longitudinal study by Snowdon (2002) beginning in 1986 that focused on Catholic nuns. All 700 subjects were Sisters of Notre Dame who agreed to annual assessments of cognitive and physical function, medical examinations, have blood drawn, allow full access to medical records and donate their brain at the time of death for neuro-pathological examination.

One sub-investigation of the Catholic Sisters study sought to determine whether linguistic ability during adolescence could predict cognitive impairment in later life. Cognitive functioning was assessed for 93 nuns, from 75 to 95 years of age. Results were compared to autobiographies that were written 58 years earlier when the nuns took their vows at age 22. This was a way to gauge vocabulary strength, complex thinking, and level of intelligence. Low idea density and low grammatical complexity correlated with low cognitive scores of sisters in later life. About 80% of nuns whose writing was lacking linguistic density developed AD. In contrast, only 10% whose writing included high idea density developed the disease. Nuns scoring in the lowest third of intelligence had a rate of AD 10 to 15 times greater than college educated sisters who remained teachers most of their lives. Researchers concluded this outcome had more to do with cognitive ability in early life than lifestyle because nuns had the same reproductive and marital histories, did not drink or smoke, engaged in similar social activities, jobs, income, ate the same foods, lived in the same housing, and shared the same medical care from early adulthood (Snowdon et al., 1996).

Most nuns never retire but instead moderate their activities as they age. Collectively, they sustain roughly the same rate of Alzheimer's as the general population. Still, the good news for them is that their onset of AD occurs at a later age and symptoms seem less severe. Their active lifestyle does not prevent AD but could be a factor related to postponing it. David Snowdon (2002), the University of Minnesota founder of the Nuns Study, speculated that, if the onset of AD could be delayed five years, incidence would be reduced by half almost immediately because it develops at such a late age that half of those impaired would have died before there was evidence of impairment.

What Are the Modifiable Risk Factors for Alzheimer's Disease?

The Alzheimer's Association (2023) estimates 6.7 million Americans suffer from dementia. Alzheimer's disease and other forms of dementia are the main reason for individual placement in long-term care facilities. A majority of nursing home residents (60%) are diagnosed with dementias. These patients, on average, live 4 to 8 years but some live as long as 20 years. Most of this time involves severe stages requiring special care (Dassel et al., 2020). So-called memory care units represent only 4% of the beds in nursing homes. As a result, residents suffering moderate cognitive impairment usually are not housed in separate sections of the facility and can sometimes wander into the rooms of non-dementia patients and bother them.

Dementias are diseases, not aspects of normal aging. The Alzheimer's Association (2023) reports estimates that between 40% to 65% of people diagnosed with Alzheimer's have certain risk genes in common. Family history is not necessary for a person to develop the disease; however, those who have a parent or a sibling with the disease are more likely to develop the disease than those who do not have a first-degree relative with AD.

Alzheimer's disease is thought to begin 20 or more years before the evidence of symptoms such as memory loss, problems with language, and problem solving. There are a greater number of cases of AD currently than earlier in history because more people live long enough to be stricken. The successive incidence of AD is less than 1% among people who are 40 years old, 6% among 65 years old, 40% at age 80, and 50% by 85. Rates of dementia actually decline among people who are in their late 80s so that, by age 95, the prevalence is only 30%, less than half the rate of 80-year-olds for reasons that remain unknown. Blacks are twice as likely to be stricken by AD as Whites; Hispanics are one-and-one-half times more likely than Whites. Two-thirds of all victims are women (Alzheimer's Association, 2023).

The United States national plan formulated in 2021 to address Alzheimer disease and related dementias include a goal to accelerate action that can promote healthy aging and reduce risk factors. Omura et al. (2022) studied the status of subjective cognitive decline with data collected from 161,941 adults age 45 and older in 31 states and Washington, D.C. Based on self-reports, the respondents were classified as experiencing subjective cognitive decline if their response was "Yes" when asked if they had experienced worsening or more frequent confusion or memory loss in the previous 12 months. Results showed that the most common potentially modifiable risk factors were (a) high blood pressure (49.9%), (b) not meeting aerobic physical activity guidelines (49.7%), (c) obesity (35.3%), (d) diabetes (18.6%), (e) depression (18%), (f) current cigarette smoking (14.9%), (g) hearing loss (10.5%), and (h) binge drinking (10.3%). These factors should become the focus for prevention and control efforts to enable more healthy aging for specific populations.

Can Short-term Memory be Revived?

One troublesome aspect of cognitive decline involves deficit in working memory that prevents retention of information that is needed to guide current tasks. Working memory is where information is kept for a matter of only seconds while people perform a task like recalling a phone number or e-mail address that has just been given them. Problem-solving and decision making rely on working memory. Can efficiency of short-term memory be revived as people become older?

A study by Reinhart and Nguyen (2019) involved 42 people between 60 to 76 years of age and 42 people who were in their twenties. Both groups engaged in a game of "spot the difference" between two images shown on a screen in immediate succession. Young adults responded faster and were more accurate than elders. Then the researchers examined the communication link between temporal and prefrontal regions of the brain and found there was a synchronization of brain waves in the two regions for younger people. However, activity rhythms in the two brain regions of older people showed they had become uncoupled, fallen out of sync with each other. So, electrical stimulation was applied to nudge activity cycles back to the matching pattern. After only 25 minutes of mild stimulation, brain synchronicity normalized. As a result, older adults were able to perform as well as younger people for the test period that lasted 50 minutes. In effect, electrical stimulation removed effects of aging on transcranial connection. Reinhart and Nguyen speculated, "Someday, people might be able to visit clinics to boost ability that declines in normal aging and in dementias such as Alzheimer's disease."

At What Age Does Normal Cognitive Decline Begin?

The timing of onset for normal cognitive decline has long been a subject of speculation with little evidence about loss reported before age 60 (Bermúdez, 2023). To explore incidence a study in England was conducted with 7,390 civil servants between the ages of 45 and 70. Over a period of ten years, all subjects were tested three times to evaluate their memory, reasoning, and visual comprehension skills. Separate analyses were performed for five year categories—ages 45–49, 50–54, 55–59, 60–64, and 65–70 (Singh-Manoux et al., 2012).

Results showed cognitive scores declined in each of the five-year categories, except for vocabulary, and rate of decline increased as people grew older. For example, there was a 3.6% decline in mental reasoning of men ages 45–49; that decline rate was 9.6% for people aged 65–70. Corresponding figures for women ages 45–49 showed a decline of 3.6% (same as men) and 7.4% for those who were 65–70 (less than men). This robust evidence showing that capacity of the brain can begin to deteriorate as early as 45 years old underscores the need to promote healthy lifestyles including access to mentally stimulating education classes. Cardiovascular health is also relevant, particularly for people with one or more heart disease risk factors, such as obesity, blood pressure, high cholesterol levels, and diabetes (Omura et al., 2022; Singh-Manoux et al., 2012; World Health Organization, 2023).

How Can Alzheimer's Disease Be Predicted?

Fifty million people across the world suffer from dementia, with Alzheimer's disease (AD) as the most common form. There is no cure and medicines only temporarily ease symptoms. Researchers speculate that prior studies may have enrolled subjects after too much brain damage had occurred or included too many individuals who had other problems besides Alzheimer's (Anstey et al., 2020). Two proteins are linked to AD-beta amyloid that forms plaque in the brain and *tau* that forms tangles in brain cells. When abnormal tau begins to spread neurons start dying and the affected persons begins to notice the initial symptoms, usually mild memory impairment. Early detection for abnormal versions of tau up to twenty years prior to symptoms could identify the right people to participate in therapy trials and track the impact of therapies that are being tested (Aronson, 2021; Gutchess, 2019).

Nakamura et al. (2018) from the National Center for Geriatrics and Gerontology in Obu, Japan, developed a blood test to screen for Alzheimer's disease and other forms of dementia. A discovery set of data from Japan ($N = 121$) and validation data set from Australia ($N = 252$) were applied. Both data sets included three groups, cognitively normal subjects, people with mild cognitive impairment, and individuals with AD. The test correctly identified 92% of those with AD and correctly ruled out 85% who did not, for an overall accuracy rate of 88%.

A study of 1,400 subjects conducted by an international team from Sweden and Arizona discovered a highly accurate blood-based marker for detection of AD by measuring tau levels in blood and validated the findings using multiple diverse populations (Mattsson-Carlgren et al., 2020). The diagnostic precision of blood was as high as established methods for determining AD including PET Imaging and spinal fluid biomarkers that are invasive, costly, and less available. Findings showed that the blood test has great sensitivity and specificity; it detects 90% of all cases of AD. The main result was blood tau distinguished AD from other neurogenerative disorders with high diagnostic accuracy between 89 and 98%. In addition, among the non-demented patients, those with elevated tau levels had a ten-fold increased risk of developing AD. The new test can be used to predict who will develop AD in the next four to six years (World Health Organization, 2023).

What Are the Gender Differences in Alzheimer Disease?

Two-thirds of the 6 million Americans suffering from Alzheimer Disease are women. In the past, it was supposed women were at increased risk because age is the main risk factor and women typically live four to six years longer than men. However, at age the 65 the chances for AD among women is 1 in 5 compared to 1 in 11 for men (Alzheimer's Association, 2023). In addition to age, there must be some unknown biological or social determinant. Many studies are underway to find out why a disproportionate number of women suffer from the disease.

Consider two examples. Women typically outperform men on verbal memory tests even in the early stages of Alzheimer's. This means test results of verbal memory may not detect mild cognitive impairment in women until the disease has progressed further, thereby preventing them from advantages of intervention or therapies. To further explore gender differences, Sundermann et al. (2020) at the University of California in San Diego School of Medicine conducted brain scans of 1,022 older adults (453 women and 569 men). The purpose was to compare brain ability to metabolize glucose, an index of brain function, between men and women at different stages of pathology and assess if a difference contributes to women's verbal memory advantage. Focus was on how well brains metabolized glucose in regions affected by AD. Glucose is the main energy source for the brain; poor metabolism is a sign of brain cell dysfunction. Memory skills were also assessed. Women outperformed men on verbal memory tests in the early AD stages but not the later severe stages. This result suggests women may be more able than men to compensate for early brain damage of AD and this may contribute to female verbal memory advantage at this stage of the disease.

Another study considered sex differences about tau pathology in the brain. Alzheimer's is characterized by an abnormal accumulation of tau, a toxic protein that, when clumped in tangles, causes brain cell death. Shokouhi et al. (2019) examined positron emission tomography (PET) scans to model the brain as a network of tau connected to regions. They examined the architecture of these networks to identify global pathways of tau propagation and test for gender differences. Subjects were healthy (123 men, 178 women) and others with mild cognitive impairment (101 men, 60 women). Results revealed the tau network of women with mild cognitive impairment had the highest network density and hubs connecting different brain regions across the entire network. Researchers speculated that this could favor an accelerated brain-wide tau spread that leads to cognitive decline. Observed differences suggest a strong possibility of sex differences in the brain structural and functional connections that may contribute to women's greater risk for AD.

How Does Cognitive Reserve Contribute to Mental Sustainability?

Cognitive reserve is defined as the ability to tolerate progressive damage to the brain without showing clinical cognitive symptoms. One view is that mental activity can develop a surplus of brain tissue that compensates for tissues damaged by dementia. The hypothesis is that, for people with more formal education, greater brain reserve in the form of increased synaptic density in the neo-cortex might delay onset of AD and reduce prevalence of dementia. Formal school is not the only determinant of cognitive reserve. Having mentally stimulating employment also builds cognitive reserve (Grzywacz et al., 2016).

Studies suggest that the more complex and resonant a brain becomes through interaction, the better protected a person is against AD. Mental stimulation appears to provide a safety net so people have further to fall before the disease process reveals itself by showing symptoms. Persons advantaged by education while growing up are more protected in later life than their peers with less schooling. Individuals disadvantaged in the first two decades of life are the same people who are exposed to greater suffering again in old age. This tragedy begins with inadequate education, then later a poor work position that does not require much thought, and greater vulnerability to dementia during old age (Stern et al., 2020). Schools should do all they can to motivate students to continue studying, graduate, and then keep on learning. The main goal of education in the past was to prepare for employment. But, in a longevity society, this goal should expand to include building the cognitive reserve needed later in life to delay onset of dementia and provide adult education to foster adjustment (Anstey et al., 2020; Montine et al., 2019).

A review of literature on brain reserve concluded men and women who remain mentally active throughout life reduce their risk to become victims of Alzheimer's disease. Global data drawn from 22 studies of 29,000 subjects examined influence of education, job complexity, and mentally stimulating lifestyle. Valenzuela and Sachdev (2005) reported that the assertion of "Use it or lose it" was confirmed. Results showed persons with high brain reserve had a 46% lower risk of dementia compared to those with low brain reserve. Instead of assuming brain reserve is a static property, fixed by early education and income, mental stimulation can continue to support brain health even during old age.

Mentally stimulating activities are modifiable lifestyle factors that are easily available to anyone at no or limited cost. Given the absence of an effective treatment or cure for Alzheimer's disease, there has been a growing interest in the investigation of lifestyle factors in the context of brain aging. In a Mayo Clinic Study of Aging (Krell-Roesch et al., 2019) involving 2,000 middle aged and later life subjects who were cognitively unimpaired at baseline were followed for five years. The participants completed a self-reported survey on timing, number, and frequency of their engagement with five mentally stimulating activities: (a) reading books, (b) computer usage, (c) social activities, (d) playing games, and (e) craft activities. The conclusion was that participating in a higher number of mentally-stimulating activities is associated with a decreased risk of mild cognitive impairment among community-dwelling older persons (Krell-Roesch et al., 2019).

Social Health

How Does Social Isolation and Loneliness Relate to Brain Health?

Julianne Holt-Lunstad (2017, 2021) was the first American to publish a large-scale analyses finding that poor social support and loneliness are major contributors to mortality. Two meta-analyses were conducted to identify how social isolation and loneliness pose risks for premature mortality. The first analysis centered on 148 studies involving 300,000 participants. Findings showed having more social connections was associated with a 50% lower risk of death (Holt-Lunstad, et al., 2015). A subsequent analysis examined 70 studies, accounting for 3.4 million people who were followed over seven years to assess how social isolation, loneliness, and living alone might affect mortality. All three factors had a significant influence on risk of premature death equal to or greater than other well documented risk factors like obesity, smoking, blood pressure, diabetes, and lack of physical activity. Having friendships and strong emotional ties forecasts greater longevity.

Crowe et al. (2021) examined a sample of 11,302 male and female participants (ages 50–95) in the national health and retirement study followed over eight years to measure the persistence of experiences with loneliness and social isolation. Those experiencing persistent loneliness and social isolation were at 57% increased hazard of mortality compared with those who had never experienced loneliness. For social isolation the increase was 28%. Researchers concluded that deficits in social connectedness were associated with morbidity, disability, mortality, and more advanced biological aging. A recommendation was to bolster social connectedness that interrupt loneliness and could promote more healthy aging. A similar set of recommendations were made by the National Academies of Sciences, Engineering, and Medicine (2020).

The U.S. Surgeon General Dr. Vivek Murthy (2023) has raised alarm regarding the devastating impact of loneliness and isolation. He stated:

> Our epidemic of loneliness and isolation has been an underappreciated public health crisis that has harmed individual and societal health. Our relationships are a source of healing and well-being hiding in plain sight – one that can help us live healthier, more fulfilled, and more productive lives. Given the significant health consequences of loneliness and isolation, we must prioritize building social connection the same way we have prioritized other critical public health issues such as tobacco, obesity, and substance use disorders. Together, we can build a country that's healthier, more resilient, less lonely, and more connected.

The global loneliness crisis has been reflected by countries establishing a Minister of Loneliness governmental position. These countries include United Kingdom, Japan, Australia, and France, all giving attention to initiatives for addressing isolation and loneliness (Ending Loneliness Together, 2021; Hertz, 2021; John, 2018; R. D. Strom & Strom, 2021).

How Do Social Networks Influence Mortality?

The National Social Life, Health and Aging Project is a longitudinal effort which began in 2005 at the University of Chicago (National Institute on Aging, 2023). Researchers are continuing to identify crucial elements of social networks that influence mortality. Over 3,000 people, born between 1920 and 1947 were interviewed in 2005 (when they were 57 to 85 years old) and again in 2011, at ages 62 to 90. A third wave was completed in 2016. By then the participants were ages 67 to 95. Subjects were asked to list up to five of their closest confidants, describe each relationship in detail, and make known how close they felt to each confidante. Excluding their spouses, participants had an average of three close confidants and most reported high support from social contacts. In the beginning most were married, in good health, and not lonely.

The initial findings reported by Iveniuk and Schumm (2016) for this project revealed that close family relationships are more important than friendships in extending the lifespan. Those extremely close to family, other than their spouses, had a 6% risk of dying over the next five years compared with 14% among peers who reported not being close to relatives. The factors most consistently associated with reduced mortality that mattered about the same extent were (a) being married, (b) having a larger social network, (c) greater involvement with social organizations, and (d) feeling closer to confidants. People are more likely to move in and out of someone's social network, especially when the person is not easy to be around. But, family seems more important because they are expected to take care of us when necessary. Everyone can choose friends but it is the people we cannot choose to be with and have little option about choosing us that may provide the greatest benefit for a lengthy lifespan. Family relationships can be troublesome but forgiveness is possible and so is recognition that maturity is shown by repeated efforts for reconciliation.

Do Older Adults Remain Able to Adjust to Social Change?

An important requirement for social health is readiness to change. There are four conflicting hypotheses regarding this capacity (Cacioppo et al., 2005; Visser & Krosnick, 1998). One assumption suggests openness to new ideas is greatest in early adulthood and thereafter declines steadily for the rest of life. This view suggests that elderly hold unyielding opinions so they are seen as being stubborn and set in their ways. The explanation is that, with the passage of time, people acquire habits that provide a sense of stability but at the price of becoming more resistant to new ways of looking at things. Age-segregation also enters an effect by restricting the social network so elder communication is mostly with others whose similar experiences reinforce rather than challenge attitudes and beliefs.

A second set of assumptions maintain that readiness to change is highest during the late teenage years and early adulthood when, for the first time, people can participate in the political process, join the workforce full time, or enlist in the military. The speculation is that attitudes about life adopted during this period tend to become fixed, causing a sharp decline in openness to change that remains in place from middle age onwards.

A third assumption accepts that susceptibility to attitude change is the highest in early adulthood and bottoms out in middle age but rises again in later life. This U-shaped experience curve comes about because older adults are confronted with the need to redefine themselves, owing to retirement or death of a spouse. These and related experiences diminish social support for long standing attitudes and force older people to alter perceptions about the world. A fourth assumption is that, because certain mental skills are known to decline, older adults become less able to present counter arguments to those who would persuade them to change their mind.

To examine the relationship between age and susceptibility to change, Visser and Krosnick (1998) exposed 8,000 adults of differing ages to the same set of change-inducing situations. During multiple experiments, opinions of men and women were reviewed on topics like gun control, death penalty, defense spending, environmental protection, and racial politics. For example, persons interviewed by phone were asked to express their views on using tax dollars to assist minority students and use of racial preferences in admissions policies at universities. Immediately after expressing an answer, each respondent was given a counter attitudinal challenge to assess whether they were willing to change their mind.

Those who favored preferential admission to college for Black students were asked if they would still feel the same even if it meant a reduction in opportunities for qualified Whites. Those who expressed opposition to racial preferences were asked if they would feel the same if it meant that hardly any Blacks would be able to attend the best schools. The researchers found that readiness to change attitudes declined after early adulthood but rose again in later life. It seems that the transition experienced by many older adults present them with new demands and expectations leading to a resocialization. In addition, more than younger groups, elders find it difficult to generate counter arguments when they are presented with persuasive appeals, thereby increasing their susceptibility to attitude change.

Conclusion

The mental dysfunction associated with Alzheimer's disease and other dementias are forecast to increase because the oldest population is growing rapidly and living longer. Elementary and secondary school is recognized as necessary preparation for employment and also because it provides cognitive protection for old age and higher education contributes to a longer life. In contrast, learning needs of older adults have not been well defined even though they share with younger people the continual difficulties of adjusting to social change. It seems a contradiction to assert older relatives have a significant role in the family and society while failing to provide instruction they need to applaud their capacity for learning without making curriculum available that identifies their responsibilities and ways to improve personal influence. Grandparents need to learn from younger relatives, understand goals parents have for children, and get to know each grandchild as individuals. Besides education, other factors can impact healthy brain functioning. Research has found a reduced risk of dementia when older people frequently engage in social activities. Isolation and loneliness are risk factors for dementia that should be addressed by local policies to ensure inclusion of older adults in community activities.

In the past, people believed that aging would be accompanied by a more comprehensive perspective. This assumption remains sensible in cultures where there is a slow pace of change. However, getting older does not produce insights about building relationships in a technological society. In a generation-separated environment, being aware of how younger generations see things and interpret events is needed to be responsive to their needs, and help attain their goals.

Key Concepts

1 All communities should provide the education everyone needs early in life. The amount of formal education while growing up influences relative risk for Alzheimer's disease. Dementia may be delayed by 7–10 years because of protective effects of education. Little is known about whether formal learning during later life can stimulate cognitive functioning and mental health.

2 Linguistic density identified during adolescence in writing samples has been identified as a predictor of risk for dementia. Encourage grandchildren to write grandparent letters or email to augment text messages. There has been a decline of verbal skills for youth over the past two decades and, while the cost of this loss cannot be determined, it is estimated to be considerable.

3 If Alzheimer's could be delayed five years, the number of victims would be diminished by half because this disease develops at such a late age in life that half the people

afflicted would have died before mental impairment and consequent difficulties became evident as symptoms.

4 The risk of mental confusion increases with a rise in incidence of social isolation. This condition has implications for interaction as an important aspect of mental health care in assisted living facilities and long-term care. Having high school or college students visit residents, read to them, and interview them using structured question agenda could be helpful for all parties.

5 Friendships and strong social ties are predictive of greater longevity. Men and women who participate more often in social activities show less cognitive decline and a decreased risk for dementia. Arranging cooperative learning classes is one way to build friendships in old age.

6 The companionship of friends may ward off depression, elevate self-esteem, provide emotional support, encourage continued effort, and help confront adverse events. Friendship building should become a priority in education programs that are designed to serve older adults.

7 Cognitive reserve is defined as ability to tolerate progressive dementia-related damage without showing clinical symptoms. This means that brains with more connections can afford to lose more to Alzheimer's disease before memory loss or other symptoms becomes noticeable.

8 The purposes of education in a longevity society must go beyond preparation for a job. Building the cognitive reserve that is needed following years of employment can help to delay dementia, while also preserving individual sense of purpose, meaning, and self-esteem.

9 Three generational studies have demonstrated that grandparents are able to learn and can improve their influence within the family as observed by younger relatives. Older adults lacking family or friendship connections and meaning demonstrate less motivation to continue learning.

10 Studies have shown that amount of time children spend with parents and grand-parents has the greatest impact on grandchild perceptions of parent and grandparent success. Arranging time with younger relatives should become a goal for all men and women.

Generational Perspectives Activities

13.1 Team Discussion
13.2 Team Discussion: Getting along by Forgetting
13.3 Agenda for Interviews with Grandparents
13.4 Agenda for Interviews with Adolescents
13.5 A Scenario: Reasoning and Problem Solving
13.6 Team Chapter Review
13.7 Criteria for Self-Evaluation of Grandparents

13.1 Team Discussion

1 How will you arrange for mental stimulation during the years of retirement?
2 Why do you suppose intergenerational communication is so uncommon?

3 What do you think older adults should be expected by society to learn?
4 What is your reaction to research about cognitive differences in gender?
5 What research findings about people over age 90 were a surprise to you?
6 Why would you want to know if blood test results indicated Alzheimer's?
7 How do you feel about research findings on loneliness and social activity?
8 What are your observations about the ability of older adults to think about the future?
9 Do you think having a job that is demanding can help sustain cognitive functioning?

13.2 Team Discussion: Getting along by Forgetting

The two men nodded as they entered the cafeteria line at their long-term care center. John and Howard have been acquainted three years and enjoy daily conversation and support.

John: I saw on the news that some people are getting an operation on the memory region of their brain. The idea is to erase long-term negative memories so it will become easier to get along with groups you have always disliked.

Howard: When we were growing up people were less exposed to integration so perhaps most of us could benefit from the operation. Before coming to this care center I had no regular contact with minorities. All I knew about them came from stories I later learned were wrong. In fact, I seldom spoke to anyone from a minority group until I came here and found they provide most of my care.

John: What do you suppose the residents would do if told that, for a limited time, anyone could get this memory removal operation for free and the result would make them a better person?

Howard: My guess is they would miss the point and see it as an invasion of their privacy. Many people seem to cherish the right to choose the groups they want to dislike, racial, religious or income. What about yourself? How do you like the idea of possibly undergoing the operation?

John: Well, there is usually sympathy for older adults who can no longer remember things. But I feel more sorry for those of any age who cannot get along because they are unable to forget the misleading lessons handed down to them by family or taught by peers. I mean it is sad to see someone with dementia struggle with their loss of memory but the greater longer-term tragedy may be rejecting strangers throughout life because our memory retains biases we were taught at an early age and still rely on for the way we perceive and treat groups other than our own.

Howard: Ok, I think my decision is to skip the operation but reflect more on ridding myself of mistaken assumptions about outsiders that should be corrected and require revision. Let's eat.

13.3 Agenda for Interviews with Grandparents

1 How do you suppose expectations for later life learning will change in the future?
2 Compare the ways you learn best with the preferences you favored at a younger age.
3 In what ways has learning become easier and more difficult for you than in the past?
4 What are some important things that people your age learn mainly from their peers?
5 What activities do you participate in that help to maintain your mental well-being?

6 What sources do you look to for understanding about age groups of younger relatives?

7 What education opportunities were there for older adults when you were growing up?

8 What personal observations can you describe about the behavior of people with AD?

9 Why do you suppose society does not provide relevant education for retired people?

10 How should public schools meet the educational needs of immigrant grandparents?

13.4 Agenda for Interviews with Adolescents

1 What lessons do you recommend grandparents learn to help them adjust to social change?

2 What changes would you make in education so going to school could be more interesting?

3 How do you feel about requiring older people to attend classes like younger students do?

4 What misbehavior at school got you into trouble with classroom teachers or the principal?

5 How do your grandparents differ from one another in willingness to continue learning?

6 How have friends helped you make progress in required subjects of school curriculum?

7 What report card grades do you receive from teachers for each of the curriculum subjects?

8 What kinds of lessons do you think should be the focus of learning for retired people?

9 What are some things you think younger people might be able to teach older people?

10 What do you suppose your life will be like years from now when you are an old person?

13.5 A Scenario: Reasoning and Problem Solving

Problem solving scenarios present a look at dilemmas in families and think about solutions. Your task is to consider the pros and cons of stated choices, think of additional options, identify relevant information that may be missing, find out how teammates see options, and defend your reasoning about the advice that you consider best.

Claire has been attending a discussion group on International Affairs at the senior center. She thought this experience would be mentally stimulating and help enlarge her social network. However, one colleague dominates conversations, and another person wanders away from the assigned topic. What do you recommend for Claire to do?

a suggest the group consider guidelines for their discussion

b give up on this set of people and try to join another group

c state her complaints privately to each offender in the group

d tell the course leader and hope that s/he will do something

e Other _____

13.6 Team Chapter Review

Efforts to assess participant learning, provide feedback, and improve quality of instruction is enhanced by a group review of each chapter. *All* members should answer at least one of these question and more if time permits.

1 What ideas in the lesson changed the way I think about this topic?
2 What insights from the lesson will I try to apply in my relationships?
3 What is the most important point for me presented in this lesson?
4 What are some aspects of this lesson I would like to better understand?
5 Which aspects of this lesson do I wish that I had known about earlier?

13.7 Criteria for Self-Evaluation of Grandparents

Directions: For each question, put a check beside statements that describe your feelings. You may want to give several answers on some items. If your feelings are not on the choices list, write them on the line marked 'other.' Results are anonymous so do not write your name. Place your sheet in the homework box next session. After results are tallied, feedback will be given on proportion of class members giving each answer on every item for comparison with your own.

1 How do you evaluate your capacity to learn?

  a I have considerable ability and intend to keep learning.
  b I can still learn most things if I am not being hurried.
  c I feel capable of learning but often lack the motivation.
  d I do not have much confidence about my ability to learn.
  e Other _____

2 What do daughters/sons say about your efforts to continue learning?

  a They complement me about my willingness to keep on learning.
  b They say that I am fine and don't need to learn or make changes.
  c They encourage physical exercise but not mental development.
  d They don't express interest in my learning or personal growth.
  e Other _____

3 What do grandchildren say about your efforts to continue learning?

  a They complement me about my willingness to keep on learning.
  b They say that I am fine and don't need to learn or make changes.
  c They encourage physical exercise but not mental development.
  d They don't express interest in my learning or personal growth.
  e Other _____

4 The kinds of learning I feel the greatest need to acquire involve

  a understanding my family and improving relationships with them
  b financial management and being able to protect my investments
  c health-related concerns and attempting to stay in good condition

    d becoming more capable in the various hobbies that I've chosen
    e Other _____

5 Group discussions with people of my own age

    a provides company and sharing so I enjoy it
    b does not provide new ideas for my reflection
    c seldom remain on track but instead wander
    d are stimulating since they offer new ideas
    e Other _____

6 Changing attitudes I have held for a long time is

    a difficult for me because I am set in my ways
    b unacceptable because I want to be consistent
    c possible when new information is persuasive
    d necessary because I cannot defend my views
    e Other _____

7 Spending time having conversation with peers

    a helps me to remain mentally alert
    b counteracts feelings of loneliness
    c offers feedback about my thinking
    d supports the building of friendships
    e Other _____

8 When I think about spending time with my grandchild

    a I would like us to talk about national current events
    b I wish we could each share the challenges we face
    c I like doing things that involve just the two of us
    d I want each of us to learn what the other values most
    e Other _____

9 When a grandchild does not stay in touch with me

    a I challenge the low priority s/he has assigned me
    b I withdraw and don't question the poor manners
    c I accept that it is normal to ignore older relatives
    d I tell the parents that my feelings have been hurt
    e Other _____

10 Knowing how relatives view my attitudes and behaviors

    a would help me determine ways to improve my behavior
    b could encourage greater motivation for my development
    c would enable me to identify topics for future learning
    d could impact my self-esteem and support adjustment
    e Other _____

References

Alzheimer's Association. (2023). *Alzheimer's disease facts and figures*. https://www.alz.org/alzheimers-dementia/facts-figures

Anstey, K., Peters, R., Zheng, L., Barnes, D., Brayne, C., Brodaty, H., Chalmers, J., Clare, L., Dixon, R. A., Dodge, H., Lautenschlager, N., Middleton, L., Qiu, C., Rees, G., Shahar, S., & Yaffee, K. (2020). Future directions for dementia risk reduction and prevention research: An international research network on dementia prevention consensus. *Journal of Alzheimers Disease*, *78*(1), 3–12. 10.3233/JAD-200674

Apted, M. (Director). (2023). *The Up Series*. United Kingdom. [Series of 9 documentary films about ages 7 to 63+ originally released 1964 to 2019] https://en.wikipedia.org/wiki/Up_(film_series)

Aronson, L. (2021). *Elderhood: Redefining aging, transforming medicine, reimagining life*. Bloomsbury.

Beker, N., Ganz, A., Hulsman M., Klausch, T., Schmand, B., Scheltens, P., Sikkes, S. A., & Holstege, H. (2021, January 15). Association of cognitive function trajectories in centenarians with postmortem neuropathology, physical health, and other risk factors for cognitive decline. *Journal of the American Medical Association Network Open*, *4*(1), e2031654. 10.1001/jamanetworkopen.2020.31654

Bermúdez, J. (2023). *Cognitive science: An introduction to the science of the mind* (4th ed.). Cambridge University Press.

Biswas, R., Kawas, C., Montine, T. J., Bukhari, S. A., Jiang, L., & Corrada, M. M. (2023). Superior global cognition in oldest-old is associated with resistance to neurodegenerative pathologies: Results from the 90+ study. *Journal of Alzheimer's Disease*, *94*(2). 10.3233/JAD-221062

Blazer, D. G., Yaffe, K., & Liverman, C. (Eds.). (2015). *Cognitive aging: Progress in understanding and opportunities for action*. National Academies Press. 10.17226/21693

Bloomberg, M., Dugravot, A., Dumurgier, J., Kivimaki, M., Fayosse, A., Steptoe, A., Britton, A., Singh-Manoux, A., & Sabia, S. (2021, February). Sex differences and the role of education in cognitive ageing: Analysis of two UK-based prospective cohort studies. *The Lancet Public Health*, *6*(2), e106–e115. https://www.sciencedirect.com/science/article/pii/S2468266720302589

Buettner, D. (2015). *The Blue Zones solution: Eating and living like the world's healthiest people*. National Geographic.

Buettner, D. (2017). *The Blue Zones of happiness: Lessons from the world's happiest people*. National Geographic.

Cacioppo, J. T., Visser, P., & Pickett, C. (Eds.). (2005). *Social neuroscience: People thinking about thinking people*. Bradford.

Calhoun, D. (2022, November). Rethinking the education potential of older adults to delay the onset of dementia. *Journal of Adult and Continuing Education*, *28*(2), 414–425. 10.1177/14779714211026939

Coscarelli, J. (2021, January 14). What happens now to Michael Apted's lifelong project 'Up'? *The New York Times*. https://www.nytimes.com/2021/01/14/movies/michael-apted-up-series-future.html

Crowe, C. L., Domingue, B., Graf, G., Keyes, K., Kwon, D., & Belsky, D. W. (2021, November). Associations of loneliness and social isolation with health span and life span in the U.S. Health and Retirement study. *The Journal of Gerontology Medical Sciences, Series A*, *76*(11), 1997–2006. 10.1093/gerona/glab128

Dassel, K., Butler, J., Telonidis, J., & Edelman, L. (2020). Development and evaluation of Alzheimer's disease and related dementias (ADRD) best care practices in long-term care online training program. *Educational Gerontology*, *46*(3), 150–157. 10.1080/03601277.2020.1717079

Daviglus, M. L., Bell, C., Berrettini, W., Bowen, P., Connolly, E. S., Cox, N., Dunbar-Jacob, J. M., Granieri, E. C., Hunt, G., McGarry, K., Patel, D., Potosky, A. L., Sanders-Bush, E., Silberberg, D., & Trevisan, M. (2010, August 3). National Institutes of Health State-of-the Science

Conference statement: Preventing Alzheimer disease and cognitive decline. *Annals of Internal Medicine, 153*(3), 176–181. 10.7326/0003-4819-153-3-201008030-00260

Ending Loneliness Together. (2021, January). A national strategy to address loneliness and social isolation. RUOK? and Australian Psychological Society. https://treasury.gov.au/sites/default/files/2021-05/171663_ending_loneliness_together.pdf

Feder, K. L. (2019). *The past in perspective: An introduction to human prehistory* (8th ed.). Oxford University Press.

Gao, S., Hendrie, H., Hall, K., & Hui, S. (1998). The relationship between age, sex, and the incidence of dementia and Alzheimer Disease: A meta-analysis. *Archives of General Psychiatry, 55*(9), 809–815. 10.1001/archpsyc.55.9.809

Grzywacz, J., Segal-Karpas, D., & Lachman, M. (2016, June). Workplace exposures and cognitive function during adulthood: Evidence from National Survey of Midlife Development and the O*NET. *Journal of Occupational and Environmental Medicine, 58*(6), 535–541. 10.1097/JOM.0000000000000727

Gutchess, A. (2019). *Cognitive and social neuroscience of aging*. Cambridge University Press.

Hertz, N. (2021). *The lonely century: How to restore human connection in a world that is pulling apart*. Penguin Random House.

Holstege, H., Beker, N., Dijkstra, T., Pieterse, K., Wemmenhove, E., Schouten, K., Thiessens, L., Horsten, D., Rechtuijt, S., Sikkes, S., Poppel, F., Meijers-Heijboer, H., Hulsman, M., & Scheltens, P. (2018). The 100-plus study of cognitively healthy centenarians: Rationale, design and cohort description (2018, October). *European Journal of Epidemiology, 33*(12), 1229–1249. 10.1007/s10654-018-0451-3

Holt-Lunstad, J. A. (2017, April 27). *Testimony before the United States Senate Aging Committee, 115th Congress*. https://www.aging.senate.gov/imo/media/doc/SCA_Holt_04_27_17.pdf

Holt-Lunstad, J. A. (2021, January 12). A pandemic of social isolation? *World Psychiatry, 20*, 55–56. 10.1002/wps.20839

Holt-Lunstad, J. A., Smith, T. B., Baker, M., Harris, T., & Stephenson, D. (2015). Loneliness and social isolation as risk factors for mortality: A meta-analytic review. *Perspectives on Psychological Science, 10*(2), 227–237. 10.1177/1745691614568352

Iveniuk, J., & Schumm, L. P. (2016, August 21). *Social relationships and mortality in older adulthood* [Paper presentation]. American Sociological Association 111th Annual Meeting, Seattle, WA, United States.

John, T. (2018, April 25). How the world's first Loneliness Minister will tackle 'the sad reality of modern life'. *Time*. https://time.com/5248016/tracey-crouch-uk-loneliness-minister/

Katzman, R. (1993). Education and the prevalence of dementia and Alzheimer's disease. *Neurology, 43*(1), 13–20. 10.1212/WNL.43.1_Part_1.13

Kawas, C. H. (2022, June 2). *"Clinical and pathological studies of the oldest-old" Claude Kawas, MD discusses 90+ Study [Lecture]*. The Science of Aging, Institute on Aging. https://penninstituteonaging.wordpress.com/2022/06/02/kawas/

Kawas, C. H., Legdeur, N., & Corrada, M. (2021, April). What have we learned from cognition in the oldest-old. *Current Opinion in Neurology, 34*(2), 258–265. 10.1097/WCO.0000000000000910

Krell-Roesch, J., Syrjanen, J., Vassilaki, M., Machulda, M., Mielke, M., Knopman, D., Kremers, W., Petersen, R., & Geda, Y. (2019, August). Quantity and quality of mental activities and the risk of incident mild cognitive impairment. *Neurology, 93*(6), e548–e558. 10.1212/WNL.0000000000007897

Lövdén, M., Fratiglioni, L., Glymour, M., Lindenberger, U., & Tucker-Drob, E. (2020). Education and cognitive functioning across the lifespan. *Psychological Science in the Public Interest, 21*(1). 10.1177/1529100620920576

Maccora, J., Peters, R., & Anstey, K. (2020 December). What does (low) education mean in terms of dementia risk? A systematic review and meta-analysis highlighting inconsistency in measuring and operationalising education. *SSM-Population Health, 12*. 10.1016/j.ssmph.2020.100654

Mattsson-Carlgren, N., Janelidze, S., Palmqvist, S., Cullen, N., Svenningsson, A., Strandberg, O., Mengel, D., Walsh, D. M., Stomrud, E., Dage, J., Hansson, O. (2020 October). Longitudinal plasma p-tau217 is increased in early stages of Alzheimer's disease. *Brain*, *143*(11). 3234–3241. 10.1093/brain/awaa286

McDonald, R. B. (2019). *Biology of aging (2nd ed.)*. Garland Science.

Montine, T. J., Cholerton, B. A., Corrada, M. M., Edland, S. D., Flanagan, M. E., Hemmy, L. S., Kawas, C. H., & White, L. R. (2019, March). Concepts for brain aging: Resistance, resilience, reserve, and compensation. *Alzheimer's Research & Therapy*, *11*(22), 22. 10.1186/s13195-019-0479-y

Murthy, V. (2023, May 3). *New surgeon general advisory raises alarm about the devastating impact of the epidemic of loneliness and isolation in the United States*. U. S. Department of Health and Human Services. https://www.hhs.gov/about/news/2023/05/03/new-surgeon-general-advisory-raises-alarm-about-devastating-impact-epidemic-loneliness-isolation-united-states.html

Murtin, F., Mackenbach, J., Jasilionis, D., & d'Ercole, M. (2017, January 14). *Inequalities in longevity by education in OECD countries: Insights from new OECD estimates*. Organization for Economic Cooperation and Development Statistics Working Papers, No. 2017/02, OECD Publishing, Paris, France. 10.1787/18152031

Nakamura, A., Kaneko, N., Villemagne, V. L., Kato, T., Doecke, J., Doré, V., ... & Yanagisawa, K. (2018, January 31). High performance plasma amyloid-β biomarkers for Alzheimer's disease. *Nature*, *554*(7691), 249–254. 10.1038/nature25456

National Academies of Sciences, Engineering and Medicine. (2020). *Social isolation and loneliness in older adults: Opportunities for the health care system*. Consensus Study Report. National Academies Press.

National Institute on Aging. (2023). *National Social Life, Health, and Aging Project*. NORC at the University of Chicago. https://www.norc.org/research/projects/national-social-life-health-and-aging-project.html

Ngandu, T., von Strauss, E., Helkala, E.-L., Winblad, B., Nissinen, A., Tuomilehto, J., Soininen, H., & Kivipelto, M. (2007). Education and dementia: What lies behind the association? *Neurology*, *69*(14), 1442–1450. 10.1212/01.wnl.0000277456.29440.16

Omura, J. D., McGuire, L. C., Patel, R., Baumgart, M., Lamb,, R., Jeffers, E., Olivari, B. S., Croft, J. B., Thomas, C. W., & Hacker, K. (2022, May 20). Modifiable risk factors for Alzheimer disease and related dementias among adults aged ≥45 Years -- United States 2019. US Department of Health and Human Services/Centers for Disease Control and Prevention. *Morbidity and Mortality Weekly Report*, *71*(20), 680–685. 10.15585/mmwr.mm7120a2

Pierce, A. L., & Kawas, C. H. (2017). Dementia in the oldest old: Beyond Alzheimer disease. *Public Library of Science Medicine*, *14*(3), e1002263. 10.1371/journal.pmed.1002263

Population Reference Bureau. (2023). *Fact sheet: U.S. Dementia trends*. https://www.prb.org/resources/fact-sheet-u-s-dementia-trends/

Rebok, G. W., Ball, K., Guey, L. T., Jones, R. N., Kim, H.-Y., King, J. W., Marsiske, M., Morris, J. N., Tennstedt, S. L., Unverzagt, F. W., & Willis, S. L. (2014). Ten-year effects of the advanced cognitive training for independent and vital elderly cognitive training trial on cognition and everyday functioning in older adults. *Journal of the American Geriatrics Society*, *62*(1), 16–24. 10.1111/jgs.12607

Reifegerste, J., Verissimo, J., Rugg, M., Pullman, M., Babcock, L., Glei, D., Weinstein, M., Goldman, N., & Ullman, M. (2021). Early-life education may help bolster declarative memory in old age, especially for women. *Aging, Neuropsychology, and Cognition*, *28*(2), 218–252. 10.1080/13825585.2020.1736497

Reinhart, R. M. G., & Nguyen, J. A. (2019). Working memory revived in older adults by synchronizing rhythmic brain circuits. *Nature Neuroscience*, *22*, 820–827. 10.1038/s41593-019-0371-x

Roser, M. (2021, November 2). Access to basic education: Almost 60 million children of primary school age are not in school. United Nations Educational, Scientific and Cultural Organization (UNESCO). https://ourworldindata.org/children-not-in-school

Schaie, K. W. (2013). *Developmental influences on adult intelligence: The Seattle longitudinal study* (2nd ed.). Oxford University Press.

Schaie, K. W., & Willis, S. (2017). History of cognitive aging research. In N. Pachana (Ed.), *Encyclopedia of Geropsychology* (pp. 1068–1086). Springer. 10.1007/978-981-287-082-7_99

Seblova, D., Berggren, R., & Lövdén, M. (2020). Education and age-related decline in cognitive performance: Systematic review and meta-analysis of longitudinal cohort studies. *Ageing Research Reviews*, 58. 10.1016/j.arr.2019.101005

Shokouhi, S., Conley, A. C., Baker, S. L., Albert, K., Kang, H., Gwirtsman, H. E., Newhouse, P. A., & Alzheimer's Disease Neuroimaging Initiative. (2019, September). The relationship between domain-specific subjective cognitive decline and Alzheimer's pathology in normal elderly adults. *Neurobiology of Aging*, *81*, 22–29. 10.1016/j.neurobiolaging.2019.05.011

Singh-Manoux, A., Kivimaki, M., Glymour, M. M., Elbaz, A., Berr, C., Ebmeier, K., Ferrie, J. E., & Dugravot, A. (2012, January 5). Timing of onset of cognitive decline: Results from Whitehall II prospective cohort study. *British Medical Journal*, 344. 10.1136/bmj.d7622

Snowdon, D. A. (2002). *Aging with grace: What the nun study teaches us about leading longer, healthier, and more meaningful lives*. Bantam Books.

Snowdon, D. A., Kemper, S. J., Mortimer, J. A., Greiner, L. H., Wekstein, D. R., & Markesbery, W. R. (1996). Linguistic ability in early life and cognitive function and Alzheimer's disease in late life: Findings from the Nun Study. *Journal of the American Medical Association*, *275*(7), 528–532. 10.1001/jama.1996.03530310034029

Stern, Y., Arenaza-Urquijo, E. M., Bartrés-Faz, D., …Vuoksimaa, E. (2020 September). Defining and investigating cognitive reserve, brain reserve, and brain maintenance. *Alzheimers Dementia*, *16*(9), 1305–1311. 10.1016/j.jalz.2018.07.219

Strom, R. D., & Strom, P. (2021). Learning throughout life about the needs of all generations: Prevention of generational alienation. In M. London (Ed.), *Oxford handbook of lifelong learning* (pp. 182–206). Oxford University Press.

Sundermann, E. E., Panizzon, M. S., Chen, X., Andrews, M., Galasko, D., & Banks, S. J. (2020, June). Sex differences in Alzheimer's-related Tau biomarkers and a mediating effect of testosterone. *Biology of Sex Differences*, *11*(33). 10.1186/s13293-020-00310-x

Valenzuela, M. J., & Sachdev, P. (2005). Brain reserve and dementia: A systematic review. *Psychological Medicine*, *36*(4), 441–454. 10.1017/S0033291705006264

Visser, P., & Krosnick, J. (1998). Development of attitude strength over the life cycle: Surge and decline. *Journal of Personality and Social Psychology*, *75*(6), 1389–1410. 10.1037/0022-3514.75.6.1389

World Health Organization (2023, March 15). *Dementia*. https://www.who.int/news-room/fact-sheets/detail/dementia

14   Abuse Across the Life Span

Mental Health and Abuse

Long-term Effects of Being Bullied

Most adults remember bullies from their school days and still wonder what motivated them to find satisfaction in harassing classmates. Similarly, opinions vary about the normality of bullying, the kinds of students who become involved, and quality of their relationships with relatives and friends. There is also speculation about the influence of bullies on classmates who observe them while they harass and intimidate peers.

One way to bring positive change is to abandon the misconception that bullying is normal, just a stage that some children go through but will outgrow as adults. Research supports the opposite conclusion and suggests ways must be found to help bullies change while they are still young. Huesmann et al. (2009) carried out a longitudinal study of 500 students, from age 8 until they reached age 30. Assessments revealed that bullies had greater adjustment problems than peers as they grew up. About 25% of students who started fights in elementary school by pushing, hitting, or stealing the belongings of others had a criminal record by age 30; the comparable record was less than 5% among non-bullies. Elimination of bully behavior that threatens normal child and adolescent development should be the primary focus of social and emotional curriculum for elementary and secondary school students (U.S. Department of Health and Human Services, 2023).

More than thirty years ago Dan Olweus (1993) was the first researcher to evaluate lasting effects of being bullied. He found that young male victims were more depressed and experienced lower self-esteem in early adulthood than non-bullied peers. Few studies have followed the mental health of victims as they grow up. A notable exception by Takizawa et al. (2014) is the British National Child Development study, a 50-year prospective cohort of the births that occurred in a single week in 1958. Parents of these 7,771 children reported on their exposure to being bullied (never, sometimes, or frequently) at ages 7 and 11. Students who were bullied in childhood had increased levels of psychological distress determined at age 23 and again at age 50. Those who were bullied often experienced much higher rates of depression, anxiety disorder, and thinking about suicide decades after they were exposed to peer abuse.

Numerous studies have shown evidence that the long-term negative effects of bullying have been underestimated, and patterns of bullying behavior continue with dire negative consequences (U. S. Department of Health and Human Sciences, 2023). A nationwide poll by the Pew Research Center (Minkin & Horowitz, 2023) of 3,757 parents of children aged 18 and younger have identified mental health concerns at the top of their list of

DOI: 10.4324/9781003401261-19

worries. Specifically, the most prominent worry (extremely worried or somewhat worried) of parents is about their children struggling with anxiety or depression (76%), followed by fears of being bullied (74%).

Bully and Peer Relationships

When they grow up, bullies generally have unstable relationships. In comparison with the general population, male bullies abuse their wives more often, drive cars erratically, often are fired from their jobs, commit more felonies, and less often have successful careers. Females who bully classmates in childhood are more inclined to severely punish their own children. Male and female bullies have higher than average rates of alcoholism, more often exhibit personality disorders, and require more mental health services (Cohen & Espelage, 2020; Pillemer, 2020).

Bullies receive considerable attention at school but responses rarely center on corrective instruction for rehabilitation. Later, the same patterns of misbehavior that make bullies troublesome for classmates are portrayed on a broader scale in the employment histories when rejection by co-worker becomes their most common response. The parents of school-age bullies should be aware that harassing others eventually harms perpetrators as well as their victims. Helping bullies develop healthy internal guidance is the best way to reduce violence (Morin, 2022; Segal, 2018).

Contrary to popular opinion, bullies are usually intelligent, receive good grades, and express self-confidence (Cohen & Espelage, 2020). These abilities can cause teachers to underestimate the dangers that may occur when children grow up lacking empathy and continue their mistreatment of others. Schools have to take the problems of bullies as seriously as other issues they attempt to remediate. When students have reading problems, tutoring is provided with an expectation that improvement will follow. However, when a student lacks self-restraint or demonstrates a disregard for the feelings of others, the school response more often focuses on punishment than recuperation.

Low self-esteem is speculated as an explanation for the motivation of bullies. Research does not support this opinion. On the contrary, there is a strong correlation between high self-esteem and violence. Persons engaging in violent behavior usually have high self-esteem. This troublesome group includes bullies, racists, gang members, people who are associated with crime, rapists, and psychopaths. Interventions that focus on self-control rather than self-esteem have been found to be more effective (de Becker, 2021).

The favorable self-impression of bullies is based on lack of awareness about what their peers really think of them until late adolescence. While bullies are growing up, they usually hang out with one or two companions, often lackeys who feel obligated to help them implement their hostile wishes. Bullies mistakenly suppose that their own social situation is normal. Owing to the social blind spot that makes them oblivious to the way they are perceived by peers, bullies typically lack empathy. Acquiring empathy is essential for long-term healthy development of bullies.

Female bullies also require rehabilitation. Male bullies rely on physical aggression such as shoving, hitting, and kicking while females resort to relational aggression. To get even they spread rumors about someone so classmates will reject the victim. The way female bullies often strive for domination is threatening social exclusion, "You cannot come to my party unless you …" Threats are made to withdraw friendship in order to get one's own way, "I won't be your friend unless …" The silent treatment is applied to produce social isolation. Expressions of coercion are effective because they place in jeopardy what females value most, relationship with other females. Social exclusion is especially powerful when females transition to adolescence (Lamanna et al., 2020).

Child Neglect and Abuse

About 4 million cases of child abuse and neglect are reported annually (American Academy of Pediatrics, 2022; Centers for Disease Control and Prevention, 2022). The highest rate of child abuse occurs with infants less than 1 year of age, and 25% are under age 3. This is likely an underestimate because many cases are unreported. In a single year, about 1,750 children die of abuse and neglect in the United States. Parental depression, parental substance abuse, domestic violence, poverty, and other mental health issues contribute to the risk factors for child abuse and neglect.

The Center on the Developing Child (2022) at Harvard University provides a report and visual resources about the effects of parent neglect and abuse of young children. Extensive biological and developmental research shows significant neglect can cause more lasting harm to a young child's development than overt physical abuse. This video explains the science behind why significant deprivation of neglect or non-responsive parenting can negatively impact the developing brain. [See the website and video at: https://developingchild.harvard.edu/resources/inbrief-the-science-of-neglect-video/].

Bullies and Their Families

Bullies generally learn about coercion and intimidation at home where they are frequently mistreated during childhood. Research has determined that parents of bullies interact with children differently than families of nonviolent children. Parents of bullies do not use praise, encouragement, or good humor like other parents do when communicating with their children. Within the family of the bully, the children generally experience put-downs, sarcasm, and criticism. The punishment of a young bully may depend more upon the mood of a parent than on the gravity of misconduct. If a parent is angry, harsh punishment is likely. If the parent is in good spirits, a child may get away with most misbehavior (Smith, 2022).

Dysfunctional parents often convey the impression that life is a battleground and threats can be anticipated from any direction at any time. Even when bullies become too strong for parents to physically abuse them, they continue to witness a similar mistreatment of their younger siblings. The lesson is always the same-- whoever has the greatest physical power is right. Based on erratic attacks from parents, bullies become wary and misinterpret motives of others. They see hostility where there is none, and this suspicion produces conflicts with classmates (Ripley, 2021). Schools should be given authority by the district to educate dysfunctional families as a unit by providing instruction for parents of bullies as well as bullies themselves. This approach could help parents adopt constructive goals while learning reasonable discipline methods. In the long-term, counseling cannot compensate for failing to offer parents the skills needed to provide suitable child guidance. A description of how aggression is learned by modeling at an early age was determined in Albert Bandura's psychological lab at Stanford University (Mcleod, 2023; Nolan, 2023).

Bully Impact on Bystanders

Students who are spared from becoming targets of bullies can still be harmed by negative social lessons they teach observers. Evidence about the impact of bullies comes from research where peers have been observers in more than 80% of bully episodes that took place at school. Coloroso's (2016) study of 1,000 elementary students found an experimental group provided guidance about ways to respond to bullies later reported more frequent engagement in fulfilling their responsibility as bystanders and less acceptance of bullying and aggression than their peers assigned to an untreated control group. The willingness to remain spectators and acquiesce often fuels more intimidation (U.S. Department of Health and Human Services, 2023).

It is important to identify conditions that motivate bystanders to intervene in behalf of peers being bullied. Few students challenge bullies but most who take action have high social status. To increase peer intervention, it is necessary to acquaint students with their individual responsibility to demonstrate empathy and respond on behalf of anyone being mistreated. In addition, all students should acquire intervention strategies and be urged to show courage to offset a silent majority whose lack of caring can deprive victims of support while jeopardizing their own future to become compassionate individuals (de Becker, 2021).

When bully behavior is viewed as a group phenomenon, the participant role of observers is recognized and attention should be given to training them to initiate social change by reporting incidents. Besides victims (who suffer humiliation, anxiety, and pain), bullies (who harm others and endanger their social and emotional development), the witnesses (who are in the process of forming lifelong responses to injustice) deserve consideration. Bully behavior may begin with minimal harm but can escalate to devastating mistreatment (Salmivalli, 2023).

When parents and students discuss school safety, the fear that someone will bring a weapon is mentioned most often (National Center for Education Statistics, 2022). A sense of fear is attributed to murders by middle school and high school students. More than 6,000 students are expelled each year for bringing a weapon to their school. Nevertheless, nearly half of students report they would not tell teachers or principals if they knew that a classmate had brought a weapon. The reason given is fear of possible retaliation, that the bully would "Get them back." Clearly, unwillingness to report peer abuse is a perilous adolescent norm. Following cases of violence, it has often been found that students knew about threats but did not take them seriously or chose not to inform teachers or parents (United States Department of Justice and Federal Bureau of Investigation, 2023). The Centers for Disease Control and Prevention (2023) reports that the number one cause of death of children and teens is firearms, reaching the highest rate since 2008.

Cyberbullies and Teasing

For the first time, cyberbullying has surpassed face-to-face bullying as the most common form of harassment in school (Gordon, 2020; U.S. Department of Health and Human Services, 2023). Students have always tried to avoid bullies but the digital era has presented concerns about enemies that are unseen. A rise in cell phones and social media has placed a growing number of students at risk for being cyberbullied. Nearly half (46%) of adolescents report they regularly have to cope with messages that are meant to intimidate them (Vogels, 2022). Messages from the cyberbullies involve name-calling with 42% of students reporting they have been called offensive names online. About a third of students report someone has spread rumors or gossip about them online. Sexting takes place less often but represents a concern for 57% of parents who worry about their children sending or receiving sexually explicit images (Morin, 2022).

Detection and rehabilitation of cyber bullies is complicated because of the way teasing is generally perceived. Many people consider teasing just making fun of someone in a playful manner. Teasers usually explain their motivation by saying "I was just kidding." In contrast, students who have been teased report that it is a stressful experience. When students report physical abuse by peers, teachers urge them to identify the classmates who hurt them. However, when students report they have been teased, they are given a different response. The dilemma involves a false assumption that teasers are not motivated to harm someone and they would stop if the individual being made fun of expressed disappointment. Consequently, victims are urged to suck it up, try to ignore the incident, consider this an aspect of life people must learn to cope with, and consider their ordeal as an opportunity to build character. Studies of teasing have found two-thirds of cases involve name-calling, focusing on physical appearance or dress, followed by attention to deviance from group norms, deficits in academic skills, and other perceived imperfections (Vogels, 2022).

Students identified by peers as the most active teasers were also identified as most popular individuals and having the most friends. Given the adult reluctance to condemn teasing in the same way that physical bullying is renounced, it is not surprising to find students adopt the same outlook. Many trivialize teasing mistreatment as they harass classmates on the Internet. In effect, students are led to believe that physically hurting someone is unacceptable behavior while teasing them is relatively harmless and could benefit the victims by helping them learn how to manage adversity (Gordon, 2020).

There can be a high emotional cost when students are called undesirable names. The name callers are seldom referred to as bullies even though their behavior undermines the mental health of others. When some teasing victims reach the end of their tolerance and respond with violence, their reasons more often relate to being teased than to being physically bullied. Teenage murderers have reported they could no longer bear being called nasty names; they identified being ridiculed as their main motivation for resorting to desperate actions. United States Department of Justice and Federal Bureau of Investigation (2023) tracked school shooters and found they had been bullied by peers for a long time. Over 70% reported being persecuted, threatened, and sometimes injured before they decided violence was the best solution. Over three-fourths of school shooters have also announced suicidal thoughts that were ignored by friends or family.

Adults remember hearing, "Sticks and stones can break my bones but names will never hurt me." This statement is false and research has found that being called names hurts and extent of harm depends in part on the age of the victim. Before adolescence, students cannot access the powerful defense mechanism called rationalization. Consequently, they are inclined to believe any negative comments others say about them. Parents struggle to convince children that such insults are false and should just be dismissed. Consider 8-year-old John who, in tears, tells his mother that Roger keeps calling him a "retard," John's mother might point out that you, John, are in the highest reading group for your grade level but Roger is in the lowest reading group. This means that for Roger to call you a retard is foolish. However, John is not old enough to rationalize so he remains convinced that he is whatever Roger calls him. This sad story implicates education to avoid name-calling in favor of treating other students with respect and kindness. Abuse has long-term consequences for self-esteem and confidence about capacity for success (Matthews et al., 2017).

Recommendations for Schools to Reduce Bullying

In 2018, the Florida Department of Education (2023) became the first state to provide an escape for K–12 students reporting they were being harassed or bullied in their public school. The Hope Scholarships allow parents to obtain a voucher good for full tuition costs at a private school. Program advocates explain that this approach gives parents leverage to ensure safety of their children when schools fail to protect them. Opponents of the law contend that, while the new practice allows mistreated students to leave the scene of their mistreatment, bullies remain and can turn attention to harassment of others, so the problem is only partially solved. Moreover, bullying rates in private schools are similar to rates that occur in public schools so there is no guarantee that moving elsewhere will terminate intimidation. But public schools with 10 or more students who request a Hope Scholarship in a year are monitored by the Florida State Department of Education to examine their bully prevention programs to assess needs for policy reforms.

The following initiatives by students, faculty, and parents can reduce bullying:

1 Use healthy self-evaluation criteria so demeaning others is not a basis for confidence.
2 Urge students to periodically identify the positive qualities that they observe in peers.
3 Portray social maturity as an achievement that is shown by acceptance of differences.
4 Help students realize that teasing shows an inability to care about feelings of others.
5 Show courage in challenging the mistreatment of others when they are observed.
6 Build feelings of belonging and mutual support for the cooperative learning teammates.
7 Place reminders on the walls about no name-calling, eye rolling, or laughing at peers.
8 Teach students to process comments from teasers presented in situations at all ages.
9 Discuss how being teased can be harmful no matter what the intention of the teaser.
10 Create a list of words that students agree not to use when talking about each other.
11 Encourage students to identify who they wish to become and set personality goals.
12 Ask students about a time when they teased someone, their reasons, and the outcomes.
13 Invite students to share an incident when they were teased and how they felt then.
14 Enable students to learn conflict resolution skills instead of using negative remarks.
15 Suggest that parents talk with their child who is a teaser or is teased by someone.

Scope of Older Adult Abuse

Over the long term, children who are abused or neglected are at increased risk for experiencing future emotional and psychological problems, violence victimization, substance abuse, sexually transmitted infections, lower educational attainment, and limited employment opportunities (Centers for Disease Control and Prevention, 2022). Some people are abused throughout their lives and are denied the fundamental attitudes of optimism and resilience which are essential for mental health. In some cases, abuse occurs within families and is cyclical; this means that when children are abused at an early age by parents, later the aging parent is likely to be abused by the adult-aged child. The National Institute on Aging (2023) provides an online help guide for elder victims of abuse. Most victims are women, average age of 78 (Office of Violence Against Women, 2023). Two-thirds of the 5 million cases recorded each year implicate mistreatment by adult relatives including spouses whose frustration, stress, and impatience accounts for failure to fulfill their roles as compassionate caregivers. Elder abuse affects mental and physical health of victims, and triples their risk of premature death as compared with mortality rates of peers with similar medical conditions but who are not abused by caregivers (National Council on Aging, 2021; Phelan, 2021).

Types of Abuse

William Barr, former U.S. Attorney General, handled the largest number of elder fraud cases in history. His office prosecuted criminals who collectively swindled over two million Americans, most of them retired. Barr explained that vulnerability of this age segment and their increased targeting by predators caused his office to assign priority to the identification and prosecution of anyone taking advantage of older adults (United States Department of Justice, 2019).

Criminals who promote fraudulent financial schemes choose older adults as targets because they are easier to mislead with confusing messages through postal mail, email, and phone scams related to alleged financial investment opportunities, soliciting monetary contributions for charities that do not exist, and related efforts meant to appeal to those who show poor judgement (Consumer Financial Protection Bureau, 2021; Robinson et al., 2023). A common scheme is a fraudulent phone call introducing themselves as representing Medicare (or other income source institutions) and asking for personal information; for example, "This is Medicare calling. I need to check your information for our records. Please tell me your birthday so I can verify you are the correct person I am talking to. … This will only take a minute." Scammers are aware that the elderly population control more than 70% of national disposable income (American Association of Retired Persons, 2023).

A related problem of extortion takes place in families where younger relatives annually steal an estimated $2.6 billion from elderly relatives (American Association of Retired Persons, 2023; Dong, 2017; Phelan, 2021). This financial exploitation accounts for 12% of elder abuse cases. The misconduct can include forgery, stealing social security checks, taking advantage of joint signature bank accounts, misusing ATMs or credit cards, taking pension funds, causing elders to turn over their stocks or savings, sign a deed or will, arrange for power of attorney by using deception or coercion. Guilty relatives often justify their misconduct by explaining they are sharing family resources.

Physical abuse represents 16% of elder abuse cases. Physical signs of elder abuse could be (a) dehydration or unusual weight loss; (b) missing daily living aids, such as eye glasses or a toothbrush; (c) unexplained injuries, bruises, cuts, or sores; (d) unsanitary living conditions and poor hygiene; and (e) misuse of prescriptions, such as excessive medication of tranquilizers and sleeping pills that disable patients making them easier to control (National Institute on Aging, 2023; National Council on Aging, 2021).

Signs of emotional/behavioral elder abuse represent 7% of cases, and include (a) increased fear or anxiety, (b) isolation from friends or family, (c) unusual changes in behavior or sleep, and (d) withdrawal from normal activities. Calling older people insulting names, threatening to institutionalize them, denying them companionship, and imposing conditions of social isolation reflect emotional abuse. Active neglect means withholding food, medicine, personal care or access to essential supports such as hearing aids and dentures. Passive neglect is defined as being ignored, left alone, and forgotten – this is the most prevalent form of elder abuse (58%) perpetrated by relatives. Only 4% of older adults reside in assisted living or long-term care centers. This means elder abuse takes place far more often for those who live at home than in an institution (Conrad et al., 2019; National Council on Aging, 2021).

Detection of Abuse

Societal impressions about families present an obstacle to the detection of elder abuse. The way relatives get along has historically been considered a private matter that bars interference by outsiders. This view is sustained by a belief that, as the basic unit of society, the family is a support system capable of providing all of its members the affection, guidance, and protection needed. In families where this normative behavior is absent, older relatives are kept from being monitored by external sources that are needed to ensure they are not being subjected to inhumane treatment.

Finding out whether individuals are abused is further complicated because many elders are relatively isolated. Most are no longer employed so there is no interaction with co-workers. They do not go to school so there are no classmates to observe them. As a result, outsiders have no windows of observation to discover whether someone is being abused in a private residence. Unlike children whose teachers can report suspicious physical conditions and try to help them, elders lack such resources and neighbors may be reluctant to check on them. When elders are in poor health and housebound, this further prevents detection of abuse by restricting their contact with outsiders (National Institute on Aging, 2023; National Council on Aging, 2021).

Detection also depends on the willingness of victims to admit mistreatment. When abuse has been verified, only 25% were reported by the victims. One-third of women and men abused deny visible evidence of their physical harm (Dong, 2017; Office of Violence Against Women, 2023; Wright, 2017). Why do victims refuse to talk about the abuse they experience?

1 They may depend on the abusers for survival and fear retaliation.
2 They accept blame for being the cause of their own mistreatment.
3 They worry about being forced to move away from their home.
4 Bonds of affection for the abuser are stronger than a desire to leave.
5 They feel guilty about having a relative who exposes them to abuse.
6 They are concerned about family status if their abuse became known.

Abuse in Care Facilities

Long-term care facilities are home for nearly three million patients; many of them are frail (National Institute on Aging, 2023). Ninety percent of nursing facilities lack enough staff to adequately perform their responsibilities. The federally recommended ratio is one staff member for six patients but, in most institutions, the usual ratio is one staff member for 15 to 25 patients. Anonymous reports given by nurse assistants indicate they sometimes neglect to provide patients with oral/dental care, not change their clothes each time residents are wet following an episode of incontinence, skip regularly scheduled baths, fail to be sure patients are hydrated, not perform required range of motion exercises, and turning off a call button light without responding to a resident's request (Bieber, 2023).

The Nursing Home Abuse Justice (2023) stated that while nursing home abuse statistics can be disturbing, it is essential to understand that this problem is quite common. This is especially true if you have a loved one living in a nursing home or assisted living facility. Serious harm involves rough handling, yelling and expressing anger, making threats, punching, or slapping a resident. One in three adults in U.S. nursing homes have been a victim of abuse; in addition, two in three staff members surveyed by the World Health Organization (2022) admitted to abusing or neglecting residents (Bieber, 2023).

Research has determined that low social support significantly increases patient risk for all forms of mistreatment in long-term care. Regular visits by relatives and friends should be seen by them as an effective way to reduce the likelihood of elder abuse. Making unexpected visits and understanding the tasks required of staff helps identify concerns before they escalate to become emotional or physical abuse (Wright, 2017).

Bullying by Older Adult Peers

Public awareness about bullying of residents in nursing homes is meager as compared with attention to the bullying problem when it involves children and adolescents. Teresi et al. (2016) observed and interviewed over 2,000 residents in 10 nursing homes across the state of New York. Twenty percent of residents reported they had been involved in at least one aggressive encounter with other residents in the four weeks prior to being interviewed.

Robin Bonifas (2016) is a social worker. She is the author of a book entitled *Bullying among older adults: How to recognize and address an unseen epidemic.* Bonifas considers bully behavior by residents of long-term care to be a result of frustrations characteristic of institutional living along with age-related issues. Elderly residents recognize their loss of independence and sense of control, so, for some, becoming a bully makes them feel as if they regain lost power. When an elderly man is excluded from a card game, there are not many ways for him to escape rejection; laundry rooms can be places where individuals have detergent stolen, and their clothes thrown on the floor. Bingo locations can become battlefields whenever lucky newcomers find themselves accused of cheating. Lesbians and gays are typically rejected by fellow residents.

In response, many elder victims of bullying stop going to social events or even visiting the dayroom. They tend to eat alone in the cafeteria and refuse the facility bus that goes to the mall, grocery store, or pharmacy. Bonifas (2016) studied a group of older adults who reported they were bullied in the preceding year. They obtained higher scores on measures of depression and lower scores on measures of self-esteem compared to peers who did not report being bullied. Working in a facility where patient bullying and other negative social behaviors exist also undermines morale of the staff.

Young adults are often surprised that in a long-term care setting there is violence and verbal aggression, screaming, yelling, and physical incidents such as hitting, biting, and kicking. Another category of abuse that becomes a source of fear is when a patient makes an unwelcome entry to someone else's room and begins to rummage through their possessions claiming to be looking for something. This abuse occurs most often in facilities that do not separate dementia patients from the space of viable patients. Neglect is a problem with 10% of residents suffering from pressure ulcers, from bed sores, and urinary tract infections (Herman et al., 2022).

Reliance on Adult Day Care

The 7,500 adult day care centers across the nation serve 300,000 older adults. Eighty percent of participants attend full day sessions; half are involved five days a week while their family caregiver is at work or engaged with other tasks. From the view of a daughter or son, the much lower-cost of day care as a form of long-term care than placing a relative in an institution allows them to remain employed and have peace of mind knowing their parent receives attention, gets a hot meal, takes medication on time, socializes with peers, has reality training, exercise, help as needed, and supervision to ensure safety. The average cost for 12 hours of daycare service is $78 although there is a wide variance among the states. Adult day care provides great relief to wives responsible for care of their often older and less self-sufficient husbands. Having these men attend day care and return home at night contributes to mental health of the family (Eldercare Locator, 2023; Hipp, 2023; National Adult Day Services Association, 2023).

Adult day care offers relief for family caregivers so they can complete their own chores. In a study of 50 families day care relief allowed caregivers to prevent or delay moving a parent into a long-term care facility. Older people should be made aware that adult day care is a better option than staying home alone and watching television, lacking socialization or chances to speak with others, and access to special supervision care when this is needed. Adult day care services reduce family stress. One study found two-thirds of caregivers reported less stress on the days that their loved ones attended day care compared to days they did not attend. Older adults also showed fewer symptoms of depression than peers who did not have adult day care services. One year later the benefits were retained. Loved ones who rely upon day care report elder parents become easier to manage, are more active and alert, show less anxiety, decreased symptoms of depression, and enjoy more social interaction with peers (Eldercare Locator, 2023; Hipp, 2023; National Adult Day Services Association, 2023).

Domestic Abuse, Child Abuse, and Older Adult Abuse

Some couples in a marital or cohabitation arrangement abuse their partner to maintain control over the behavior of that person. The scope of domestic violence can include physical abuse, sexual abuse, emotional abuse, financial abuse, technological abuse, and psychological abuse. Each day over 20,000 calls are received by domestic hotlines from individuals reporting cases of abuse. The most common solution to ensure safety of the victim and others in their household is to obtain a restraining order from the court (Herman et al., 2022). The victims and those who witness intimidation, including children, are often traumatized. The Office of Violence Against Women (2023) reported that partner violence accounts for 15% of all violent crimes in the United States; women who suffer from intimate partner violence are most likely to be young adults between the ages of 18 to 24.

There are several similarities between elder abuse and child abuse. First, adults who were abused by parents are far more likely to behave the same way later on toward their aging parents. This reverse cycle suggests that revenge can be a powerful motive for abuse. Studies have found that people who were not treated violently while growing up mistreated their parents in later life by a ratio of 1 in 400; in comparison, adults who were abused early in life mistreated their parents by a ratio of 1 to 2 (Dong, 2017).

Another similarity relates to the explanation given by perpetrators to explain their behavior. Usually abuse takes place because prior efforts to control unacceptable conduct of an elder did not achieve the desired result. Non-compliant elders are unaccustomed to accepting the authority of adult children, spouse or other caregivers show an unwilling-ness to comply with demands and expose themselves to increased risk for abuse. When children oppose the demands of parents by refusing to eat, have toilet accidents, or decide to cry, these reactions are generally interpreted as signs of defiance. On the other hand, when frail elders demonstrate similar forms of resistance, the caregivers are presented with unanticipated problems. In exasperation, a caregiver who strikes an aging parent sounds like the abusive parent of a child who says, "She made me hit her. She's been asking for it all day" (Pillemer, 2020).

Figures regarding elder abuse are underestimated because victims do not typically self-report (Burnes et al., 2019). Also, the figures regarding child abuse are underestimated because many cases are unreported. According to the Centers for Disease Control and Prevention (2022), at least 1 in 7 children have experienced abuse or neglect in the past year in the United States. Most victims are young, from birth to age 5. Child abuse and elder abuse are experienced in a society that does not acknowledge the widespread existence of family violence. Some people feel physical punishment of children is needed as a method to correct misbehavior. However, using the same strategy to manage the noncompliant behavior of elders is seen as a violation of their rights. As a result, people who mistreat elders are less likely to admit their abuse, recognizing others may disagree with their correction effort (Weir, 2017).

Differing expectations of the young and old are also implicated. Generally, children are considered more vulnerable and require greater protection than older adults who are more often viewed as a burden to their family. Older people have more legal, economic, and emotional independence than children, including the right to refuse help or intervention from professionals. Consequently, government agencies involved with protection of families usually give higher priority and resources for prevention of child abuse (Centers for Disease Control and Prevention, 2022, 2023).

Victims of elder abuse are frequently mentally and physically frail whereas children who are abused, although dependent, typically do not have disabilities. Then too, it becomes more difficult to detect abuse of older people. They do not live public lives as other age groups so there is limited contact with agencies or maybe anyone other than the abusers. They do not go to school and are not required to have regular medical checkups. In addition, norms of development for children are well established so deviation from these patterns triggers investigation. However, situations are more complex with older people. The differing extent of acute and chronic illness in later life means there are less accurate indicators to define normal. Therefore, it is frequently medically difficult to assess the difference between exposure to a deliberate injury or an accidental fall.

Another distinction implicates perceptions about the future. Most child caregivers can look forward to a time when dependency will end as youth gain independence to provide self-care. In contrast, aging people become increasingly more dependent and place greater demands on those responsible for their care. It is not always possible for caregivers of older relatives to foresee a satisfactory outcome or know how long it will be before they can expect to get relief. Death of a dependent elder may be only a partial solution if the caregivers are left with unresolved guilt and remorse (Jantz & McMurray, 2017).

In a longevity society, some caregivers for aging parents are elderly themselves and may have to deal with poor health or physical disabilities. It is becoming common for people in their 50s and 60s to care for parents in their 70s and 80s, some of whom are in better health and could outlive daughters or sons. Finally, in child abuse, the relationship has a recent origin whereas the abuse of elders is based on a relationship that could have spanned many years. Elder abuse can be based on long-standing conflicts (Pillemer et al., 2016).

Families should be aware that most elder abuse cases involve self-neglect by individuals who live alone and lack motivation to properly care for themselves. Many are malnourished widows who prefer not to cook because no one eats with them. They seldom change their clothes or bathe, and fail to keep the residence clean. In such situations, family caregivers should arrange for home health care and personal mainte- nance. When this help is not enough, day care or long-term care are options to preserve health and safety (National Institute on Aging, 2023).

Conclusion

In the past children learned civil behavior and etiquette from rules they were expected to follow and reinforced by adult observers. This is not the way many students now learn how to treat others in cyber space. While grownups agree that student safety should have priority in schools and families, the current scope of bullying suggests the need for greater societal attention to this goal. Feeling safe is an aspiration that society must strive to arrange for everyone from all age groups.

The population of retired persons is increasing at a more rapid rate than it is for younger generations. Protection for this vulnerable group depends on caregivers who demonstrate patience, willingness to spend time and listen, and exercise self-restraint when the difficulties of caring lead to frustration. The personality attributes that contribute to maturity should be nurtured by all families so middle-aged people will be equipped to provide the care expected of them. Elder abuse is less likely to occur when siblings share responsibility, friends and neighbors step up to relieve family caregivers, regular visits to long term care are made by church members and other organizations, and initiatives are taken by youth to show they value older adults, want to teach them and learn from them about experiences that are associated with aging. Local, state, and federal government are responsible to combat fraudulent schemes meant to exploit older people and supervise long-term care facilities so that health and safety standards are maintained in all of the states.

Key Concepts

1 Victims of bullying early in life, including those who bully others, are at an increased risk as adults for poor health, lower income, and less satisfying relationships. The long-lasting negative effects for victims make it clear that their suffering should not be seen as harmless or considered an inevitable aspect of growing up that they should feel expected to endure.

2 Abuse is often learned at home where bullies are mistreated. Studies have found that parents of bullies interact with children much differently than families of non-violent children. Parents of bullies do not use praise, encouragement, or humor as other parents for communication and guidance about methods of getting along with others.

3 There can be a high emotional cost if people are called undesirable names. The name callers are seldom referred to as bullies even though their behavior undermines the mental health of others. When some name calling victims cannot take it anymore and respond using violence, their reasons more often involve incessant teasing than being subjected to physical abuse.

4 Senior centers should provide workshops for retirees about fraudulent schemes meant to target their age group. These education initiatives should acquaint elders with how

scams operate, what to look out for, how to get information, and where to report their observation or exposure.

5 Persons who abuse elders are usually relatives who require help so they can carry out their caregiver tasks without being overwhelmed by frustration. Siblings, neighbors, friends, and volunteers should provide relief and emotional support that main caregivers need to retain the resilience and maturity required for their demanding role.

6 Unannounced visits to nursing homes by relatives, neighbors, or friends are helpful ways to diminish any potential for patient mistreatment. More benefits happen when people outside the family also spend time visiting to ensure required procedures are being followed by the staff.

7 Some elders have reason to distrust relatives and try to avoid them having personal financial information. Social workers from adult protective services should have private conversations with older adults to assess whether anyone is asking them for money, soliciting donations for charitable causes, or wants to have control of their finances.

8 When visiting a long-term care facility, inquire about whether the patient has seen residents bully others. Invite them to describe incidents they are aware of and if they personally experienced harassment by anyone else. This anecdotal information should be brought to the attention of the administrator and ombudsman who serve the facility.

9 Adolescent and young adults should recognize they have a stake in prevention of elder abuse. They should periodically visit their older relatives and other residents in assisted living and long term care facilities. Unless youth become motivated to be part of a community effort to prevent elder abuse, their development of maturity can be jeopardized.

10 Older adults cared for at home should know that expressing their gratitude means a lot to their younger family members. Failing to acknowledge help can be interpreted as a form of abuse that takes a toll when it leads caregivers to feel unappreciated and justifies mistreatment of elders.

Generational Perspectives Activities

14.1 Team Discussion #1
14.2 Team Discussion #2
14.3 A Scenario: Reasoning and Problem Solving
14.4 Team Chapter Review
14.5 Criteria for Self-Evaluation of Team Members

14.1 Team Discussion #1

1 What kinds of financial schemes do you know about that try to exploit elders?
2 How does your church participate in helping caregivers fulfill their obligation?
3 What conditions have you observed when visiting patients in long-term care?
4 If elders do not trust family with financial information, who should they trust?
5 What incidents are you aware of about patients who bully their fellow residents?
6 What role should society expect of young people in terms of elder caregiving?
7 What have you been told by elder caregivers about difficulties they encounter?

8 How should caregivers of relatives with dementia be helped by the government?
9 What do you think about installing cameras in long-term care patient rooms?
10 What has been your experience with providing care for older family members?

14.2 Team Discussion #2

1 What do you think society should do to minimize elder abuse?
2 When family members abuse older relatives, how should the community respond?
3 Why do you suppose women are more often abused during old age than men?
4 What methods have you seen used by media to target elders for financial abuse?
5 How can people your age be part of the solution for curbing abuse of elders?
6 How can society know if elderly people are being abused by their caregivers?
7 Why do you think abused elders are unwilling to tell what happened to them?
8 What have been your observations when visiting patients in a nursing home?
9 Why should dementia patients be prevented from non-dementia patient rooms?
10 How is bullying by nursing home patients similar to bullying by your peers?

14.3 A Scenario: Reasoning and Problem Solving

Christine attended the women's weekly Bible study class at a local church for almost a year but then stopped coming a month ago. She did not contact the teacher or fellow students. The women are wondering what should be done. They know Christine's daughter is the main caregiver but the status of their relationship is unknown. What actions do you think should be taken by the group?

a Pray for Christine and hope that she will soon return to class.
b Choose one person to phone or visit Christine to check on her.
c Assign someone to visit unannounced and observe the situation.
d Call the daughter to inquire about Christine and ask if help is needed.
e Other _____

14.4 Team Chapter Review

Efforts to assess participant learning, provide feedback, and improve quality of instruction is enhanced by a group review of each chapter.

1 What ideas in the lesson changed the way I think about this topic?
2 What insights from the lesson will I try to apply in my relationships?
3 What is the most important point for me presented in this lesson?
4 What are some aspects of this lesson I would like to better understand?
5 Which aspects of this lesson do I wish that I had known about earlier?

14.5 Criteria for Self-Evaluation of Team Members

1 Lessons I have learned from conversations with elder caregivers are that

    a providing care is difficult and rarely includes expression of gratitude
    b I have not spoken with an elder caregiver to learn about their needs
    c they feel socially isolated and disconnected from their community
    d they would welcome having visitors stop by to talk with the elders
    e Other _____

2 I feel like the community sense of responsibility toward elderly neighbors

    a is decreasing and we are not interested in knowing about their needs
    b is indifferent because we are trying to cope with our own priorities
    c is most people care for their families and expect others to do it too
    d Other _____

3 When elders believe they cannot trust relatives with financial information

    a adult protective services should be contacted for a financial advisor
    b they should choose a confidante who can be trusted with information
    c the senior center can contact a pro bono attorney to prepare a will
    d organizations serving elders should provide social companionship
    e Other _____

4 My awareness of conditions in local long-term care facilities is based on

    a I have no experience in visiting patients residing in long-term care
    b my limited understanding comes from the observations of friends
    c documentaries I have seen on social media
    d going with a friend to explore long-term care together
    e Other _____

5 I believe youth should have some role in efforts to curb the abuse of elders

    a passive neglect of being ignored and lonely is reduced by visitors
    b school assignments should involve learning about caring for elders
    c lifespan development and its challenges should be a course in school
    d adolescents should be expected to stay in touch with elder relatives
    e Other _____

6 Because some patients in long-term care are bullied by other patients

    a facilities need volunteers acting as observers to detect and report abuse
    b all patients should know that not telling on bullies means hurting others
    c patients should be visited personally and urged to make abuse known
    d families should ask relatives who are patients to tell them about abuse
    e Other _____

7 I believe communities should help caregivers with their role by

    a recruiting volunteers from churches to provide periodic relief
    b informing siblings of main caregivers their contribution is needed
    c having volunteers provide free lawn care and other related jobs
    d giving an extra income tax deduction for service to the society
    e Other _____

8 When the time comes that my parents may need caregiver assistance

    a I know I can depend on one or more of my siblings for help
    b finding a community agency to help me will be necessary
    c I will seek advice from my church group or pastor
    d I will try to enroll them in day care
    e Other _____

9 My personal experience with taking care of elderly relatives is

   a I took care of my parents before they passed away
   b My siblings and I shared responsibility for elder care
   c My parents died before there was a need for elder care
   d I depended on a sibling to provide care for our parents
   e Other _____

10 I believe elderly relatives abused by family members should be

   a moved to a safe place where they will receive proper care
   b urged to disinherit relatives from receiving financial benefit
   c informed that not telling about abuse increases the behavior
   d encouraged to forgive and adjust to life in another setting
   e Other _____

References

American Academy of Pediatrics. (2022, March 16). *Child abuse and neglect: What parents should know*. https://www.healthychildren.org/English/safety-prevention/at-home/Pages/What-to-Know-about-Child-Abuse.aspx

American Association of Retired Persons. (2023). *Elder financial abuse*. https://states.aarp.org/maine/elder-financial-abuse#:~:text=Visit%20the%20AARP%20Fraud%20Watch,help%20with%20a%20fraud%20encounter.&text=Contact%20information%20and%20more%20from%20your%20state%20office

Bieber, C. (2023, January 12). *Nursing home abuse lawsuit guide 2023*. Forbes. https://www.forbes.com/advisor/legal/personal-injury/nursing-home-abuse-lawsuit/

Bonifas, R. (2016). *Bullying among older adults: How to recognize and address an unseen epidemic*. Health Professionals Press.

Burnes, D., Acierno, R., & Hernandez-Tejada, M. (2019). Help-seeking among victims of elder abuse: Findings from the National Elder Mistreatment Study. *The Journals of Gerontology: Series B*, 74(5), 891–896. 10.1093/geronb/gby122

Center on the Developing Child. (2022). *InBrief: The science of neglect [Video]*. Harvard University. https://developingchild.harvard.edu/resources/inbrief-the-science-of-neglect-video/

Centers for Disease Control and Prevention (2022, April 6). *Fast facts: Preventing child abuse & neglect*. https://www.cdc.gov/violenceprevention/childabuseandneglect/fastfact.html

Centers for Disease Control and Prevention. (2023, June 13). Children are dying at the highest rate in 13 years. USA Facts. https://usafacts.org/data-projects/child-death

Cohen J., & Espelage, D. (Eds.). (2020). *Feeling safe in school: Bullying and violence prevention around the world*. Harvard Education Publishing Group.

Coloroso, B. (2016). *Bully, the bullied, and the not-so innocent bystander: From preschool to high school and beyond: Breaking the cycle of violence and creating more deeply caring communities*. William Morrow.

Conrad, K., Liu, P., & Iris, M. (2019). Examining the role of substance abuse in elder mistreatment: Results from mistreatment investigations. *Journal of Interpersonal Violence*, 34(2), 366–391. 10.1177/0886260516640782

Consumer Financial Protection Bureau. (2021). *Preventing elder financial abuse: Guide for family and friends of people living in nursing homes and assisted living communities*. https://files.consumerfinance.gov/f/documents/cfpb_preventing-elder-financial-abuse_friends-family-guide.pdf

de Becker, G. (2021). *The gift of fear: Survival signals that protect us from violence*. Back Bay Books.

Dong, X. (Ed.). (2017). *Elder abuse: Research, practice and policy*. Springer.

Eldercare Locator. (2023). *Welcome to the Eldercare Locator.* Administration for Community Living and Administration on Aging. https://eldercare.acl.gov

Florida Department of Education. (2023). *K-12 Scholarship Programs: The Hope Scholarship.* https://www.fldoe.org/schools/school-choice/k-12-scholarship-programs/hope/

Gordon, S. (2020, June 11). Cyberbullying surpasses bullying as most common type of harassment: An inside look at cyberbullying from a teen's perspective. https://www.verywellfamily.com/how-common-is-cyberbullying-4570942

Herman, C., Anetzberger, G., Brandl, B., & Breckman, R. (2022, June). *Social work roles in elder abuse prevention and response.* National Association of Social Workers. https://www.socialworkers.org/LinkClick.aspx?fileticket=f7ruO-rd0rI%3D&portalid=0

Hipp, D. (2023, May 5). *What is adult day care?* Forbes. https://www.forbes.com/health/healthy-aging/what-is-adult-day-care/

Huesmann, L., Dubow, E., & Boxer, P. (2009, March-April). Continuity of aggression from childhood to early adulthood as a predictor of life outcomes: Implications for the adolescent-limited and life course-persistent models. *Aggressive Behavior, 35*(2), 136–149. 10.1002/ab.20300

Jantz, G., & McMurray, A. (2017). *Healing the scars of child abuse: Moving beyond the past into a healthy future.* Revell.

Lamanna, M., Riedmann, A., & Stewart, S. (2020). *Marriages, families, and relationships: Making choices in a diverse society* (14th ed.). Cengage Learning.

Matthews, K., Jennings, J., Lee, L., & Pardini, D. (2017). Bullying and being bullied in childhood are associated with different psychosocial risk factors for poor physical health in men. *Psychological Science, 28*(6), 808–821. 10.1177/0956797617697700

Mcleod, S. (2023, June 14). *Bandura's bobo doll experiment on social learning.* Simply Psychology. https://www.simplypsychology.org/bobo-doll.html

Minkin, R., & Horowitz, J. M. (2023, January 24). *Parenting in America today: Mental health concerns top the list of worries for parents; most say being a parent is harder than they expected.* Pew Research Center. https://www.pewresearch.org/social-trends/2023/01/24/parenting-in-america-today/

Morin, A. (2022, July 20). *Cyberbully statistics everyone should know: From threat to rumors, cyberbullies use a variety of tactics.* Verywellfamily. https://www.verywellfamily.com/cyberbullying-statistics-4589988

National Adult Day Services. (2023). *Welcome to National Adult Day Services Association.* https://www.nadsa.org/

National Center for Education Statistics. (2022). *The condition of education 2022: Students carrying weapons and students' access to firearms.* https://nces.ed.gov/programs/coe/pdf/2022/a13_508.pdf

National Council on Aging. (2021, February 23). *Get the facts on elder abuse.* The Council. https://ncoa.org/article/get-the-facts-on-elder-abuse

National Institute on Aging. (2023, July 21). *Elder abuse.* https://www.nia.nih.gov/health/elder-abuse

Nolan, J. (2023). Bobo doll experiment. *Encyclopaedia Britannica.* https://www.britannica.com/event/Bobo-doll-experiment

Nursing Home Abuse Justice. (2023). *What is nursing home abuse?* https://www.nursinghomeabuse.org/nursing-home-abuse/

Office of Violence Against Women. (2023, March 17). *What is domestic violence?* U. S. Department of Justice. https://www.justice.gov/ovw/domestic-violence

Olweus, D. (1993). *Bullying at school: What we know and what we can do.* Blackwell.

Phelan, A. (2021). *Advances in elder abuse research: Practice, legislation, and policy.* Springer.

Pillemer, K. (2020). *Fault lines: Fractured families and how to mend them.* Avery.

Pillemer, K., Burnes, D., Riffin, C., & Lachs, M. S. (2016, April). Elder abuse: Global situation, risk factors and prevention strategies. *The Gerontologist, 56* (Supplement 2), S194–S205. 10.1093/geront/gnw004

Ripley, A. (2021). *High conflict: Why we get trapped and how we get out.* Simon & Schuster.

Robinson, L., Saisan, J., & Segal, J. (2023, June 5). *Domestic abuse: Elder abuse and neglect.* HelpGuide.org. https://www.helpguide.org/articles/abuse/elder-abuse-and-neglect.htm

Salmivalli, C. (2023). Focus on targeted interventions addressing bullying: What explains their success or failure? *European Journal of Developmental Psychology.* 10.1080/17405629.2022.2156857

Segal, E. (2018). *Social empathy: The art of understanding others.* Columbia University Press.

Smith, J. (2022). *Why has nobody told me this before?.* HarperOne.

Takizawa, R., Maughan, B., & Arseneault, L. (2014, July 1). Adult health outcomes of childhood bullying victimization: Evidence from a five-decade longitudinal British birth cohort. *The American Journal of Psychiatry, 171*(7), 777–784. 10.1176/appi.ajp.2014.13101401

Teresi, J., Burnes, D., Skowron, E., Dutton, M., Mosqueda, L., Lachs, M., & Pillemer, K. (2016). State of the science on prevention of elder abuse and lessons learned from child abuse and domestic violence prevention: Toward a conceptual framework for research. *Journal of Elder Abuse, 28*(4-5), 273–300. 10.1080/08946566.2016.1240053

United States Department of Health and Human Services (2023). *Prevention: Learn how to identify bullying and stand up to it safely.* https://www.stopbullying.gov

United States Department of Justice. (2019, March 7). *Attorney General William P. Barr delivers remarks at press conference regarding elder fraud law enforcement announcement.* Office of Public Affairs. https://www.justice.gov/opa/speech/attorney-general-william-p-barr-delivers-remarks-press-conference-regarding-elder-fraud

United States Department of Justice and Federal Bureau of Investigation (2023, April). *Active shooter incidents in the United States in 2022.* https://www.fbi.gov/file-repository/active-shooter-incidents-in-the-us-2022-042623.pdf/view

Vogels, E. (2022, December 15). *Teens and cyberbullying 2022.* Pew Research Center. https://www.pewresearch.org/internet/2022/12/15/teens-and-cyberbullying-2022/

Weir, D. (2017). *Aging in the 21st century: Challenges and opportunities for Americans.* University of Michigan Survey Research Center, Institute for Social Research. https://hrs.isr.umich.edu/about/data-book

World Health Organization. (2022, June 13). *Abuse of older people.* https://www.who.int/news-room/fact-sheets/detail/abuse-of-older-people

Wright, T. (2017). *The family guide to preventing elder abuse: How to protect your parents – and yourself.* Skyhorse Publishing.

15   Social Connections in Later Life

Social Needs and Aging

Over 2 million Americans reside in assisted living facilities or nursing homes across the United States. Most are females (71%); males are (29%) (Johnson & Dey, 2022). Until recently the cognitive and social needs of this population were overlooked (Fulmer et al., 2021). But evidence has been mounting that policy reforms are necessary to improve the quality of care. Shippee et al. (2015) at the School of Public Health for the University of Minnesota interviewed 13,000 elderly patients regarding the quality of their care. The inquiry covered six aspects of health: physical environment, personal attention, individual engagement, enjoyment of food, negative mood, and positive mood. The average amount of time staff spent with each patient was 20 minutes a day. Yet, despite the brevity of these contacts across all six domains, the amount of time that staff interacted with patients was positively associated with quality of life as perceived by patients. The research team concluded that mental health and quality of life could improve by going beyond regular nursing care to also provide mental stimulation activities to build social connections.

A subsequent report by the same team from the University of Minnesota confirmed that changes in the culture of care by increasing the amount of staff time spent with patients was positively correlated with quality of life reported by the patients (Duan et al., 2022). A more balanced approach than the traditional medical model would allow greater attention to social, emotional, and cognitive needs. The reason so little is understood about promotion of health in later life is because studies have focused only on physical needs of patients using a minimum of staff to maximize economic profits. More than 80% of nursing homes are owned and operated by for-profit organizations (Samuels, 2022). The American Health Care Association and the National Center for Assisted Living (2023) forecast that the age 80 and over population will increase 9% by the year 2027. Meanwhile, the number of unpaid caregivers, such as family and friends, is expected to decrease over the next four years, resulting in a greater need for paid long term caregivers.

Peer Teaching in Assisted Living

The large assisted living and nursing care facility in Arizona invited the Office of Parent Development International at Arizona State University to tour their facility, talk with some residents, and discuss a possibility for collaboration. The 800 residents, average age 81, were mainly female (70%) and widowed (62%). Three hundred staff worked at the facility. Most of the residents lived independently in their own apartment and were

DOI: 10.4324/9781003401261-20

required to eat one meal a day in the common dining room to ensure that dietary needs were met. Patients in the recuperation unit were cared for by onsite nurses and physicians; one-third of the residents lived in a separate facility where they received complete care because of their dementia (R. D. Strom & Strom, 2016).

The Director of the facility told us his staff was familiar with our education projects for older adults from different ethnic backgrounds (R. Strom & Strom, 1995, 2017, 2018). During our tour of the assisted living facility the resident guides shared their enthusiasm about the possibility of having a course designed especially for them on family relationships and ways to improve their personal influence. They felt the concept of *life-long learning* had overlooked them because it did not include family-related curriculum. They believed that, unless their education needs were met, influence in the family was bound to decline, they would experience greater social isolation and loneliness, and their sense of purpose would continue to erode. Older adults gauge their importance by the amount of attention that younger relatives give them and their perceived impact on loved ones.

The director shared findings of a survey conducted by his administration. Results showed that 80% of residents identified themselves as being grandparents and/or great-grandparents. Some residents had no family relatives but had close relationships with younger people. The request was that the university consider providing a free course for the residents wanting to improve their relationships with younger relatives and friends. The decision was made to collaborate on condition that enough residents could be recruited and trained to become indigenous leaders who would guide classes provided by a team from the university.

The project goals for residents were to participate in mental stimulation, establish social networks, improve awareness about the hopes and concerns of younger relatives and learn about group dynamics that would meet the conditions for success of cooperative learning teams. Goals for the university team were to experiment with teaching students of an advanced age, provide a relevant family-oriented curriculum, explore ways to support indigenous peer instruction, and implement a model education program that could be observed and replicated by professional visitors who wanted to improve access to education for residents at their own facility.

All independent living residents were invited to a meeting where content and procedures to guide an innovative course on "Becoming a Better Grandparent" was discussed. This course would describe current goals of parents, explain what growing up is like for children and adolescents in the present setting, and recognize how social change implicates what families expect of grandparents. By exploring the experiences of three successive generations, we hoped a broader perspective could emerge to support mental health and relationships. Residents agreed to work in small teams of four or five members. Each group would be led by residents trained to perform a leadership role.

Training Insiders as Volunteer Leaders

After the general orientation meeting, a letter was sent to all independent living residents inviting them to consider becoming a part of the leadership team. Twenty residents (15 women and 5 men), aged 77 to 91years old volunteered to undergo training. Most of them had retired from careers as teachers, social workers, nurses, or business personnel. The insiders agreed they would establish a Grandparent Education Council with the following responsibilities (R. D. Strom & Strom, 2017):

- Participate in weekly training to lead and monitor groups;
- Recruit students by personal invitation and with publicity;
- Apply cooperative learning as a new form of instruction;
- Explore methods to evaluate the outcomes of instruction;
- Identify topics of interest for lessons offered to participants;
- Recommend ways to improve any class procedures; and
- Orient other institutions wishing to observe the program.

The team leaders expressed concern that unforeseen situations might arise which would require them to be absent from a class session. This possibility was seen as troubling because it meant that a leader could not always meet the commitment s/he promised to fellow residents. Therefore, working in pairs was recommended since this would reduce anxiety because both leaders shared the same preparation for each of the lessons. Then, in the event that one leader could not attend a session the partner would take over and the lesson could proceed.

Social Isolation and Loneliness

At the beginning of the class, participants were asked to estimate the number of friends they had at the facility. Most participants reported lack of friends and admitted they often felt socially isolated and lonely. We were aware that people can feel lonely even if they have lots of peers living around them because loneliness is about quality of personal connections. We wanted the program to motivate individuals to recognize their need to build a supportive social network. By adapting principles and procedures of cooperative learning as the method for instruction we hoped this strategy would encourage people to be comfortable disclosing feelings to teammates, developing trust relationships, and encouraging more interaction with others outside the class.

Each class participant received a free guidebook containing lessons, principles to apply, and activities for discussion with peers (R. D. Strom & Strom, 1991, 1992). The lesson topics included giving and seeking family advice, understanding child and adolescent development, setting goals and expectations of modern families, recognizing parent success, sharing fears and worries, managing conflicts, understanding mental stimulation and aging, and promoting social health.

Orientation to Educational Change

Emphasis on Learning in Groups

When grandparents were growing up they attended public schools where their teachers required them to work alone in class and do the homework assignments alone. This emphasis on individual productivity reflected the prevailing view that development of independence is the key to success. Managing personal affairs without depending on others and knowing ways to move forward on your own was a national goal. Interdependence, collaborating with others to solve group problems, was given little attention. Consequently, teachers seldom arranged time in the schedule to work in groups and to practice teamwork skills. Then, beginning around the year 2000, businesses began to encounter considerably more global competition that caused them to find ways to improve productivity. The shift led employers to expect newcomers to provide evidence of independence and show interdependence abilities as demonstrated by teamwork skills. Getting adolescents ready for employment calls for having opportunities that require cooperative attitudes and skills. Educators are currently expected to ensure their students are competent in the basic academic skills and teamwork skills (Kellerman & Seligman, 2023).

During early adolescence, around age 10 or 11, most students become capable of looking at ideas and situations from the viewpoint of others. These abilities to act objectively and to think critically are accompanied by a decline in narcissism, self-absorption, in favor of considering the welfare of others. In addition, most students become capable of introspection, looking within themselves to improve attitudes and behavior based on self-examination. They like conversations with peers and frequently turn to them for approval and advice (Carter, 2020). In an information-driven society, some lessons that are fact-based may be relevant for only a short time. However, the teamwork skills acquired can be relied on as an asset to enrich relationships throughout life.

Benefits of Learning in Teams

The traditional way to organize learning activities has been to invite competition among students. This approach motivates individuals most likely to perform well but also ensures that other students become candidates for poor grades. To offset adverse effects of competition on low achievers, educators have used individualized instruction. This strategy allows students to work alone at their own pace using their past and current performance levels as a basis to assess individual progress. The competitive and individualized orientations to teaching provide benefits but share a limitation of minimizing opportunities for students to learn through interaction.

Cooperative learning, a movement that has been popular for more than a generation, has been the focus of many experiments to assess how social relationships influence student behavior and achievement. Studies of cooperative learning have compared effectiveness of teachers using cooperative, competitive, and individualistic goal structures. One meta-analysis examined 685 studies involving 52,000 students in 26 countries. Results showed that students in classes where cooperative learning goals were the focus earned higher scores for problem-solving, reasoning, and critical thinking compared to other classes that emphasized competitive or individualistic goals (Johnson et al., 2014).

Guidelines for Older Adult Learning in Groups

David Johnson and Roger Johnson (2019) from the University of Minnesota have been long time leaders in cooperative learning development in public schools and universities. They believe the way students interact with one another in small groups remains a neglected aspect of peer instruction for productive learning. The way teachers guide group dynamics can enrich or impede learning, self-esteem, and peer appreciation (Tannenbaum & Salas, 2020).

Previous observations of group discussions by older adults motivated us to develop guidelines to increase benefits of education. We recommend the following 26 guidelines to monitor student behavior and improve team performance for middle-aged and older adults. The numbers assigned to guidelines do not reflect their order of importance but are intended to easily identify a reference for team discussions.

Guideline 1. Maximize Participation of Team Members

Adult education classes can proceed best when students work together in teams of four to five members. During the time scheduled for team reflection and discussion, each student chooses one question from a provided agenda that s/he is willing to answer. Anyone who has not spoken when the time for discussion is nearly over should be invited by the leader to comment. Full participation can often be achieved by asking non-speakers to react to views already expressed by others. For example, "Jim, how do your views compare with what Amy told us?" Unless all students participate, some people's views remain unknown so they cannot benefit from group feedback.

Guideline 2. Respect the Opinions Expressed by Individuals

Some older adults are accustomed to being ignored so they believe their opinions have little value. They may suppose passive behavior is acceptable as shown by this remark "I don't have anything important to say." Negative self-impressions undermine the worth that everyone should experience and prevent teammates from knowing them as an individual. An important way to show respect for others is to acknowledge their ideas, feelings, suggestions, and concerns. All students are encouraged to support the principle that the ideas of everyone should be valued.

Guideline 3. Consider Physical Conditions for Hearing

About one-third of older adults experienced some hearing loss (National Institute on Aging, 2023). They have trouble understanding what people say over the telephone, find it hard to follow conversations where two or more persons are talking, often ask people to repeat what they are saying, need to turn up the television volume so loud that others complain, and believe that many people seem to mumble. Therefore, it is important in planning a class to have physical conditions that support listening and comprehension. Comfortable chairs with participants seated at round tables allows teammates to look at each other while they speak and listen. Noisy air conditioning or other distracting sounds should be avoided near the location of class meetings. Many religious institutions have poor physical arrangements that detract from the possibilities for successful cooperative learning in old age.

Guideline 4. Limit the Time Each Person Can Speak

Some individuals monopolize conversations. To ensure that each person has an equitable opportunity to speak, students should be told that comments by individuals are limited to three minutes as estimated by team leaders. Establishing a time limit determines how long someone is expected to talk and, in most cases, three minutes is more than enough. If an individual continues speaking beyond the time limit, a team leader can gently interrupt by stating "Your time is up" and call on someone else to make their views known. The prevention of group domination is an important responsibility of team leaders.

The responses of older adults to teammates who ignore courtesy are predictable. Most of them do not want to be with someone who talks too much or shows unwillingness to hear what others have to say. Students usually expect team leaders to confront the offenders who disregard civil behavior. While the team leader is responsible to ensure guidelines are followed the whole team should consider themselves accountable to support group learning processes by monitoring the behavior of peers. The influence of constructive peer norms can become a powerful force to persuade individuals to leave poor communication habits behind in favor of more respectful interaction.

Guideline 5. Strive for Equity in Team Conversations

Older adults are likely to be more upset than younger people when they have to manage interpersonal conflict. Some students contact the team leaders outside of class to tell them about someone who dominates conversations. This behavior can motivate some students to consider withdrawing from a course or request a transfer to another team. These complaints about group dynamics should be taken seriously. Fortunately, the class leaders made good progress in being able to deal with class management.

We created a new tracking method to promote greater equity in team discussions. One of the class leaders or a volunteer helper observes each team discussion for ten minutes. The visitor keeps a "frequency of speech" tally for each group member. For example, John speaks four times, Mary once, Larry once, and Michelle not at all. In a later visit to the same team, perhaps the next session, the visiting observer notes John speaks five times, Mary twice, Larry once, and Michelle not at all. Because John is inclined to take over discussions the team leaders should talk to him privately about valuing the ideas and opinions of teammates. Michelle, the individual who never spoke, was encouraged privately to realize that peers cannot learn from her views unless she expresses them. Most leaders were able to guide teams to achieve conversational equity. Reciprocal learning occurs when all students are encouraged to speak and respond to ideas of others. Listening to teammates is a valuable asset that provides a more comprehensive outlook about ideas and interpretations of events.

Guideline 6. Accept Spontaneous Expression by Students

Reacting spontaneously can be preserved by team leaders who allow individuals to speak when they are ready instead of controlling speech based on where people are seated in a group. The acceptance of spontaneity means allowing occasional interruption, balanced by willingness of a leader to intervene when anyone exerts dominance. Discussions can be more stimulating when there is spontaneity than when the order of speaking is pre-established. Otherwise, people are inclined to think about what they are going to say when it is their turn to talk. The consequent lack of listening to others prevents being able to process their ideas and learn from them.

The anxiety that accompanies ordered speech can be overcome by encouraging everyone to decide when they want to enter a conversation to communicate their observations or points of view. Students should read the discussion agenda ahead of time to decide question(s) they want to give an answer for and reflect on ideas they want to express. Everyone should have an opportunity to speak so that no one is left out.

Guideline 7. Monitor the Thinking Process of Teammates

Older adults are not accustomed to challenging assertions made by peers. Perhaps it seems courteous to allow someone to say what they want without monitoring their message. However, the actual effect is to approve poor thinking and condone unwarranted generalizations. When older adults behave this way outside the team, they reduce the opportunity to be considered by relatives as a favorable influence. People who resent having peers monitor aspects of their behavior and consider challenges to their opinion as an insult deprive themselves of authentic conversations and undervalue the benefit that can be provided by friendship. There is value in encouraging a speaker to substantiate statements that seem exaggerated. For example, John commented, "You can't trust the government."

The leader could respond, "Sometimes this may seem to be true, but can you think of cases where trusting the government has been a good practice?"

Candace is a middle-aged nurse. She observed that her mom, who resides in an assisted living facility, challenges statements by her companions whenever she thinks they are unfounded. The result is some patients interpret mom's challenges as evidence of insensitivity. Leaders should help grandparents graciously accept challenges to their remarks by reminding them this practice can help each of us remain mentally on track. Monitoring someone's assertions should not be seen as rude behavior or impolite. Older adults dislike it when they are patronized by young people so they should avoid acting the same way when they are challenged by peers.

Guideline 8. Use Examples that Support Conclusions

Some people have difficulty with discussions that are meant to explore ideas or concepts. They prefer conversations that focus on people and situations that are usually unknown to teammates. This approach might seem to qualify the speakers as authorities on the conditions they describe, but comments should be related to the questions identified as discussion agenda. When someone makes a personal observation but does not provide clarification the team leader should restate the remark to check for accuracy. For example, "Nancy, I think the point that you are making is ..." Nancy can then further elaborate or confirm the re-statement offered by the leader is an accurate rendition of her intended meaning and implications.

Guideline 9. Stay Focused on the Lesson Topic

When a discussion wanders from the designated theme of a conversation and is lost, teammates or the leader should re-introduce the topic. By repeating an agenda question and summarizing what team members have said so far, the group remains on target without embarrassment or placing undue reliance on memory. Everyone should know that distractions can prevent teams from being able to maintain the focus needed for effective dialogue.

Gloria Mark (2023) specializes in a new field called Interruption Science, study of effects of disruption on workplace performance. Surveys by Mark have determined that, in a typical day, office personnel shift tasks on average every three minutes. Email, texts, instant messages, phone inquiries, and questions from co-workers can present a continued stream of interruptions. Once interrupted people, on average, take 25 minutes to return to devoting full attention to their mental tasks such as writing reports after they had responded to incoming e-mail. The delay is usually attributed to straying away from the agenda to answer messages or browse the Web.

Michael Posner (2014) has studied how attention is critical for perception, language, and memory. He urges reflection about the possibility that we may be evolving to become a society that prizes frenetic movement, accepts fragmented work, and craves instant answers. Such conditions will do more than just speed up the pace of living. A social environment that puts excessive emphasis on the present and avoids reflective consideration of the future can restrict the scope of focus, awareness, planning, and judgment that comprise attention.

Guideline 10. Reinforce Insights Expressed by Teammates

Wisdom routinely surfaces during discussions. One way to magnify impact of valuable insights is draw attention to them. The leader can turn to speakers and reinforce their views by asking, "Would you please say that again?" "Tell us more," or "Will you clarify that position?" Alternately, anyone can contribute to the self-esteem of peers by saying, when it seems deserved: "What an interesting way to look at this particular situation," or "Thank you for letting us know that insight. I had not thought about the issue in that way before." This kind of reaction calls attention to and honors the expression of creative thinking.

Guideline 11. Encourage Risk-taking by Self-disclosure

The willingness to take risks declines with age (Cassidy, 2021). Consequently, older people might need some encouragement to share feelings and make their points of view known. When individuals believe their cooperative learning team is a safe environment to express personal opinions, there can be a common benefit. For this to occur, a group norm should be established that encourages the acceptance of self-disclosure by peers without making judgmental responses. Reluctance to reveal experiences about situations and events can cause people to become socially isolated and exposes them to greater loneliness. A desire to prevent teammates from being aware of certain conditions in our past is a reason some people become guarded, shown by meager sharing during discussions. This behavior prevents relatives and peers from recognizing when someone needs emotional support (National Academies of Sciences, Engineering, and Medicine, 2020).

Guideline 12. Wait for Teammates Who Are Slow to Give Responses

Older adults typically need more time than younger students to evaluate situations. This is particularly the case when someone has been the victim of a stroke or has acquired a disability that impacts speech and causes halting responses that appear to reflect confusion (King, 2020; Seale, 2020). This behavior is exhibited by individuals who say, "I forgot the point that I was going to make … ," or says "Well, ah, the, … ah … ." reactions. Impatient teammates sometimes try to anticipate what a slow spokesman is wanting to say so they attempt to complete sentences for the person as if prompted by clues in a game of charades. This second-guessing type behavior often causes the speakers to feel rushed, denies individuality of expression, and contradicts the benefits of groups learning to wait. When a leader observes such behavior, just say, "Please, let him/her finish his thought. This example of how peers should behave usually sets a future pattern for group reaction when it is time to listen to slow respondents. As length of the lifespan increases, there will be larger numbers of people whose halting speech warrants greater patience of teammates.

Guideline 13. Discourage Reliance on Repetitious Comments

Listening to people tell interesting stories can be a source of satisfaction for teammates. There are also times when people repeat stories they have told before. By privately reminding a storyteller that s/he has become repetitious, this can motivate a more diligent self-monitoring of conversation. For example, "John, your story about the flat tire was interesting but you told us that before. Try to think of other examples that illustrate the same point you want to make. Reminding someone about repetitious speech that can be misinterpreted should be seen by recipients as important evidence of support from peers instead of being considered an insult.

Some people say, "So, what if Harold has told that same story five times? He obviously likes to tell it so just listen and don't say anything that might cause him to become embarrassed." Decline in mental ability in later life is often shown by repetitious storytelling and lapses of memory. Teammates should feel responsible to help one another by monitoring speech that can undermine relationships with younger relatives and other people in their social network.

Guideline 14. *Avoid Rushing Others in Favor of Reflection*

Adult education classes are typically held weekly for 90 to 120 minutes. The amount of time assigned to each group activity should be flexible, depending on discretion of the team and their leaders. Some activities may take longer than were planned and provide benefit for everyone. In that case, it is possible to defer an activity until the next weekly session or eliminate the activity from further consideration. The most important factor is to avoid imposing feelings of being hurried that can cause someone to feel pressured about completion of an activity. As individuals learn to appreciate that the main purpose of the class is to be responsive to personal needs instead of to complete a rigid schedule, they feel more comfortable when activities sometimes have to be extended or remain incomplete.

Guideline 15. *Listen to Younger Generations for Learning*

Grandparents should get to know each grandchild as an individual. The way to attain this goal is by scheduling regular conversations in person, by text, e-mail, Skype, Zoom, or cell-phone. Some of the agenda questions that accompany each lesson provide a focus for use in family dialogue. In class grandparents should report to teammates outcomes of interviews with their grandchildren whose ideas and impressions are usually poorly understood by their aging grandparents. The entire class benefits from interviews the individuals on a team conduct with younger relatives.

Guideline 16. *Improve Reasoning and Problem-solving Skills*

Reasoning and problem-solving skills are among the cognitive abilities that decline earlier than other mental functions. Research on the enduring benefits of instruction related to reasoning and problem-solving underscores a common need to continue emphasizing this context. A study with the National Institute of Health evaluated long-term effects of training for specific cognitive abilities (Rebok et al., 2014). The 2,800 men and women in a culturally diverse sample, average age 73, lived independently in six regions of the nation. Subjects were divided into three groups, each with a separate focus for training. Group 1 emphasized reasoning and problem solving; Group 2 dealt with speed of processing information; and Group 3 focused on memory. The orientation consisted of ten weekly sessions of 60 minutes. Follow-up tests were administered when training was finished and annually thereafter. When the clinical trials ended ten years later, at an average age 83, groups trained in reasoning, problem-solving, and processing information speed but not memory, continued to retain the effects of instruction provided a decade earlier.

Relatives unintentionally contribute to cognitive loss when they leave older adults out of discussions that are related to family concerns. One way to offset this limitation is by practicing reflective thinking skills in class. When confronting hypothetical situations, it becomes easier to evaluate choices and generate alternatives than when someone must assume the risks of real life. Every lesson contains a scenario that teams consider and individuals make known the way they would respond to the situation. Older adults like to discuss pros and cons about each of the given options or one of their own and share reasoning about the advice they think is best.

A scenario approach enlarges the range of solutions people are able to see and discourages reaching hasty conclusions. There are several ways to proceed with a discussion about reasoning and problems in each lesson. The leader can start by asking, "Which of the four opinions given do you favor most?" or "What are your reasons for recommending a particular option?" or "Tell us why you think one of the stated options is inappropriate." Another alternative is to invite new options not on the list – "Tell me an answer you think could be option E." Or, read aloud each of the stated solutions and ask people to raise their hands when the option that most appeals to them is stated. Have a team member count hands and state number of people favoring each option.

Guideline 17. Review Key Concepts for Personal Application

Few students are able to master note-taking skills. The common practice of adolescents and young adults is to underline some aspects of the text and later identify points to remember before taking a test. As older adults carefully read lessons, it can be helpful for them to mark margins beside passages they consider most important. These priorities can later be compared with key concepts of a lesson. This practice improves the detection of significant issues. A reader may discover that s/he has found an important idea not included in the list of key concepts concluding each lesson. For group review of a lesson each person can be asked to identify two concepts that were important for them and explain their choices.

Guideline 18. Participate in Self-evaluation to Promote Growth

Self-evaluation is essential for personal development so everyone should get to practice this task (Dunning, 2005). Each lesson includes ten multiple-choice questions that are accompanied by four or five options. The questions enable team members to make known their feelings and expectations. Participants can write down their choices for each item before class. When they get to class, their self-evaluation sheet is placed in the homework box. They do not write their name on their sheet so that the homework remains anonymous. This prevents anxiety and encourages self-disclosure. When group responses are tallied, feedback is announced as older adults record the percentage of peers who gave each response. Older adults like to find out how their perceptions resemble and differ from classmates.

Guideline 19. Maintain an Optimistic Outlook on Life

Attitudes of optimism and pessimism are explanatory styles people rely on to interpret troublesome situations. While a pessimistic individual may consider their experiences of defeat to be permanent, overwhelming, and evidence of personal weakness, an optimist could look at the same situation as a temporary setback, an obstacle that can be overcome by approaching the problem in another way. More is involved than just the difference of personal opinion. Research has determined that optimists perform better in class, athletics, and at work since they cheerfully persist when faced with setbacks while pessimists having equal ability may decide to give up (Odom, 2018; Purkiss, 2020).

Studies have found that negative thinkers have weaker immune systems, higher rates of infectious disease, greater health problems from the middle of life onward, and are much more likely to suffer from depression (Kellerman & Seligman, 2023). They are also uncomfortable to be around. Together these factors suggest positive thinking should become more common among older adults. When pessimism is expressed in a team, acknowledge the individual's experience by stating "Some people have endured a lot and experienced a bad time." Then, invite peers to share some positive experiences that illustrate the need to sustain a pattern of optimistic thinking.

Guideline 20. Acknowledge the Importance of Unlearning

When new ways of doing things and thinking about situations are necessary, unlearning presents a significant challenge. This obstacle is experienced by people of all ages. Unlearning is defined as a willful activity to abandon or revise strong habits of mind that necessitate attitude or behavior change being able to adjust to unfamiliar events or situations. In many cases unlearning is considered more difficult than new learning and people often fail as they try to leave behind their customary forms of response. Unlearning is particularly difficult for older adults because they have a lifetime of habits, some of which no longer serve them well. Periodically, ask the class to comment on long held lessons they have been able to unlearn and also identify other lessons that continue to present obstacles for unlearning.

Guideline 21. Accept all Colleagues on Your Team

Some people reject being around anyone they consider to be unpleasant. They reason that their choice to avoid communicating with such people, a behavior not allowed while they were in the workforce, does not apply in retirement. However, cooperative learning requires changes in everyone. There may be students who are not well liked because they talk too much, like to pry into the affairs of others, bring up the same topics for every lesson regardless of the designated agenda or generally seem to interfere with group procedures. You might prefer to ignore these individuals or want them to recognize that their behavior is offensive. Another way to see the situation is to view it as an opportunity to help someone who obviously needs support so they can grow. The way a team leader treats such persons can establish the norm for group members. Always take the high road and everyone will be better off. Remember that it may be necessary from time to time to remind the team about some cooperative learning guidelines and their obligations. The leader should call aside anyone who offends others and talk about positive behaviors expected in class and that change will favorably influence their status in relationships.

Guideline 22. Remind Students about Interdependence

Most older adults have learned to equate self-respect with independence and failure with dependence. This means they are bound to be at war within themselves. During their earlier role as parents, they insisted children learn and practice self-reliance. Consequently, many middle-aged and older adults believe that dependence is a sign of weakness, except among young children or the disabled (Minkin & Horowitz, 2023). Yet these same advocates of independence, if they live long enough, will find they need help from others. This situation presents a serious problem in our society that does not exist in some other cultures. In effect, self-concept and even physical survival can be threatened if we maintain an exclusive commitment to the prominent values of a former individualistic society instead of the current more interdependent social environment (Tannenbaum & Salas, 2020). Acquainting older adults with the advantages of cooperative learning can sustain independence while adding to appreciation of interdependence. Reliance on cooperative learning methods that reflect how grandchildren learn in school now can help grandparents improve communication skills needed for adjustment to transformation of the family.

Guideline 23. Maximize the Benefits of Team Lesson Reviews

Individual students share impressions about one of five questions they select for group lesson review. Consider some benefits each question can make to personal growth.

1. What ideas in the lesson changed the way I think about this topic?

The willingness to admit new ideas have led us to change our thinking is evidence of learning. This favorable attitude can improve elder status with younger relatives too. Daughters, sons, and grandchildren should know we are able to consider new information, we can change our mind, and it is possible for them to favorably persuade our ways of thinking about situations.

2. What insights from the lesson will I try to apply in my family relationships?

The intentions are to learn that more productive ways of responding to loved ones deserve recognition as well as reinforcement by teammates and the team leader.

3. What is the most important point for me presented in this lesson?

When grandparents draw attention to aspects of a lesson that offered new insights, they identify personal growth and encourage others to make known improvement in their self-evaluation. These comments show the connections individuals make and how they feel new information applies to them. This item shows an ability to identify important points of a lesson and reach decisions about revision of priorities.

4. What are some aspects of the lesson I would like to better understand?

This expression of curiosity, willingness to admit uncertainty, and desire for clarification is basic to being a self-directed learner. Sometimes several students identify the same aspects of a lesson they would like to better understand. This response urges leaders to figure out better options for further instruction about the issue.

5. What aspects of this lesson do I wish I had known about earlier?

The practice of retroactive self-evaluation allows people to admit limitation and failure in prior understanding. This can be useful to confirm that learning is necessary for growth at every age.

Guideline 24. Accept Flexible Planning and Amend Some Goals

Some students get upset when cooperative tasks require more time than was planned. In such cases students should recognize they can return to incomplete tasks at the next session if they choose before starting the next lesson. What matters most is everyone has an opportunity to express their views, listen carefully to what others have to say, and do not feel rushed. Unlike homework in elementary and secondary school, education for older adults allows each student to decide what to expect of themselves. Accepting incompleteness and over-choice can foster personal adjustment and enable a healthy revision of goals.

Guideline 25. Importance of a Support Network

A growing body of evidence reveals that social connections make a valuable contribution to mental and physical health. However, as people grow older, most are alone more often than when they were younger, leaving them vulnerable to the effects of social isolation and loneliness (Cacioppo & Patrick, 2009). A meta-analytic research review was conducted by Holt-Lunstad et al. (2015) involving nearly 300,000 men and women. The results of the research study showed that lack of social connections elevated the health risks for cognitive decline, depression, and premature mortality; having more social connections was associated with a 50% lower risk of death (Holt-Lunstad, 2022).

Dr. Vivek Murthy, Surgeon General of the United States, has warned that the epidemic of loneliness and isolation has profound consequences for our individual and collective physical health, including a 29% increased risk of heart disease, 32% risk of stroke, and 50% increased risk of developing dementia for older adults (Office of the Surgeon General of the United States, 2023). In addition, a lack of social connection increases risk of premature death by over 60%. Besides physical health, loneliness and isolation contribute substantially to mental health issues. The risk of developing depression among adults who report feeling lonely often is more than double that of people who rarely or never feel lonely. We must prioritize building social connections in the same way we have prioritized other critical public health issues like tobacco, obesity, and substance abuse disorders. Together we should strive to build a country that is healthier, more resilient, less lonely, and more connected (Hertz, 2021).

Guideline 26. Encourage Community Service

The Grandparent Education Council found that many residents felt disconnected from the community outside their institution and wanted to be helpful if practical opportunities could be arranged (R. D. Strom & Strom, 2016, 2017). In response, the superintendent of a nearby school district was contacted. Most of the residents who wanted to volunteer were unable to transport themselves to schools. Therefore, volunteers were driven in minivans offered by community agencies. The volunteers attended training provided by the school district about ways to help teachers in the classroom. Some grandparents were incontinent or had other health limitations that prevented them from going to an elementary school and working directly with students. Consequently, their assignments were to check student practice sheets in mathematics and reading. Teacher time was saved when the practice sheets were returned with corrections for feedback to individuals.

Conclusion

Most older adults want close relationships with children, grandchildren, and younger friends. The chance to achieve this goal improves when cooperative learning team members help one another acquire communication skills and teamwork principles which were not taught in the past but needed now for collaboration at work and at home. Orienting older adults to adaptive cooperative learning practices can reinforce the value of independence while adding appreciation for interdependence. The one-year project in this assisted living facility had an average weekly attendance of 65 older adults. The results confirmed that older adults can remain capable of learning, and provide indigenous leadership to maximize benefits from classes.

A long-standing assumption has been that aging is accompanied by a more comprehensive perspective on life. However, the perspective needed in a technological society requires more than just getting older. Living in a generation-separated culture means some aspects of wisdom can emerge with awareness about the opinions and values of younger relatives. During the past, patronizing older adults by referring to them as wise was intended to convey respect but the actual consequence was failure to identify their learning needs, ignore potential for development, and deny instruction to support adjustment. Education for the participants at this assisted living facility was effective in reinforcing individual sense of importance, building social connections, finding satisfaction in community volunteer service, and gaining awareness about the concerns of younger generations.

Key Concepts

1 Providing education for assisted living residents improves their quality of life because of mental stimulation and social engagement. Recruiting indigenous leadership makes it possible for residents to feel a greater sense of control over their program and rely on the talents of peers.

2 Developing a comprehensive schedule for classes is important to allow for a wide range of conditions that can impact grandparent attendance. Residents appreciate having multiple options so they can make up missed sessions by attending at an alternative time and place.

3 Indigenous leaders can be trained to work in pairs so neither party has worry or anxiety if it is sometimes necessary to be absent sometimes. By preparing lessons together, either partner is ready to assume leadership for a session alone and making it unnecessary to cancel a class meeting.

4 There is benefit in introducing older adults to cooperative learning practices they were never exposed to while in school. Conversations with classmates and relatives are enriched when collaborative attitudes and skills are applied to guide discussions that take place in small teams.

5 Self-evaluation is needed to guide development and know when personal changes in attitudes or behavior should be made. Grandparents benefit from anonymous peer feedback that informs them of how their experiences resemble and differ from other members of their class.

6 Some individuals monopolize conversations. To ensure each student has an opportunity to speak, everyone in class should know remarks are limited to three minutes as estimated by the leader. When someone continues speaking beyond the limit, the leader should gently interrupt and call on someone else to share their views.

7 Teammates can help one other by monitoring their thinking processes. Older adults less often challenge poor thinking habits and unwarranted generalizations. If people behave this way when they are with relatives, they risk having their views ignored. Individuals who regard challenges to their opinion as an insult deprive themselves of having authentic conversations and friendships.

8 When a group discussion wanders from the designated topic or theme of a conversation is lost, teammates and the leader should re-introduce the focus. By repeating an agenda question and summarizing what has already been said, the team is able to stay on target without causing embarrassment. Everyone should be aware that distractions can prevent the needed focus.

9 Some people are stroke victims or have another disability that interferes with their speech and causes halting responses. Impatient teammates sometimes try to anticipate what a slow student is intending to say. This second-guessing of intention denies individual expression and discourages participants from learning how to wait patiently for a response.

10 Some older adults unknowingly repeat the same stories. By calling this annoying behavior to their attention, such learners are reminded to monitor their conversations. Everyone should feel obligated to help teammates by monitoring expression of repetitious speech. The actions younger people often associate with mental decline are repetitious stories and memory lapse.

Generational Perspectives Activities

> **15.1 Team Discussion**
> **15.2 Conversations with Adolescents**
> **15.3 Agenda for Interviews with Grandparents**
> **15.4 A Scenario: Reasoning and Problem Solving**
> **15.5 Team Chapter Review**
> **15.6 Criteria for Self-Evaluation of Team Members**

15.1 Team Discussion

1 What are your concerns about the relationships among peers in assisted living facilities?
2 How do you suppose the cost of care will be managed with the increase of older adults?
3 What advantages can you see in training insiders to become indigenous education leaders?
4 What curriculum focus should be emphasized in the education for those who are retired?
5 What obligations should adolescents have toward older relatives who are institutionalized?
6 How can educators help older students learn about current teaching and learning practices?
7 Why do you suppose there are no large-scale curriculums available for education of elders?
8 How could college students help older people to identify and meet their learning needs?
9 How could churches experiment with reciprocal learning between generational groups?
10 What can be done to ensure older adults are well informed about needs of younger people?

15.2 Conversations with Adolescents

1 What have you found to be the benefits of working in cooperative learning teams?
2 What are some things about working in teams that you would like to see changed?
3 What are some teamwork skills you perform well and others you need to work on?
4 How can teachers know the teamwork skills demonstrated by individual students?
5 Why do you suppose there are report card grades for subjects but not teamwork?

6 What problems prevent younger and older relatives from talking more together?
7 How much of a problem is distraction when students work in cooperative teams?
8 Why would you favor or disapprove of giving students grades for teamwork skills?
9 How do you feel about encouraging students to compete with other class members?
10 How do you suppose employers feel about students learning teamwork skills at school?

15.3 Agenda for Interviews with Grandparents

1 What habits do you want to leave behind to improve teamwork performance?
2 How often did you work in teams with classmates when you attended school?
3 What do you remember about the importance of competition in the classroom?
4 How have you seen adults respond to someone who monopolizes group discussion?
5 How should churches and senior centers improve conditions for group discussion?
6 How are people who engage in repetitive storytelling treated by their teammates?
7 How do groups react when a disabled person is slow in stating an idea or opinion?
8 How do you feel when the agenda for discussion is not finished in the time allowed?
9 How do you feel about interviewing grandchildren and reporting results to teammates?
10 Identify a cooperative learning guideline that you think is needed more than others?

15.4 A Scenario: Reasoning and Problem Solving

Problem solving scenarios present an opportunity to look at situations that might happen for a family and think about possible solutions. Your task is to look at pros and cons of choices that are stated, think of additional options, identify relevant information that might be missing, find out how teammates view the alternatives, and defend reasoning about advice you consider best.

Kathy just attended the first of six weekly discussions at church on improving relationships with other generations. At the outset all participants indicated agreement that this topic was personally important and wanted ideas about how to create better communication. However, despite common enthusiasm, the session did not go well because too much time was spent complaining about behavior of younger relatives. This left Katy frustrated and wondering what could be done next week to get the group on track. Identify a recommendation you favor and provide reasoning for your choice(s).

a Have each person describe an aspect of family relationships they find satisfying.
b Describe some self-behaviors that should be changed to support better relations.
c Interview younger relatives and report their opinions about desired family change.
d Instruct leaders to strive for a balanced expression of negative and positive views.
e Other

15.5 Team Chapter Review

1 What ideas in the lesson changed how I think about this topic?
2 What insights from the lesson will I try to apply in my relationships?
3 What are the main points and key issues presented in this lesson?

4 What are aspects of this lesson that I would like to better understand?

5 Which of the principles in this lesson do I wish I had known about earlier?

15.6 Self-Evaluation of Cooperative Team Members

1 The way(s) I could contribute more to cooperative learning discussions is

 a listen carefully to how others describe the way they manage their problems

 b monitor thinking of teammates and remind them when change is needed

 c make sure that the group stays on task instead of wandering from the topic

 d show patience when someone needs more time to finish their comment

 e Other _____

2 Some things I should unlearn to become a more effective team member are

 a avoid rushing others to prematurely finish ideas they want to explain

 b accept that it is ok when the announced agenda does not get done

 c become more willing to consider views that differ from my behavior

 d leave all group monitoring to the leader without sharing leadership

 e Other _____

3 When teammates express opinions that disagree with my own perceptions I

 a can be persuaded to change my mind if their logic seems right

 b am unlikely to take seriously any opposing position on things

 c will listen respectfully but not change my attitude or behavior

 d provide a rebuttal intended to clarify my own perspective

 e Other _____

4 Reminding a team member about their need to change behavior

 a is an initiative outside my comfort zone so I would not do it

 b I think it is a good way to help monitor behavior of my peers

 c I would tell the group leader to handle behavior corrections

 d I would ignore it and move ahead as if nothing had happened

 e Other _____

5 The way I look at academic competition for my younger relatives is to

 a encourage them to perform better than other students in the class

 b urge them to compete but also develop team skills they need

 c be conflicted about supporting both independence and teamwork

 d remind them grade point average is the most important indicator

 e Other _____

6 When some aspects of my behavior require improvement, I want peers to

 a provide feedback that will help me remain a capable teammate

 b explain it to me privately so I can think about making changes

 c keep their opinions regarding my performance to themselves

 d encourage me to modify some of my actions to increase success

 e Other _____

7 Paying attention and avoiding distraction during group discussion is

   a recognized as sometimes being a problem in my case
   b a personal limitation that I recognize must be overcome
   c not a problem for me because I am able to focus well
   d a common problem that I observe in others but not myself
   e Other _____

8 When someone in my team makes an insightful comment

   a I take note of the idea but do not say anything
   b I commend the person and thank them as well
   c my peers rarely contribute anything that is new
   d I acknowledge that this was helpful news for me
   e Other _____

9 Making an effort to achieve cooperative learning group guidelines

   a will enable me to be more in sync with how younger relatives learn
   b can help me make a greater contribution to peers in discussion groups
   c probably would not improve my relationships with peers or the family
   d should motivate me to become a better resource for the people I know
   e Other _____

10 When there is an expectation to complete all the discussion agenda questions

   a I feel that reflection and interaction do not get the attention deserved
   b I experience stress and find the group discussion to be less satisfying
   c I have observed that some points of view get overlooked for consideration
   d I am less informed because this encourages hasty information processing
   e Other _____

References

American Health Care Association and the National Center for Assisted Living (2023, June 27). *ICYMI: Median age in the U.S. reaches record high, underscoring need for long term care access.* American Health Care Association. https://www.ahcancal.org/News-and-Communications/Press-Releases/Pages/ICYMI-Median-Age-In-The-U-S-Reaches-Record-High,-Underscoring-Need-For-Long-Term-Care-Access.aspx

Cacioppo, J. T., & Patrick, W. (2009). *Loneliness: Human nature and the need for social connection.* W. W. Norton.

Carter, C. (2020). *The new adolescence: Raising happy and successful teens in an age of anxiety and distraction.* BenBella Books.

Cassidy, S. S. (2021). *Choose possibility: Take risks and thrive (even when you fail).* Mariner.

Duan, Y., Mueller, C., Yu, F., Talley, K., & Shippee, T. (2022). The relationship of nursing home culture change practices with resident quality of life and family satisfaction: Toward a more nuanced understanding. *Research on Aging, 44*(2), 174–185. 10.1177/01640275211012652

Dunning, D. (2005). *Self-insight: Roadblocks and detours on the path to knowing thyself.* Psychology Press.

Fulmer, T., Reuben, D., Auerbach, J., Fick, D., Galambos, C., & Johnson, K. (2021). Actualizing better health and health care for older adults. *Health Affairs, 40*(2), 219–225. 10.1377/hlthaff.2020.01470

Hertz, N. (2021). *The lonely century: How to restore human connection in a world that's pulling apart.* Crown Currency.

Holt-Lunstad, J. (2022, April 5). Social connection as a public health issue: The evidence and a systemic framework for prioritizing the "Social" in social determinants of health. *Annual Review of Public Health, 43*, 193–213. 10.1146/annurev-publhealth-052020-110732

Holt-Lunstad, J., Smith, T. B., Baker, M., Harris, T., & Stephenson, D. (2015 March). Loneliness and social isolation as risk factors for mortality: A meta-analytic review. *Perspectives on Psychological Science, 10*(2), 227–237. https://pubmed.ncbi.nlm.nih.gov/25910392/

Johnson, D. W., Johnson, R. T. (2019). Cooperative learning: The foundation for active learning. In S. M. Brito (Ed.), *Active learning -- Beyond the future* (pp. 59–70). Intech Open. 10.5772/Intechopen.73460

Johnson, D. W., Johnson, R. T., Roseth, C., & Shin, T. (2014). The relationship between motivation and achievement in interdependent situations. *Journal of Applied Social Psychology, 44*(9), 622–633. 10.1111/jasp.12280

Johnson, R. W., & Dey, J. (2022, September 22). *Long-term care services and supports for older Americans: Risks and financing.* Office of Behavioral Health Disability, and Aging Policy, U.S. Department of Health and Human Services. https://aspe.hhs.gov/reports/ltss-older-americans-risks-financing-2022

Kellerman, G. R., & Seligman, M. E. P. (2023). *Tomorrowmind: Thriving at work with resilience, creativity, and connection -- now and in an uncertain future.* Atria Books.

King, V. L. (2020). *When the words suddenly stopped: Finding my voice again after a massive stroke.* Author Academy Elite.

Mark, G. (2023). *Attention Span: A groundbreaking way to restore balance, happiness and productivity.* Hanover Square Press.

Minkin, R., & Horowitz, J. (2023, January 24). *Parenting in America today.* Pew Research Center. https://www.pewresearch.org/social-trends/2023/01/24/parenting-in-america-today/

National Academies of Sciences, Engineering, and Medicine. (2020). *Social isolation and loneliness in older adults: Opportunities for the health care system.* National Academies Press.

National Institute on Aging (2023). *Hearing Loss: A common problem for older adults.* https://www.nia.nih.gov/health/hearing-loss-common-problem-older-adults#:~:text=Aboutone-third of older and hearing doorbells and alarms

Odom, L., Jr. (2018). *Failing up: How to take risks, aim higher, and never stop learning.* Feiwel & Friends.

Office of the Surgeon General [Vivek Murthy]. (2023). *Our epidemic of loneliness and isolation 2023: The U.S. Surgeon General's Advisory on the healing effects of social connection and community.* U.S. Department of Health and Human Services. https://www.hhs.gov/sites/default/files/surgeon-general-social-connection-advisory.pdf

Posner, M. I. (2014). *Attention in a social world.* Oxford University Press.

Purkiss, J. (2020). *The power of letting go: How to drop everything that's holding you back.* Aster.

Rebok, G., Ball, K., Guey, L., Jones, R., Kim, H., King, J., Marsiske, M., Morris, J., Tennstedt, S., Unverzagt, F., & Willis, S. (2014). Ten-year effects of the advanced cognitive training for independent and vital elderly cognitive training trial on cognition and everyday functioning in older adults. *Journal of the American Geriatrics Society, 62*(1), 16–24. 10.1111/jgs.12607

Samuels, C. (2022, April 21). *Assisted living statistics: Population & facilities in 2022.* https://www.aplaceformom.com/caregiver-resources/articles/assisted-living-statistics

Seale, A. (2020). *With one hand tied behind my brain: A memoir of life after stroke.* Texas Christian University Press.

Shippee, T., Henning-Smith, C., Kane, R. L., & Lewis, T. (2015). Resident- and facility-level predictors of quality of life in long-term care. *The Gerontologist, 55*(4), 643–655. https://www.ncbi.nlm.nih.gov/pmc/articles/PMC4542585/

Strom, R. D., & Strom, P. S. (2016). Grandparent education for assisted living facilities. *Educational Gerontology, 43*(1), 11–20. 10.1080/03601277.2016.1231518

Strom, R. D., & Strom, P. S. (2017). Grandparent learning and cultural differences. *Educational Gerontology*, *43*(8), 417–427. 10.1080/03601277.2017.1314642

Strom, R. D., & Strom, P. S. (2018). Education for grandparents in longevity societies. *Journal of Adult and Continuing Education*, *24*(2), 208–228. 10.1177/1477971418810652

Strom, R. D., & Strom, S. (1991). *Becoming a better grandparent: Viewpoints on strengthening the family*. Sage.

Strom, R. D., & Strom, S. (1992). *Achieving grandparent potential: Viewpoints on building intergenerational relationships*. Sage.

Strom, R. D., & Strom, S. (1995). Intergenerational learning: Grandparents in the schools. *Educational Gerontology*, *21*(4), 321–335. 10.1080/0360127950210403

Tannenbaum, S., & Salas, E. (2020). *Teams that work: The seven drivers of team effectiveness*. Oxford University Press.

16   Goals and Concerns of Five Generations

Generation Z, Born 1997 to 2012

Personality, Social, and Emotional Development

Many of the youngest members of Generation Z want to become rich, famous, good looking, well-liked, and recognized as caring about the well-being of others and the planet. Their parents suggest adopting the goals of working hard, paying attention in the classroom, and earning good grades. This is also the ideal age for students to begin setting some personal goals. Adults should encourage students to choose personality goals before choosing career goals. This sequence of personality goals before occupational aspirations urges early adolescents to focus on the kind of person they want to become, ways they want to behave, and how to contribute to others. These aspects of maturing can be observed well before there is evidence about kind of work a student may one day be qualified to perform.

Goals for Consideration

Personality and social development should become prominent goals for students. This aspect of curriculum could enable greater personal success, increase the scope of civil behavior, create a more safe society, and ensure community welfare (Belsky et al., 2020). Major problems in being able to get along well with others, including abuse, divorce, crime, racism, and being fired from a job, are more often attributed to poor mental health and immaturity than to lack of academic competence. Reading, writing, and mathematics are basic skills; they are also the easiest lessons for people to learn. In addition, education should equip students with an ability to cope with stress, manage anxiety, and demonstrate resilience. Progress toward these goals can be observed by adults to confirm growth and identify further needs. Some goals suitable for early adolescents (ages 10 to 14) are presented (P. S. Strom & Strom, 2012; R. D. Strom & Strom, 1991, 1992).

- *Getting along with others* – A 14-year-old granddaughter of an 82-year-old Black grandmother told her, "Grandma Flora, I want to be just like you when I grow up." Flora replied, "Why? I have little in material things and did not make much of myself." Her granddaughter said, "Grandma, you have more friends than anybody I know." What a compliment.
- *Treat people around me fairly* – Society is struggling to get this right; it is an important lesson to learn and difficult one to teach.
- *Show a willingness to help others* – This is what growing up and maturity are all about, moving from being self-centered in favor of showing greater concern for the welfare of others.

DOI: 10.4324/9781003401261-21

- *Look at the bright side of things* – Every problem should not be seen as an unfair crisis but looking instead at the possibilities in others, situations, and ourselves. Few things are worse for adolescents than to be around cynical adults who cause them to lose their hope for the future.
- *Make time for what is important* – Setting priorities is a vital lesson that usually comes with growing older, discovering what matters most. This lesson could be learned earlier in life. Many parents do not devote time to being with their family and children suffer because of it.
- *Develop a healthy sense of humor* – As people mature, they often discover laughing at themselves is a way to support their mental health.
- *Settle arguments in a peaceful way* – Many young people are not learning this lesson and parents should not expect teachers in the classroom to be the only source of instruction.
- *Avoid making unkind comments about others* – Teenagers often report they learn values from relatives indirectly by how adults respond to characters on television, and the way they react to stories about neighbors or people in the news.
- *Be patient in dealing with others* – Impatience has become more common and generally undermines relationships.
- *Be a person others can rely on* – This is one of the greatest accomplishments a person can achieve.
- *Become self-directed* – Demonstrate capability of making decisions independently and performing tasks without outside control.

Clique groups are formed during early adolescence and high school that make peer approval a dominant goal for socialization. As more families help adolescents commit to attainment of personality goals, this shift can have a favorable influence on peer expectations, promote healthy norms for attitudes and behaviors, and diminish the scope of peer abuse (Carter, 2020; P. S. Strom et al., 2019).

Interpersonal skills on the list of personality goals could support success regardless of the occupation a student may decide to pursue. Individually chosen personality goals have a more long-term focus for self-evaluation than academic subjects. This focus allows for feedback from adults who care about them and can monitor their progress. Personality is the key to identity, the way people see themselves and are seen by others. Personality and identity are linked because both are lifelong concerns whereas having employment is not. Uniting family and school support for personality development conveys the message to everyone that emotional and social growth require attention (Iwai, 2023).

When adults are asked to identify personality attributes they want to be remembered for by family and friends, they usually mention behaviors that endear people to one another. These assets become more common when they are chosen as goals by students. The example relatives set is important. Adults can acknowledge personal shortcomings to younger relatives, describe plans to overcome them, and ask for feedback to evaluate progress. In addition to helping teenagers set their own short-term and long-term goals, wise adults review their own goals and make them known to younger relatives. Everyone should strive to improve their personality for as long as they live.

Concerns about Higher Education

Most older members of Generation Z have a broad range of career preferences. They want to prepare themselves for employment by pursuing training after high school and believe the cost of higher education tuition should be paid for by taxpayers. How does this goal compare with the opinions of adults? Quadlin and Powell (2022) wrote *Who should pay? Higher Education, Responsibility, and the Public.* They found that in 2010 the public overwhelmingly felt that students and their parents should be responsible for higher education costs. But, just one decade later, in 2020, the proportion of adults who believed government should pay for college tuition doubled. Questions are increasingly being raised about the commitment of society to the well-being of young adults (LeBlanc, 2021).

A growing proportion of undergraduate students come from low income families. Many economists maintain that the increasing income gap between the poor and affluent families is the nation's greatest problem and having equal access to higher education or technical training must be part of the solution. About 25% of White households qualify as low income compared to 50% Black and Hispanic households. Group wealth studies are defined as total assets minus liabilities. The median wealth held by White households was ten times Black households and eight times the wealth of Hispanics (Bhutta et al., 2020).

As college tuition continues to rise, more families have to borrow money. The consequent student debt crisis is estimated to be nearly two trillion dollars. Students must repay this debt to the government or other lenders. One reason the federal government is a partner is because it can spend more than it receives from income taxes whereas all of the states must balance their budget or raise taxes. The national debt exceeds $30 trillion. Young adults are the most passionate advocates for equity, fairness, and social justice. They could unite in attempting to persuade the lawmakers in each state to enact legislation for provision of free higher education.

Mike Rowe (2019) explained that the goal of college-for-all narrative emerged during the 1970s when, to increase university enrollments, high school students were told that not going to college would mean having to settle for a job reliant on using a wrench. This denigration of blue-collar positions lessened their appeal and undermined social status, a position later reinforced by the elimination of shop classes in many high schools. As a result, the talent pool of skilled workers has continued to shrink so millions of trade job vacancies remain unfilled. Rowe's observation was that over a trillion dollars in debt by 44 million students and massive skills gap are what happens when a society promotes only the single most expensive post high school education option as the right one for almost everyone.

According to Altus (2023), college enrollments have declined by 15% over the past decade while apprenticeships have increased by more than 50%. Currently, colleges and universities enroll approximately 15 million students while companies employ around 800,000 apprentices. An apprenticeship is vocational training that combines workplace learning along with practical experience under the supervision of a mentor. Programs are expanding beyond construction so 40% of apprenticeships now involve white-collar industries such as banking, cybersecurity, and consulting at companies including JPMorgan Chase & Company (Belkin, 2023). This option for apprenticeships and good paying jobs should be made known to high school students, parents, and career education counselors.

Great Britain and the United States have a poor record of orienting students and their parents to technical or trades education. However, in Germany, half of all high school students select vocational training as their first choice. Over 40% become apprentices to develop a trade skill compared to Americans where apprenticeships involve less than 1% of students (St-Esprit, 2019). Fortunately, reforms are underway to diminish the skills gap and counteract the lower status distinction assigned to students who choose technical or trade positions. In 2018, Congress passed the Strengthening Career and Technical Education for the 21st Century Act (2018). This law permits each of the 50 states to set goals for career and technical education programs without approval from the U.S. Secretary of Education and requires keeping records of student progress. Perhaps high school career education programs and apprenticeships can cause students and parents to abandon a college-for-all expectation in favor of other options to prepare for work.

Goals for Consideration

Many college dropouts quit as freshmen or sophomores because the general studies requirements prevent them from enrolling in classes that relate directly to their career preference. If students were allowed to take classes in their preferred career choice from the beginning and choose an occupation based on knowledge of personal strengths and labor market forecasts, more of them could remain in school instead of dropping out. The general studies requirement means students must first perform well in courses they may not be interested in before being allowed to enroll in classes that lead to their chosen career. The concept of general studies contradicts what is known about motivation for learning. Elimination of general studies would enable students to finish a degree in less time, and at much lower cost. Some countries including England and Australia permit students to move directly from attending high school to professional studies like law and medicine. Physicians and attorneys in these countries are considered competent, graduate at a younger age, and encumber less debt (Kirp, 2019; Quadlin & Powell, 2022).

Generation Millennials, Born 1981 to 1996

Parenting and Care of Young Children

A common goal among millennial parents is the provision of quality care for their preschool children at a reasonable cost. There are 11 million children under age 5 in group care; 60% have two parents employed outside their home. ChildCare Aware of America (2022) reported that the national average cost of child care was $10,600. This equals 10% of a married couple's average annual income and 35% of a single parent's income. In the past decade, child care costs have risen twice as fast as medium income of families.

The U.S. Department of Health and Human Services (ChildCare Aware of America, 2022, p. 41) recommended the affordable amount of family income for child care should not exceed 7%. Using this benchmark, Millennial parents in all 50 states experience difficulty paying for child care. While parents have to pay more than they can afford, workers within the child care industry are poorly paid. Most receive minimum wage. Developing a skilled workforce for early childhood should become a national goal for education. One out of four child care centers have employee turnover rates of 20% or more, a financial reality that diminishes continuity of care.

Goals for Consideration

Early childhood care and education from infancy until age 5 should become part of the existing public school structure. Parents would decide whether to take advantage of the free child care and education program offered by the public schools. Or they could home-school, pay a babysitter, or invite help from grandparents. The inclusion of early childhood into the school structure would mean teachers of young children would be paid the same salary as elementary and secondary school faculty, have the same workplace benefits, and enable more women to join the workplace and equip their children with the learning they deserve without encumbering significant expense. Colleges of Education would provide an innovative major in early childhood education. Research evidence has accumulated for years about the relative importance of early cognitive development. Estimates are that 90% of a child's brain develops by age 5 (Belsky et al., 2020; Bergen et al., 2020; Garvey, 2023).

The United States is behind in terms of child care and should try to catch up with other nations. Progress toward a better future has been demonstrated by the UNICEF report on "Where do rich countries stand on child care?" (Gromada & Richardson, 2021). Wealthy countries around the world were ranked by strengths and effectiveness of child care policies using four criteria: (a) family leave policies, (b) access to child care, (c) quality of child care, and (d) affordability of child care for working families. The United States ranked 40th out of 41 among wealthy nations for child care policies, surpassing only Slovakia for last place due to lack of paid parental leave, and rising cost of child care.

Learning Needs of Students K–12

Millennial parents want their children to perform well in school and suppose this to be a common achievement. A more accurate picture is presented by The National Assessment of Educational Progress (2022), known as The Nation's Report Card. Biannual examinations are administered to students in grades 4 and 8 throughout the United States. The most recent results for reading found that 37% of fourth graders performed below *NAEP Basic* in reading. Reading scores for eighth graders were also poor with 30% performing at or below grade level. One-quarter of fourth-graders performed below *NAEP Basic* in mathematics. Thirty-eight percent of eighth-grade students performed below *NAEP Basic* in mathematics. The gap between highest and lowest students is widening, despite a trillion dollars in federal spending over 40 years to close it. Because many students get high grades regardless of test scores, parents are misled about child competence and suppose their child is more successful than is actually the case.

The Programme for International Student Assessment (2023) is a survey meant to evaluate education systems globally, helping nations to recognize their achievements and detect needs for improvement. PISA examinations are conducted every three years. About 600,000 15-year-olds from 85 nations completed the most recent assessment. The major domain assessed was reading literacy although mathematics and science were also tested. Most of the highest ranked nations were in Asia including Singapore, China, Hong Kong, Macau, Taiwan, Japan, and South Korea. In these nations intensive tutoring is a norm because educators believe in equality, assume most students can reach high standards when provided individual help, and are willing to work hard. American students ranked 13th in reading, 37th in mathematics, and 18th in science (National Center for Education Statistics, 2019).

Goals for Consideration

Teachers of all grades struggle to provide individual help for students, allow those of different achievement levels to progress at their own pace, welcome retirees and other community volunteers to assist with tutoring, and arrange a balance between competition and cooperative teams. Academic weaknesses should be acknowledged and addressed by tutoring. Being tutored by classmates or online sources such as the Khan Academy (2023) contribute to achievement of these gains. The common gains of students who are tutored include greater interest in school, better test scores, increased persistence for difficult tasks, and greater self-confidence. For peer tutors, this activity provides a chance to help others and gain recognition. Tutoring fosters healthy attitudes and social skills that can be relied on throughout life (Strom et al., 2022).

Generation X, Born 1965 to 1980

Goals for Consideration

This is the largest generation of caregivers for their aging relatives. Goldstein (2022) estimates that they represent 73% of all employees reported having some type of current caregiving responsibility. Half of all employees who quit work before reaching the age of retirement identify caregiving as the main reason for having to leave their employment. Looking ahead, demographic forecasts indicate that the decade of the 2030s will mark the first time the population age 65 and older will be larger than the population under age 18. Businesses have to create innovative policies that link productivity and caregiving.

There are good reasons to establish innovative practices that could contribute to the retention of female employees who currently represent 61% of family caregivers (Goldstein, 2022). A disconnect between employer and employee perceptions regarding the stress of caregivers is underscored by results from the Harvard Business School (2019) Project on Managing the Future of Work, Co-chaired by Professors Joseph Fuller and Manjari Raman (2019). The survey was administered to 1,547 who identified themselves as caregivers or anticipated becoming caregivers, and 301 human resources employers. Results showed that 24% of employers reported that caregiving negatively affected employee productivity; however, over 80% of employees reported caregiver obligations undermined their productivity at work. The employers identified unplanned absences, missed days of work, late arrival at work, and early departure from work as the top behaviors that undermined career promotion. These are all behaviors that most frequently arise due to an employee's need to respond to a caregiving obligation. The employee survey revealed that nearly one-third of all employees had voluntarily left the job during their career due to their caregiving responsibilities. Fuller summarized the prevailing circumstance by stating: "U.S. firms are facing a caregiving crisis and refuse to acknowledge it. They are oblivious to the growing costs of the care economy and that is hurting them and their employees. It is clear that firms can gain a competitive advantage by investing in a care culture. But first they need to recognize the problem and implement a deliberate care strategy to support their employees" (Fuller & Raman, 2019; Harvard Business School, 2019).

Couples are also implicated. They should realize similar changes should be made in gender expectations within the family to prevent female burnout. The National Council on Aging (Body, 2022) has acknowledged women are more likely to perform significant unpaid labor costs that contribute to health and well-being of families. Building an equitable care infrastructure is necessary so women can have a choice of remaining in the labor force and caring for loved ones. Equalizing the care burden is essential to better support household financial stability and well-being. Even in heterosexual relationships where both partners work full time, women still spend 40% more time caregiving than their male partner. All adults should become aware that equity in caregiving is better for women and better for everyone.

Grandparent Assumptions

There are approximately 70 million grandparents in the United States (American Association of Retired Persons, 2019). They usually assume this important role for the first time when they are in their early fifties, can expect in time to have several grandchildren, and anticipate continued involvement in this family position for another twenty years. Fulfilling grandparent responsibilities depends on being well-informed about the ever-changing ages of each grandchild and corresponding concerns of their parents. Accordingly, knowledge about the development of young family members should be the continuous focus for education until all of the grandchildren have become young adults (R. D. Strom & Strom, 2018). The Strom Theory of Grandparent Development is based on these five assumptions (R. D. Strom & Strom, 1997).

1. Grandparent Responsibilities Should be More Clearly Defined

Mothers and fathers can attend parenting courses to help maintain competence with their role as children get older but no corresponding opportunities are available for the grandparents. Instead, they are left alone to wonder. What are my rights and my responsibilities? How can I become a favorable influence on grandchildren as they grow older? How well am I performing in the grandparent role? These questions will persist until common guidelines are established for setting goals and guiding self-evaluation. Grandparents have difficulty defining their function and knowing how to be a more valued resource. Consequently, for an increasing number of families, the task of guiding children has become disproportionate with grandparents assuming less obligation than is in everyone's best interest.

2. Grandparents Need to Learn How to Improve Their Influence

Parents who can count on grandparents to help share the load of child care and guidance less often seek support from outside the family. Grandparent success requires awareness of the parenting goals of their daughters and sons, and acting as their partner in reinforcing these goals. However, even though research has shown that people remain capable of adopting new attitudes and skills during middle and later life, grandparent development is not considered a priority for courses in adult education. This reduces the possibility of a meaningful life for grandparents.

3. Relevant Grandparent Education Should Be Widely Available

Older adults have been led to believe that learning should focus on whatever topics they find interesting without regard for societal expectations as we insist on for younger learners. However, as people age, they should also continue to grow, and not just in leisure-oriented skills. Some of education in later life should focus on responsibilities and roles, just as the curriculum for younger students. Senior citizens are the only age group whose learning needs have not been defined; consequently, a suitable curriculum for them is lacking. Because demographic forecasts indicate this population segment will grow at a more rapid rate than others, education should be available to help them contribute to their family.

Society should understand that learning remains important after people complete the employment stage of their lives. This contradicts a belief that whatever grandparents need to know will be revealed by wisdom which comes naturally with aging. Such an assumption permits communities to ignore the education needs of older adults and causes them to underestimate their need for further learning. Educational psychologists should support the concept of lifelong learning by discovering suitable methods of instruction and procedures to evaluate learning that are effective in promoting grandparent development.

4. Society Should Set Higher Expectations for Grandparents

By themselves grandparents may be unable to generate the motivation that is needed to stimulate widespread educational commitment by their peer group. This task is difficult because so many people think about retirement as a time when they should withdraw from community responsibility. Peers reinforce the impression that being carefree and without obligation is an acceptable goal for the final stage of life. The problem is compounded by age-segregation. When older adults are limited to peers for conversation, they can adopt behaviors that are not in accord with what society as a whole believes is best.

To revise the existing grandparent norms so they include more learning, younger people should raise their expectations of older relatives and make them known. The talent and potential of grandparents could enrich the lives of everyone. Society should expect them to demonstrate a commitment to personal growth, spend time with loved ones, show community concern through volunteerism, and support public schools to ensure a better future for children. When educational expectations are established for older adults, they are bound to experience greater influence and self-esteem.

5. The Benefits of Grandparent Education Should Be Evaluated and Made Available

Public support can be anticipated for programs that help grandparents enlarge their scope of influence, improve their ability to communicate with relatives, become more self-confident, and experience greater respect in the family. When grandparent class participants report they have achieved some gains, they express satisfaction. However, self-reports on success are more credible when they are corroborated by other generations. Children and grandchildren can confirm when grandparent attitudes and behaviors improve as a result of attending educational programs. Benefits could also be evaluated by three-generational instrumentation such as the *Grandparent Strengths and Needs Inventory* (R. D. Strom & Strom, 1997, 2017; R. D. Strom et al., 1995, 1999 ; Watson & Koblinsky, 2000).

Grandparent Education Goals

We collaborated with 400 grandparents in a program to determine their educational needs. The topics participants chose as most relevant became the design for the nation's first grandparent education program. Two courses were successfully field-tested with support from the American Association of Retired Persons (R. D. Strom, 1989). Two books on curriculum were published, *Becoming a Better Grandparent* (R. D. Strom &

Strom, 1991), and *Achieving Grandparent Potential* (R. D. Strom & Strom, 1992). Each course included 12 lessons presenting family issues as viewed by grandparents, parents, and grandchildren. This broad frame of reference with attention also paid to ethnic backgrounds enabled older adults to understand how younger relatives see their purposes and concerns. The goals of the educational program were to:

1 Increase the satisfactions of being a grandparent.
2 Improve how well grandparents perform their role.
3 Enlarge the scope of guidance expected of grandparents.
4 Enable grandparents to understand their common difficulties.
5 Provide support for grandparents in coping with frustrations.
6 Help grandparents to have their information needs met.

Boomers, Born 1946 to 1964

Retaining a Sense of Purpose

As volunteers in the community, older adults are significant contributors to the mental health of society. Yet, it has been unclear how unpaid productive activities implicate loneliness. Cho and Xiang (2022) conducted a study using data from the Health and Retirement Study at the University of Michigan. The sample consisted of 5,000 individuals age 60 and older who reported at the outset of their participation in the 12-year-longitudinal study (2006 to 2018) that they did not experience loneliness. A majority (52%) of the subjects were women. Self-reported involvement in formal volunteer work were classified into three levels: (0) no volunteering, (1) less than 100 hours of volunteering a year, and (2) more than 100 hours of volunteering a year. Volunteering more than 100 hours a year was statistically associated with a lower risk of loneliness compared to the non-volunteers. The protective effect was not observed for those who volunteered less than 100 hours per year. The benefits of volunteering in mitigation of loneliness did not differ by gender.

Marital Relationships and Health

Many Boomers reported concerns about being able to sustain a long-term marriage. National data indicate that 36% of divorces in the United States involve people age 50 and older; their divorce rate nearly doubled over the period 1990 to 2010 (Brown & Lin, 2022). The only age group with an increasing divorce rate are ages 65 and older, raising questions regarding how they will navigate their years of old age (Carr & Utz, 2020; Upham, 2023). The usual explanation of couples is that they have grown apart, the stigma of divorce no longer exists as it did in previous years, and their children are old enough to adjust to separation (Levin & Van Haren, 2022). This so-called *gray divorce* typically occurs after couples become empty nesters, and they are less concerned about how splitting up will influence their reputation. According to family relationship experts, marriages in recent years have become individualized with spouses focusing on their own fulfillment and satisfaction rather than trying to prove they can stay in a legal arrangement that does not provide them satisfaction (Smock & Schwartz, 2020).

Epidemiological studies that examine large populations to compare outcomes associated with various factors suggest that most older married couples experience better physical and mental health along with greater longevity than people who are unmarried in their cohort. Analysis of a longitudinal sample included 164,597 respondents, from ages 65 to 85, to the Medicare Health Outcomes Survey found that married men and women had lower mortality rates and longer life expectancy than unmarried persons (Jia & Lubetkin, 2020). For example, at age 65, the total life expectancy for married men was 2.2 years longer than unmarried men. Similarly, at age 65, life expectancy for married women was 1.5 years longer than for unmarried women. One reason for the differences is the influence marital partners have on healthy behaviors; they take fewer risks, eat better, look after each other in times of need, and are less inclined to smoke and drink excessively.

Mental health of married couples is also better because of social support they give that is less available for single persons who have higher rates of depression, loneliness, and social isolation. Instead of viewing grey divorce as a path to fulfillment during retirement, the English poet Robert Browning (1812–1889) urged his wife Elizabeth Barrett (1806–1861) to "Grow old along with me! The best is yet to be, the last of life, for which the first was made. Our times are in his hands who saith, 'A whole I planned, youth shows but half; trust God. See all, nor be afraid!'" (Browning, 1895).

Silent Generation, Born 1928 to 1945

Intergenerational Religious Education

Spiritual growth, ethical behavior, character development, and seeking wisdom are goals for many in the Silent Generation. They look to churches, parishes, synagogues, and temples for guidance. Religious educators should consider innovative teaching methods that can implicate intergenerational learning. Consider an outline that could motivate this reciprocal exchange.

Purpose

In many religious institutions, people of all age groups come to the sanctuary for worship led by a minister, priest, rabbi, or layman. Sometimes a short sermon is given to children who gather around the altar with adults acting as observers. Following the lesson, everyone leaves to convene again in a few minutes elsewhere at church where age-segregated groups meet. Young children meet in a room with a teacher, adolescents get together in a different room, and adults, categorized by age, meet in other places for lessons to young adults, middle aged, and retirees. The purpose of intergenerational religious education would be to broaden the perspective.

Participants

Individuals could be placed in teams of five, with each member representing a different age group, balanced for gender. One member could be an adolescent ages 14 to 20, another is 20 to 30 years old, one person is 30 to 40, another is 40 to 60, and one is over age 60.

Focus

The curriculum should emphasize social and emotional development, a context that receives little attention even though this context for learning can contribute to ethical and spiritual development. Some possible topics to get started could include the following.

- Knowing right and wrong (factors that influence character development)
- Managing social and emotional stress (in school, at work, and the family)
- Improving communication in relationships (forgiveness, gratitude, and regrets)
- Defining success for different age levels (goal setting and amending goals)
- Dealing with failure and resilience throughout life (perseverance, disappointment)
- Coping with fears in a hurried and distracted environment (regrets)
- Helping people with feelings of loneliness and social isolation (volunteering)

Format

Everyone is provided four discussion questions a week ahead of time. This homework encourages reflection, allows individuals to make notes, and reduces concern for those who prefer structure to uncertainty. Participants bring their agenda questions with answers to the next class. For example, a discussion about the topic of honesty and dishonesty might acknowledge survey results that show adolescents (ages 10–20) are satisfied with their ethical development even though many of them readily admit they cheat in school.

Question 1. Make some guesses as to why students might not recognize this contradiction.

Question 2. Some reasons for cheating are "I didn't have time," "Everyone else is cheating and I must get good grades for college." Provide your reactions to each of these or other excuses.

During discussions of some topics one age group could be invited to speak while others listen. For example, people over 65 may be asked to share concerns about feelings of loneliness and concerns about personal safety. This emphasis on listening to a single age cohort can inform others. Everyone is reminded that no one can speak for an entire generation but their familiarity with peer norms can help outsiders become better informed.

Agenda

Depending on the topic and ease of discussion, there could be several questions.

1 Can you share knowledge about cheating reports that really bothered you?
2 Why do you suppose so many people become involved with cheating or lying?
3 How would relatives react if they knew that you cheated to get a better grade?
4 How does artificial intelligence impact the reports students submit to teachers?

In addition, anyone who wants to can share verses from a religious source- old or new testament the Torah, or Book of Mormon, a story, or observation for reflection. This allows those familiar with religious literature to share their knowledge in this context.

Presentation

One or more team members could volunteer to offer a short presentation on a topic for the next session or devise an outline of common consideration. For some topics additional discussions could take place during the week in sessions attended mostly by older adults who choose to spend time socializing with peers at their place of worship.

Novelists and playwrights have written stories that feature courage and illustrate the danger of reaching premature conclusions. An example of a lesson reflecting the importance of honesty for all generations comes from Norwegian author Henrik Ibsen (1828–1906) in his play *An Enemy of the People* (Ibsen, 1882/2021). Leaders of the town which was economically dependent on tourists who visited the resort health bathing spa were informed by Dr. Stockman that the draining system was seriously contaminated and had to be repaired to eliminate pollution. The first response of officials was gratitude for alerting them about the problem and solution. But then, Stockman's brother, the town mayor along with the newspaper editor, urged him to retract his statement because of the adverse effects it would have on the local tourism and economy. Stockman convened a town meeting to explain why the repairs were needed even though it would mean tourism must temporarily suffer. The townspeople were opposed to any decline in business so they shouted Stockman down, identifying him as an enemy of the people. The next day Stockman's home was vandalized and his landlord warned of eviction. Stockman along with his daughter, a teacher, were fired from their jobs. Everyone assumed Stockman would leave town but he chose to stay because his family supported him. In the end, Stockman remained true to his principles and stated his belief that the strongest man is the one able to stand alone.

Schedule

Intergenerational religious education would not be a replacement for existing worship. Participants would still attend regular services in the sanctuary. A schedule to unite the adults could be the time currently devoted to age-segregated Sunday school.

Goals for Consideration

Presenting a continuous example for younger relatives about the importance of spiritual development and ways to maintain an ethical lifestyle is a significant contribution to everyone. Encouraging older adults to demonstrate their wisdom and maturity in the context of religious commitment is an educational responsibility that deserves support by the collective generations.

Conclusion

Some priority purposes and concerns for each generation have been described along with goals for consideration. Generation Z can better be served by incorporating early childhood education as part of the public school structure from birth to age 5. Teachers of young children would be paid the same salary as elementary and secondary teachers. Generation Z believes the education of their children should include setting goals to choose values that can help them grow up. Goals for personality development deserve consideration. Generation Z also wants free post high school education to get ready for work. Devoting greater time to schoolwork while cutting back on social media and peer interaction would be a healthy goal for common adoption.

Millennial parents lack affordable group child care and believe public policy should make it possible. They favor transparency by schools to identify student deficiencies, provide effective tutoring, and arrange cost-free higher education. The college experience could be shortened by eliminating general studies, thereby reducing tuition and increasing relevance. Millennials need education to support adjustment attitudes and skills like time management, coping with stress, and moving from self-absorption to commitment for the well-being of others.

Generation X has children in need of cost-free college or technical vocational education to prepare for work. They also need greater support from employers to balance productivity at work and caregiving at home. Boomers want a well-defined grandparent role and recognize education is key to their adjustment. Finding support for grandparent education is difficult because adult education does not focus on understanding how to support younger generations. The scope of public education should expand beyond careers to include further maturity that is needed during retirement. Grandparent learning needs must be met or their influence is bound to decline, they will suffer from isolation, and their sense of worth will diminish. Religious institutions should provide intergenerational spiritual education.

Success in a modern longevity society requires that all age groups become aware of and responsive to the separate goals and concerns of five generations. Continual development of maturity should be the basic purpose of lifelong learning that is evident by reciprocal caring, collaborative effort, and harmonious relationships across age groups.

Key Concepts

1 Helping elementary students set personality goals enables them to acquire attributes that will make them more successful adults. This orientation can also build healthy peer group norms of behavior that contribute to safety and well-being of peers.

2 The main purpose of adult education should be to motivate further development of maturity in retirement. Progress toward this goal is evident when older adults provide support to meet the needs of younger relatives, help them attain their goals, and serve the community.

3 Federal education policy reforms are being implemented to diminish skill gaps and eliminate the lower status distinction that has been assigned to students who want to prepare themselves for employment by completing technical or trade training.

4 Only 23% of mothers and 3% of fathers can afford to stay home to take care of young children. Locating affordable child care is a major problem for millennial parents. Grandparents who live close by can sometimes assume the important task of providing care, instruction, and guidance for younger relatives.

5 Two out of three of the nation's children are not proficient readers. This situation means communities should mobilize retired volunteers to act as tutors by listening to children read, providing correction, and encouraging individual students to achieve literacy.

6 Spending time together is common among successful families. Communication, learning, and emotional support decline whenever families lose control of how time is spent. A majority of adolescents assign their parents poor ratings for spending time with them.

7 Caregivers of older relatives report feeling discouraged because parents never seem satisfied, no matter what is done to make their life more comfortable. Older adults should remind each other that their daughters and sons deserve gratitude for caregiving.

8 The longer life span poses a challenge of motivating further development of maturity in retirement instead of becoming self-absorbed and rejecting responsibilities to others. A sense of purpose requires an expression of concern for well-being of relatives and the community.

9 The main purpose for grandparent education is to become aware of experiences of children, adolescents, and young adults. This knowledge needed to become a source of guidance cannot be drawn from memory or intuition.

10 Knowing the goals and concerns of each generation should be a goal for lifelong learning. This common educational orientation can ensure that the needs of all age groups are better met and people gain personality attributes that support success in their relationships.

Generational Perspectives Activities

> **16.1 Team Discussion**
> **16.2 Conversations with Children**
> **16.3 A Scenario: Reasoning and Problem Solving**
> **16.4 Team Chapter Review**
> **16.5 Criteria for Self-Evaluation of Team Members**

16.1 Team Discussion

1 How do you feel about everyone knowing the goals and obstacles of each generation?
2 How should expectations of the retired population be modified in a longevity society?
3 How could granting adult status to adolescents impact intergenerational relationships?
4 How do you feel about polling students to learn their views on reforming the schools?
5 What sources should be responsible to pay for the cost of post high school education?
6 What do you think should be done to improve National School Report Card results?
7 What are the benefits of developing a partnership between parents and grandparents?
8 How should society respond to an increasing number of older adults who need care?
9 What things would you like to understand about experiences of your grandchildren?
10 How do you feel about the amount of time you and younger relatives spend together?

16.2 Conversations with Children

1 What do you think are the priority goals and obstacles your parents have to manage?
2 What do you think grandparents fail to understand about what life is like at your age?
3 What could be done to increase communication that takes place between age groups?
4 What do you suppose are the priority goals and obstacles your grandparents encounter?
5 Who do you believe should pay the cost of tuition at college, technical or trade school?
6 What conditions of learning would you like to see changed in classes that you attend?
7 What should younger people expect of those who are retired in a longevity society?
8 Why do you suppose most grownups are unwilling to recognize teenagers as adults?
9 How do you and your parents attempt to help older members within your family?
10 What would you like to know about some of the generations older than your own?

16.3 A Scenario: Reasoning and Problem Solving

Nancy's 70th birthday will be celebrated by the whole family. Her daughter, son, and their children, ages 13, 15, and 16 are all going to be together. Nancy is asking friends ahead of time about some possible topics to introduce for conversation. What options do you suggest?

a Have everyone tell a priority goal they hope to achieve.
b Find out the views of each teen about career exploration.
c Ask each person to share something that is worrisome.
d Describe one of their most important accomplishments.
e Other _____

16.4 Team Chapter Review

Efforts to assess participant learning, provide feedback, and improve quality of instruction is enhanced by a group review of each chapter.

1 What ideas in the lesson changed the way I think about this topic?
2 What insights from the lesson will I try to apply in my relationships?
3 What is the most important point for me presented in this lesson?
4 What are some aspects of this lesson I would like to better understand?
5 Which aspects of this lesson do I wish that I had known about earlier?

16.5 Criteria for Self-Evaluation of Team Members

1 The idea of everyone learning about the goals and concerns of other generations

  a may be unrealistic because people are too busy to arrange for this education
  b could be a way to increase social stability and help people meet their needs
  c may prevent generational self-absorption by increasing concern for others
  d appeals to me as a way to make each of us less selfish and more responsive
  e Other _____

2 My view on society granting teenagers their common goal of adult identity status is

  a they deserve to be treated as equals with the other subpopulations of adults
  b their youth status should remain the same until they get full time employment
  c their computer knowledge is a reasonable basis to qualify as being adults
  d they should not be seen as adults until they are no longer financially dependent
  e Other _____

3 My thinking about providing free college, technical, or trade school preparation is

  a each state should assume the responsibility to pay for higher education
  b parents should be expected to pay the cost of tuition for their children
  c society cannot afford another entitlement so borrowing money is best
  d older relatives should consider whether to provide financial assistance
  e the federal government should accept the obligation to pay for college
  f Other _____

4 I believe that families with young children should consider

  a having one parent stay home as the best caregiving option
  b searching for a group care center they are able to afford
  c asking a retiree or other relatives to provide needed care
  d take turns caregiving with neighbors who have children
  e Other _____

5 The amount of time I talk with my parents and grandparents

    a is enough and we know each other well
    b is not enough for me to know them well
    c is enough but we do not share our problems
    d is not enough because we are all too busy
    e Other _____

6 When I become old or frail enough to need caregiving

    a I am sure my children will provide help I need
    b I may have to enter a care facility to get help
    c I don't know who I can count on for support
    d This is a topic my family has never discussed
    e Other _____

7 The way that I schedule time

    a includes community volunteering
    b trying to help other relatives
    c pursuing my hobbies and interests
    d attending events at my church
    e Other _____

8 My experience in visiting residents at care facilities

    a includes seeing a friend on a regular basis
    b not going except for birthdays or holidays
    c I avoid visits because it feels uncomfortable
    d I don't know anyone who is in a care center
    e Other _____

9 The loneliness reported by residents in care facilities

    a is a subject that I have not discussed with others
    b is a situation younger relatives should understand
    c is a problem communities should take seriously
    d undermines their feelings of personal importance
    e Other_____

10 My grandparents

    a understand my goals and encourage attainment of them
    b are unaware of my goals and do not ask me about them
    c lack curiosity about my daily experiences and lifestyle
    d want to know about my worries and are willing to comfort me
    e Other _____

References

Altus, K. (2023, March 24). *Mike Rowe celebrates more students forgoing college for apprenticeships: 'Chickens have come home to roost'.* https://www.foxbusiness.com/economy/mike-rowe-celebrates-more-students-forgoing-college-apprenticeships-chickens-home-roost

American Association of Retired Persons. (2019, April 8). *New AARP research on grandparents busts stereotypes on attitudes, employment, finances and lifestyle.* https://press.aarp.org/2019-4-9-new-aarp-research-on-grandparents-busts-stereotypes-on-attitudes-employment-finances-and-lifestyle

Belkin, D. (2023, March 16). More students are turning away from college and toward apprenticeships. *Wall Street Journal.* https://www.wsj.com/articles/more-students-are-turning-away-from-college-and-toward-apprenticeships-15f3a05d

Belsky, J., Caspi, A., Moffitt, T., & Poulton, R. (2020). *The origins of you: How childhood shapes later life.* Harvard University Press.

Bergen, D., Lee, L., Dicarlo, C., Burnett, G., & Stone, S. J. (2020). *Enhancing brain development in infants and young children: Strategies for caregivers and educators.* Teachers College Press.

Bhutta, N., Chang, A., Dettling, L., & Hsu, J. (2020). *Disparities in wealth by race and ethnicity in the 2019 survey of consumer finances.* Board of Governors of the Federal Reserve System. https://www.federalreserve.gov/econres/notes/feds-notes/disparities-in-wealth-by-race-and-ethnicity-in-the-2019-survey-of-consumer-finances-20200928.html

Body, D. (2022, May 12). *Caregiving equity: Better for all women, better for us all.* National Council on Aging. https://www.ncoa.org/article/caregiving-equity-better-for-women-better-for-us-all

Brown, S. L., & Lin, I-F. (2022, September). The graying of divorce: A half century of change. *Journals of Gerontology: Series B*, *77*(9), 1710–1720. 10.1093/geronb/gbac057

Browning, R. (1895). *Browning's complete poetical works [Cambridge edition].* Houghton, Mifflin & Co.

Carr, D., & Utz, R. L. (2020 February). Families in later life: A decade in review. *Journal of Marriage and Family*, *82*, 346–363. 10.1111/jomf.12609

Carter, C. (2020). *The new adolescence.* BenBella Books.

ChildCare Aware of America. (2022). *Demanding change: Repairing our child care system.* https://www.childcareaware.org/demanding-change-repairing-our-child-care-system/

Cho, J., & Xiang, X. (2022). The relationship between volunteering and the occurrence of loneliness among older adults: A longitudinal study with 12 years of follow-up. *Journal of Gerontological Social Work*, *66*(5), 680–693. 10.1080/01634372.2022.2139322

Fuller, J. B., & Raman, M. (2019, January 17). *The caring company: How employers can cut costs and boost productivity by helping employees manage caregiving needs.* Harvard Business School. https://www.hbs.edu/managing-the-future-of-work/Documents/The_Caring_Company.pdf

Garvey, D. (2023). *Little brains matter: A practical guide to brain development and neuroscience in early childhood.* Routledge.

Goldstein, K. (2022, November 21). 5 Things employers get wrong about caregivers at work. *Harvard Business Review.* https://hbr.org/2022/11/5-things-employers-get-wrong-about-caregivers-at-work

Gromada, A., & Richardson, D. (2021, June). *Where do rich countries stand on childcare?* United Nations International Children's Emergency Fund (UNICEF). https://www.unicef-irc.org/publications/pdf/where-do-rich-countries-stand-on-childcare.pdf

Harvard Business School. (2019, January 16). *New research from HBS Prof: Growing caregiving crisis hurting firm profitability, employee productivity [Press release].* https://www.hbs.edu/news/releases/Pages/growing-caregiving-crisis.aspx

Ibsen, H. (2021). *An enemy of the people* (R. F. Sharp, Trans.). Musaicum Books. (Original work published 1882)

Iwai, T. (2023). *The psychology of personal growth and better relationships: Manga for success.* Wiley.

Jia, H., & Lubetkin, E. I. (2020, December). Life expectancy and active life expectancy by marital status among older U.S. adults: Results from the U.S Medicare Health Outcome Survey. *SSM-Population Health.* 10.1016/j.ssmph.2020.100642 https://www.ncbi.nlm.nih.gov/pmc/articles/PMC7452000/

Khan Academy. (2023). *For every student, every classroom. Real results.* Khan Academy. https://www.khanacademy.org

Kirp, D. L. (2019, August 1). *The college dropout scandal.* Oxford University Press.

LeBlanc, P. (2021). *Students first: Equity, access, and opportunity in higher education.* Harvard University Press.

Levin, S., & Van Haren, P. C. (2022). *70s are the new 50s: How grey divorce differs from a typical divorce. American Bar Association.* https://www.americanbar.org/groups/dispute_resolution/publications/JustResolutions/just-resolutions-march-2022/how-grey-divorce-differs-from-a-typical-divorce/

National Assessment of Educational Progress. (2022). *NAEP report card: 2022 NAEP Reading assessment.* The Nation's Report Card. https://www.nationsreportcard.gov/highlights/reading/2022/

National Center for Education Statistics. (2019, December 3). *Highlights of U.S. PISA 2018 Results Web Report.* [NCES Publication No. 2020166]. https://nces.ed.gov/pubsearch/pubsinfo.asp?pubid=2020166

Programme for International Student Assessment. (2023). Organisation for Economic Co-operation and Development. https://www.oecd.org/pisa/

Quadlin, N. M., & Powell, B. (2022). *Who should pay? Higher education responsibility and the public.* Russell Sage Foundation.

Rowe, M. (2019). *The way I heard it.* Gallery Books.

Smock, P. J., & Schwartz, C. R. (2020). The demography of families: A review of patterns and change. *Journal of Marriage and the Family, 82*, 9–34. 10.1111/jomf.12612

St-Esprit, M. (2019, March 6). The stigma of choosing trade school over college. *The Atlantic.* https://www.theatlantic.com/education/archive/2019/03/choosing-trade-school-over-college/584275/

Strengthening Career and Technical Education for the 21st Century Act, Pub. L. No. 115-224, 132 Stat. 1563 (2018, July 31). https://www.congress.gov/115/plaws/publ224/PLAW-115publ224.pdf

Strom, P. S., Hendon, K. L., Strom, R. D., & Wang, C.-H. (2019). How peers support and inhibit learning in the classroom: Assessment of high school students in collaborative groups. *School Community Journal, 29*(2), 183–202. http://www.adi.org/journal/2019fw/StromEtAlFW2019.pdf

Strom, P. S., & Strom, R. D. (2012). *Learning throughout life: An intergenerational perspective.* Information Age.

Strom, P. S., Strom, R. D., Sindel-Arrington, T., & Wang, C. (2022). Tutoring support and student voice in middle school. *School Community Journal, 32*(1), 39–62. https://www.adi.org/journal/2022ss/StromEtAlSS22.pdf

Strom R. D. (1989). *Grandparent development: Final Research Report.* Andrus Foundation of the American Association of Retired Persons.

Strom, R. D., & Strom, P. S. (2017). Grandparent learning and cultural differences. *Educational Gerontology, 43*(8), 417–427. 10.1080/03601277.2017.1314642

Strom, R. D., & Strom, P. S. (2018). Education for grandparents in longevity societies. *Journal of Adult and Continuing Education, 24*(2), 208–228. 10.1177/1477971418810652

Strom, R. D., & Strom, S. (1991). *Becoming a better grandparent: Viewpoints on strengthening the family.* Sage.

Strom, R. D., & Strom, S. (1992). *Achieving grandparent potential: Building intergenerational relationships.* Sage.

Strom, R. D., & Strom, S. (1997). Building a theory of grandparent development. *The International Journal of Aging and Human Development, 45*(4), 255–286. 10.2190/HAVE-HWKU-6BCG-9EY5

Strom, R. D., Strom, S., Collinsworth, P., Sato, S., Makino, K., Sasaki, Y., Sasaki, H., & Nishio, N. (1995). Grandparents in Japan: A three-generational study. *International Journal of Aging and Human Development, 40*(3), 209–226. https://ncbi.nlm.nih.gov/pubmed/7615350

Strom, R. D., Strom, S., Wang, C. M., Shen, Y. L., Griswold, D. L., Chan, H. S., & Yang, C. Y. (1999). Grandparents in the United States and the Republic of China: A comparison of generations and cultures. *International Journal of Aging and Human Development*, *49*(4), 279–317. https://ncbi.nlm.nih.gov/pubmed/10696817

Upham, B. (2023, June 2). Why more couples are divorcing at older ages (and after more years of marriage) than before – and what you can do to avoid it. *EveryDay Health*. https://www.everydayhealth.com/emotional-health/why-more-couples-are-divorcing-at-older-ages-than-before-and-what-you-can-do-to-avoid-it/

Watson, J. A., & Koblinsky, S. A. (2000, Summer). Strengths and needs of African American and European American grandmothers in the working and middle classes. *The Journal of Negro Education*, *69*(3), 199–214. 10.2307/2696232

Index

Pages in **bold** refer to tables.

THE ROUTLEDGE COMPANION TO APPLIED QUALITATIVE RESEARCH IN THE CARIBBEAN

This cutting-edge book provides a comprehensive examination of applied qualitative research in the Caribbean. It highlights the methodological diversity of qualitative research by drawing on various approaches to the study of Caribbean society, addressing the lack of published qualitative research on the region.

Featuring 17 chapters, the book covers five key areas, namely Overview and Introduction; Gender, Crime, and Violence; Gender and Intimate Partner Violence; Health, Management, and Public Policy; and Migration and Tourism. Throughout the course of the book, the chapters explore how different kinds of qualitative research can be used to inform public policy and help deal with a myriad of socioeconomic problems that affect Caribbean people. The book further uses distinct approaches to showcase a diverse selection of qualitative research methods, such as autoethnography, life history, narrative enquiry, participants' observation, grounded theory, case study, and critical discourse.

The book will be beneficial for students and scholars both from the Caribbean and internationally who are engaged in the conduct of qualitative empirical enquiry. It will further hold appeal to advanced undergraduate level classes and postgraduate students along with scholars in the fields of social sciences and education.

Corin Bailey is a Professor of Sociology, Crime and Social inequality at the University of the West Indies (UWI). He is the Director of the Centre for Criminal Justice and Security, located at UWI, Regional Headquarters, Mona Campus, Jamaica.

Roy McCree is a Senior Research Fellow at the Sir Arthur Lewis Institute of Social and Economic Studies at the University of the West Indies, St Augustine Campus, Trinidad and Tobago.

Latoya Lazarus is a Research Fellow at the Sir Arthur Lewis Institute of Social and Economic Studies at the University of the West Indies, Cave Hill Campus, Barbados.

Natalie Dietrich Jones is a Research Fellow at the Sir Arthur Lewis Institute of Social and Economic Studies at the University of the West Indies, Mona Campus, Jamaica.